# ACP | MKSAP® 17

## Medical Knowledge Self-Assessment Program®

# Infectious Disease

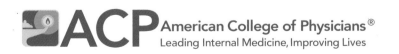

**ACP** American College of Physicians®
Leading Internal Medicine, Improving Lives

# Welcome to the Infectious Disease Section of MKSAP 17!

In these pages, you will find updated information on skin and soft tissue infection, community-acquired pneumonia, tick-borne disease, urinary tract infections, *Mycobacterium tuberculosis* and nontuberculous mycobacterial infection, sexually transmitted infection, travel medicine, infectious gastrointestinal syndromes, health care–associated infection, and many other clinical challenges. All of these topics are uniquely focused on the needs of generalists and subspecialists *outside* of infectious disease.

The publication of the 17th edition of Medical Knowledge Self-Assessment Program (MKSAP) represents nearly a half-century of serving as the gold-standard resource for internal medicine education. It also marks its evolution into an innovative learning system to better meet the changing educational needs and learning styles of all internists.

The core content of MKSAP has been developed as in previous editions—newly generated, essential information in 11 topic areas of internal medicine created by dozens of leading generalists and subspecialists and guided by certification and recertification requirements, emerging knowledge in the field, and user feedback. MKSAP 17 also contains 1200 all-new, psychometrically validated, and peer-reviewed multiple-choice questions (MCQs) for self-assessment and study, including 108 in Infectious Disease. MKSAP 17 continues to include *High Value Care* (HVC) recommendations, based on the concept of balancing clinical benefit with costs and harms, with links to MCQs that illustrate these principles. In addition, HVC Key Points are highlighted in the text. Also highlighted, with blue text, are *Hospitalist*-focused content and MCQs that directly address the learning needs of internists who work in the hospital setting.

MKSAP 17 Digital provides access to additional tools allowing you to customize your learning experience, including regular text updates with practice-changing, new information and 200 new self-assessment questions; a board-style pretest to help direct your learning; and enhanced custom-quiz options. And, with MKSAP Complete, learners can access 1200 electronic flashcards for quick review of important concepts or review the updated and enhanced version of Virtual Dx, an image-based self-assessment tool.

As before, MKSAP 17 is optimized for use on your mobile devices, with iOS- and Android-based apps allowing you to sync your work between your apps and online account and submit for CME credits and MOC points online.

Please visit us at the MKSAP Resource Site (mksap.acponline.org) to find out how we can help you study, earn CME credit and MOC points, and stay up to date.

Whether you prefer to use the traditional print version or take advantage of the features available through the digital version, we hope you enjoy MKSAP 17 and that it meets and exceeds your personal learning needs.

On behalf of the many internists who have offered their time and expertise to create the content for MKSAP 17 and the editorial staff who work to bring this material to you in the best possible way, we are honored that you have chosen to use MKSAP 17 and appreciate any feedback about the program you may have. Please feel free to send us any comments to mksap_editors@acponline.org.

Sincerely,

Philip A. Masters, MD, FACP
Editor-in-Chief
Senior Physician Educator
Director, Clinical Content Development
Medical Education Division
American College of Physicians

# Infectious Disease

## Committee

**Patricia D. Brown, MD, FACP, Section Editor[1]**
Professor of Medicine
Division of Infectious Diseases
Wayne State University School of Medicine
Associate Chief of Staff for Medicine
John D. Dingell VA Medical Center
Detroit, Michigan

**Allan R. Tunkel, MD, PhD, MACP, Associate Editor[2]**
Professor of Medicine
Associate Dean for Medical Education
The Warren Alpert Medical School of Brown University
Providence, Rhode Island

**Karen C. Bloch, MD, MPH[2]**
Associate Professor
Department of Infectious Disease and Health Policy
Division of Infectious Diseases
Vanderbilt University Medical Center
Nashville, Tennessee

**Larry M. Bush, MD, FACP[2]**
Affiliated Professor of Biomedical Sciences
Charles E. Schmidt College of Medicine
Florida Atlantic University
Boca Raton, Florida
Affiliated Associate Professor of Medicine
University of Miami-Miller School of Medicine
Comprehensive Infectious Diseases, LLC
West Palm Beach, Florida

**Elisa Choi, MD, FACP[2]**
Atrius Health
Internal Medicine/HIV Medicine/Infectious Disease
Co-Director, CME Education Conferences—Internal Medicine
Harvard Medical School—Faculty
Boston, Massachusetts

**Louise M. Dembry, MD, MS, MBA[2]**
Professor of Medicine/Infectious Diseases and Epidemiology
Yale University School of Medicine
New Haven, Connecticut

**Michael Frank, MD, FACP[1]**
Professor of Medicine
Residency Program Director
Vice Chair for Education
Department of Medicine
Medical College of Wisconsin
Milwaukee, Wisconsin

**Fred A. Lopez, MD, MACP[2]**
Richard Vial Professor and Vice Chair
Department of Medicine
Louisiana State University Health Sciences Center
New Orleans, Louisiana

**Annette C. Reboli, MD, FACP[2]**
Founding Vice Dean
Professor of Medicine
Department of Medicine
Division of Infectious Diseases
Cooper Medical School of Rowan University
Cooper University Hospital
Camden, New Jersey

## Editor-in-Chief

**Philip A. Masters, MD, FACP[1]**
Senior Physician Educator
Director, Clinical Content Development
American College of Physicians
Philadelphia, Pennsylvania

## Director, Clinical Program Development

**Cynthia D. Smith, MD, FACP[2]**
American College of Physicians
Philadelphia, Pennsylvania

## Infectious Disease Reviewers

Robert M. Centor, MD, MACP[1]
Elizabeth Cerceo, MD, FACP[2]
Mayurika Ghosh, MD[1]
Duane R. Hospenthal, MD, FACP[1]
Robert T. Means, Jr., MD, FACP[2]
Ileana L. Piña, MD[2]
Peter H. Wiernik, MD, FACP[2]

## Infectious Disease Reviewer Representing the American Society for Clinical Pharmacology & Therapeutics

Carol Collins, MD[1]

## Infectious Disease ACP Editorial Staff

**Linnea Donnarumma[1]**, Staff Editor
**Julia Nawrocki[1]**, Staff Editor
**Margaret Wells[1]**, Director, Self-Assessment and Educational Programs
**Becky Krumm[1]**, Managing Editor

## ACP Principal Staff

**Patrick C. Alguire, MD, FACP**[2]
*Senior Vice President, Medical Education*

**Sean McKinney**[1]
*Vice President, Medical Education*

**Margaret Wells**[1]
*Director, Self-Assessment and Educational Programs*

**Becky Krumm**[1]
*Managing Editor*

**Katie Idell**[1]
*Manager, Clinical Skills Program and Digital Products*

**Valerie A. Dangovetsky**[1]
*Administrator*

**Ellen McDonald, PhD**[1]
*Senior Staff Editor*

**Megan Zborowski**[1]
*Senior Staff Editor*

**Randy Hendrickson**[1]
*Production Administrator/Editor*

**Linnea Donnarumma**[1]
*Staff Editor*

**Susan Galeone**[1]
*Staff Editor*

**Jackie Twomey**[1]
*Staff Editor*

**Julia Nawrocki**[1]
*Staff Editor*

**Kimberly Kerns**[1]
*Administrative Coordinator*

**Rosemarie Houton**[1]
*Administrative Representative*

---

1. Has no relationships with any entity producing, marketing, reselling, or distributing health care goods or services consumed by, or used on, patients.

2. Has disclosed relationship(s) with any entity producing, marketing, reselling, or distributing health care goods or services consumed by, or used on, patients.

### Disclosure of Relationships with any entity producing, marketing, reselling, or distributing health care goods or services consumed by, or used on, patients.

**Patrick C. Alguire, MD, FACP**
*Consultantship*
National Board of Medical Examiners
*Royalties*
UpToDate
*Stock Options/Holdings*
Amgen Inc, Bristol-Myers Squibb,
   GlaxoSmithKline, Stryker Corporation, Zimmer
   Orthopedics, Teva Pharmaceuticals, Medtronic,
   Covidien, Inc., Express Scripts

**Karen C. Bloch, MD, MPH**
*Royalties*
First Edition
*Research Grants/Contracts*
Centers for Disease Control and Prevention

**Larry M. Bush, MD, FACP**
*Speakers Bureau*
Cubist, Sanofi-Pasteur

**Elizabeth Cerceo, MD, FACP**
*Employment*
Scientific Therapeutics, Inc.

**Elisa Choi, MD, FACP**
*Board Member*
MAP for Health
*Consultantship*
DynaMed

**Louise M. Dembry, MD, MS, MBA**
*Board Member*
Society for Healthcare Epidemiology of America
*Honoraria*
AHRQ National Advisory Council
*Stock Options/Holdings*
Advanced Technical Support/ReadyDoc

**Fred A. Lopez, MD, FACP**
*Royalties*
UpToDate
*Other (Speaker)*
PriMed with ACP

**Robert T. Means, Jr., MD, FACP**
*Consultantship*
Xenon Pharmaceuticals

**Ileana L. Piña, MD**
*Consultantship*
FDA

**Annette C. Reboli, MD, FACP**
*Other*
Merck and Co.; spousal employment at Merck,
*Research Grants/Contracts*
Merck and Co., T2 Biosystems
*Royalties*
UpToDate

**Cynthia D. Smith, MD, FACP**
*Stock Options/Holdings*
Merck and Co.; spousal employment at Merck

**Allan R. Tunkel, MD, PhD, MACP**
*Employment*
American College of Physicians
*Other*
Infectious Diseases Society of America; Committee Chair
*Research Grants/Contracts*
UpToDate

**Peter H. Wiernik, MD, FACP**
*Consultantship*
Teva Pharmaceuticals, Bristol-Myers Squibb
*Speakers Bureau*
Jansen, Novartis, Celgene

## Acknowledgments

The American College of Physicians (ACP) gratefully acknowledges the special contributions to the development and production of the 17th edition of the Medical Knowledge Self-Assessment Program® (MKSAP® 17) made by the following people:

*Graphic Design*: Michael Ripca (Graphics Technical Administrator) and WFGD Studio (Graphic Designers).

*Production/Systems*: Dan Hoffmann (Director, Web Services & Systems Development), Neil Kohl (Senior Architect), Chris Patterson (Senior Architect), and Scott Hurd (Manager, Web Projects & CMS Services).

*MKSAP 17 Digital*: Under the direction of Steven Spadt, Vice President, Digital Products & Services, the digital version of MKSAP 17 was developed within the ACP's Digital Product Development Department, led by Brian Sweigard (Director). Other members of the team included Dan Barron (Senior Web Application Developer/Architect), Chris Forrest (Senior Software Developer/Design Lead), Kara Kronenwetter (Senior Web Developer), Brad Lord (Senior Web Application Developer), John McKnight (Senior Web Developer), and Nate Pershall (Senior Web Developer).

The College also wishes to acknowledge that many other persons, too numerous to mention, have contributed to the production of this program. Without their dedicated efforts, this program would not have been possible.

## MKSAP Resource Site (mksap.acponline.org)

The MKSAP Resource Site (mksap.acponline.org) is a continually updated site that provides links to MKSAP 17 online answer sheets for print subscribers; the latest details on Continuing Medical Education (CME) and Maintenance of Certification (MOC) in the United States, Canada, and Australia; errata; and other new information.

## ABIM Maintenance of Certification

Check the MKSAP Resource Site (mksap.acponline.org) for the latest information on how MKSAP tests can be used to apply to the American Board of Internal Medicine for Maintenance of Certification (MOC) points.

## Royal College Maintenance of Certification

In Canada, MKSAP 17 is an Accredited Self-Assessment Program (Section 3) as defined by the Maintenance of Certification (MOC) Program of The Royal College of Physicians and Surgeons of Canada and approved by the Canadian Society of Internal Medicine on December 9, 2014. Approval extends from July 31, 2015 until July 31, 2018 for the Part A sections. Approval extends from December 31, 2015 to December 31, 2018 for the Part B sections.

Fellows of the Royal College may earn three credits per hour for participating in MKSAP 17 under Section 3. MKSAP 17 also meets multiple CanMEDS Roles, including that of Medical Expert, Communicator, Collaborator, Manager, Health Advocate, Scholar, and Professional. For information on how to apply MKSAP 17 Continuing Medical Education (CME) credits to the Royal College MOC Program, visit the MKSAP Resource Site at mksap.acponline.org.

## The Royal Australasian College of Physicians CPD Program

In Australia, MKSAP 17 is a Category 3 program that may be used by Fellows of The Royal Australasian College of Physicians (RACP) to meet mandatory Continuing Professional Development (CPD) points. Two CPD credits are awarded for each of the 200 *AMA PRA Category 1 Credits*™ available in MKSAP 17. More information about using MKSAP 17 for this purpose is available at the MKSAP Resource Site at mksap.acponline.org and at www.racp.edu.au. CPD credits earned through MKSAP 17 should be reported at the MyCPD site at www.racp.edu.au/mycpd.

## Continuing Medical Education

The American College of Physicians (ACP) is accredited by the Accreditation Council for Continuing Medical Education (ACCME) to provide continuing medical education for physicians.

The ACP designates this enduring material, MKSAP 17, for a maximum of 200 *AMA PRA Category 1 Credits*™. Physicians should claim only the credit commensurate with the extent of their participation in the activity.

Up to 19 *AMA PRA Category 1 Credits*™ are available from December 31, 2015, to December 31, 2018, for the MKSAP 17 Infectious Disease section.

## Learning Objectives

The learning objectives of MKSAP 17 are to:
- Close gaps between actual care in your practice and preferred standards of care, based on best evidence

- Diagnose disease states that are less common and sometimes overlooked or confusing
- Improve management of comorbid conditions that can complicate patient care
- Determine when to refer patients for surgery or care by subspecialists
- Pass the ABIM Certification Examination
- Pass the ABIM Maintenance of Certification Examination

## Target Audience

- General internists and primary care physicians
- Subspecialists who need to remain up-to-date in internal medicine and in areas outside of their own subspecialty area
- Residents preparing for the certification examination in internal medicine
- Physicians preparing for maintenance of certification in internal medicine (recertification)

## Earn "Instantaneous" CME Credits Online

Print subscribers can enter their answers online to earn instantaneous Continuing Medical Education (CME) credits. You can submit your answers using online answer sheets that are provided at mksap.acponline.org, where a record of your MKSAP 17 credits will be available. To earn CME credits, you need to answer all of the questions in a test and earn a score of at least 50% correct (number of correct answers divided by the total number of questions). Take any of the following approaches:

1. Use the printed answer sheet at the back of this book to record your answers. Go to mksap.acponline.org, access the appropriate online answer sheet, transcribe your answers, and submit your test for instantaneous CME credits. There is no additional fee for this service.

2. Go to mksap.acponline.org, access the appropriate online answer sheet, directly enter your answers, and submit your test for instantaneous CME credits. There is no additional fee for this service.

3. Pay a $15 processing fee per answer sheet and submit the printed answer sheet at the back of this book by mail or fax, as instructed on the answer sheet. Make sure you calculate your score and fax the answer sheet to 215-351-2799 or mail the answer sheet to Member and Customer Service, American College of Physicians, 190 N. Independence Mall West, Philadelphia, PA 19106-1572, using the courtesy envelope provided in your MKSAP 17 slipcase. You will need your 10-digit order number and 8-digit ACP ID number, which are printed on your packing slip. Please allow 4 to 6 weeks for your score report to be emailed back to you. Be sure to include your email address for a response.

If you do not have a 10-digit order number and 8-digit ACP ID number or if you need help creating a user name and password to access the MKSAP 17 online answer sheets, go to mksap.acponline.org or email custserv@acponline.org.

## Disclosure Policy

It is the policy of the American College of Physicians (ACP) to ensure balance, independence, objectivity, and scientific rigor in all of its educational activities. To this end, and consistent with the policies of the ACP and the Accreditation Council for Continuing Medical Education (ACCME), contributors to all ACP continuing medical education activities are required to disclose all relevant financial relationships with any entity producing, marketing, re-selling, or distributing health care goods or services consumed by, or used on, patients. Contributors are required to use generic names in the discussion of therapeutic options and are required to identify any unapproved, off-label, or investigative use of commercial products or devices. Where a trade name is used, all available trade names for the same product type are also included. If trade-name products manufactured by companies with whom contributors have relationships are discussed, contributors are asked to provide evidence-based citations in support of the discussion. The information is reviewed by the committee responsible for producing this text. If necessary, adjustments to topics or contributors' roles in content development are made to balance the discussion. Further, all readers of this text are asked to evaluate the content for evidence of commercial bias and send any relevant comments to mksap_editors@ acponline.org so that future decisions about content and contributors can be made in light of this information.

## Resolution of Conflicts

To resolve all conflicts of interest and influences of vested interests, the American College of Physicians (ACP) precluded members of the content-creation committee from deciding on any content issues that involved generic or trade-name products associated with proprietary entities with which these committee members had relationships. In addition, content was based on best evidence and updated clinical care guidelines, when such evidence and guidelines were available. Contributors' disclosure information can be found with the list of contributors' names and those of ACP principal staff listed in the beginning of this book.

## Hospital-Based Medicine

For the convenience of subscribers who provide care in hospital settings, content that is specific to the hospital setting has been highlighted in blue. Hospital icons (🄷) highlight where the hospital-based content begins, continues over more than one page, and ends.

## High Value Care Key Points

Key Points in the text that relate to High Value Care concepts (that is, concepts that discuss balancing clinical benefit with costs and harms) are designated by the HVC icon (**HVC**).

## Educational Disclaimer

The editors and publisher of MKSAP 17 recognize that the development of new material offers many opportunities for error. Despite our best efforts, some errors may persist in print. Drug dosage schedules are, we believe, accurate and in accordance with current standards. Readers are advised, however, to ensure that the recommended dosages in MKSAP 17 concur with the information provided in the product information material. This is especially important in cases of new, infrequently used, or highly toxic drugs. Application of the information in MKSAP 17 remains the professional responsibility of the practitioner.

The primary purpose of MKSAP 17 is educational. Information presented, as well as publications, technologies, products, and/or services discussed, is intended to inform subscribers about the knowledge, techniques, and experiences of the contributors. A diversity of professional opinion exists, and the views of the contributors are their own and not those of the American College of Physicians (ACP). Inclusion of any material in the program does not constitute endorsement or recommendation by the ACP. The ACP does not warrant the safety, reliability, accuracy, completeness, or usefulness of and disclaims any and all liability for damages and claims that may result from the use of information, publications, technologies, products, and/or services discussed in this program.

## Publisher's Information

## Unauthorized Use of This Book Is Against the Law

MKSAP 17 ISBN: 978-1-938245-18-3
(Infectious Disease) ISBN: 978-1-938245-27-5

Printed in the United States of America.

For order information in the United States or Canada call 800-523-1546, extension 2600. All other countries call 215-351-2600, (M-F, 9 AM – 5 PM ET). Fax inquiries to 215-351-2799 or email to custserv@acponline.org.

## Errata

Errata for MKSAP 17 will be available through the MKSAP Resource Site at mksap.acponline.org as new information becomes known to the editors.

# Table of Contents

# Infectious Disease High Value Care Recommendations

The American College of Physicians, in collaboration with multiple other organizations, is engaged in a worldwide initiative to promote the practice of High Value Care (HVC). The goals of the HVC initiative are to improve health care outcomes by providing care of proven benefit and reducing costs by avoiding unnecessary and even harmful interventions. The initiative comprises several programs that integrate the important concept of health care value (balancing clinical benefit with costs and harms) for a given intervention into a broad range of educational materials to address the needs of trainees, practicing physicians, and patients.

HVC content has been integrated into MKSAP 17 in several important ways. MKSAP 17 now includes HVC-identified key points in the text, HVC-focused multiple choice questions, and, for subscribers to MKSAP Digital, an HVC custom quiz. From the text and questions, we have generated the following list of HVC recommendations that meet the definition below of high value care and bring us closer to our goal of improving patient outcomes while conserving finite resources.

**High Value Care Recommendation:** A recommendation to choose diagnostic and management strategies for patients in specific clinical situations that balance clinical benefit with cost and harms with the goal of improving patient outcomes.

Below are the High Value Care Recommendations for the Infectious Disease section of MKSAP 17.

- Viral meningitis is managed supportively, with empiric antimicrobials given only until cerebrospinal fluid cultures exclude bacterial meningitis.
- Skin infection is usually diagnosed clinically; radiography should be reserved for when the diagnosis is uncertain, necrotizing fasciitis is suspected, or when an associated abscess or foreign body is a concern.
- In community-associated methicillin-resistant *Staphylococcus aureus* infections, the primary treatment of a cutaneous abscess is incision and drainage.
- No antibiotic treatment is needed after incision and drainage of a simple furuncle, except in patients who are immunosuppressed, who do not respond adequately to incision and drainage or antibiotics without MRSA activity, or who have systemic signs of infection (see Item 103).
- Amoxicillin-clavulanate prophylaxis is recommended only for patients with animal bites who are immunosuppressed; have moderate-to-severe wounds, particularly on the face or hand; have wounds near a joint or bone; or have wounds associated with significant crush injury or edema.
- One of several decision support tools (Pneumonia Severity Index, CURB-65/CRB-65, Infectious Diseases Society of America/American Thoracic Society criteria for severe pneumonia) should be used to assess the need for outpatient versus hospitalized patients care of community-acquired pneumonia.
- Patients treated with intravenous antibiotics for community-acquired pneumonia with an appropriate clinical response can be switched to an oral agent, generally of the same antimicrobial class and with similar spectrum of activity, when clinical stability has been attained (see Item 51).
- Continued in-hospital monitoring of stable patients following the transition from parenteral to oral therapy has not been shown to improve outcomes.
- In patients taking intravenous antimicrobial therapy, a switch to oral therapy should be considered in all patients with an intact and functioning gastrointestinal tract and whose clinical status is improving (see Item 42).
- Empiric antimicrobial therapy should be modified or de-escalated as soon as culture results become available to provide the narrowest-spectrum agent available (see Item 53).
- Treatment courses for community-acquired pneumonia longer than 5 days have not shown clinical benefit and should be avoided to minimize unnecessary antimicrobial use and avoid extra expense of care.
- The routine use of follow-up chest radiography after successful treatment of community-acquired pneumonia is not recommended because findings may linger despite clinical improvement and symptom resolution.
- Antibodies may not be present early in Lyme disease infection; documentation of erythema migrans with a compatible epidemiologic history is sufficient for diagnosis, and serologic testing is not indicated and may be falsely negative in localized disease.
- Lyme arthritis is excluded if symptoms have been present for longer than 1 month and Western blot IgG result is negative; there is no need for further evaluation or treatment for Lyme disease in these patients (see Item 82).
- Post–Lyme disease syndrome or "chronic Lyme disease" occurs in some patients despite appropriate antibiotic therapy and includes nonspecific but disabling symptoms; management focuses on amelioration of symptoms

- and prolonged administration of antibiotics is contraindicated.
- Avoid inappropriate antibiotic use wherever possible; antimicrobial resistance among urinary pathogens is increasing in frequency in the community and hospital settings because of antibiotic overuse, inappropriate treatment of asymptomatic bacteriuria, and local differences in antibiotic use.
- A culture of midstream, clean-void urine should be reserved for patients with suspected pyelonephritis, complicated urinary tract infection, recurrent urinary tract infection, or multiple antimicrobial allergies and in those in whom the presence of a resistant organism is suspected.
- Fosfomycin has lower efficacy and is more expensive than nitrofurantoin or trimethoprim-sulfamethoxazole in first-line antimicrobial therapy for women with acute uncomplicated cystitis.
- Acute uncomplicated pyelonephritis should be treated with fluoroquinolones for 5 to 7 days, complicated infections should be treated for 14 days, and hospitalized patients treated initially with parenteral antibiotics can be switched to oral agents after clinical improvement is noted and oral therapy can be tolerated.
- The interferon-γ release assay should be reserved for persons who have received bacillus Calmette-Guérin vaccine previously or are members of groups that are unlikely to return to have their tuberculin skin test interpreted.
- Routinely combining a tuberculin skin test with interferon-γ release assay to test for tuberculosis adds expense but no additional value and should be avoided.
- Nucleic acid amplification testing targeting *Mycobacterium tuberculosis* in sputum from patients with high clinical suspicion of having tuberculosis (AFB smear–positive sputum) can expedite initiation of treatment, although it is more expensive and does not provide drug susceptibility and genotyping information necessary to guide long term treatment.
- At least monthly clinical evaluations are recommended during tuberculosis treatment, and routine laboratory monitoring is recommended for patients with baseline abnormalities or increased risk for adverse effects; otherwise, laboratory studies are reserved for those who develop potential drug-associated toxicities.
- Treatment of asymptomatic candiduria is indicated only in neutropenic patients and those undergoing urologic procedures; if an indwelling catheter is present, it should be removed if possible (see Item 73).
- Conventional plain radiography lacks sensitivity and specificity for diagnosing osteomyelitis and has a limited role.
- MRI is the best imaging technique for diagnosing osteomyelitis because of its high sensitivity for bone infection and superiority at delineating bone anatomy and providing excellent resolution of surrounding soft tissues; the role for follow-up MRI is limited to patients who do not clinically improve with therapy.

- Blood cultures should be obtained in all suspected cases of osteomyelitis because cultures are positive in more than 50% of cases and may avert more invasive testing.
- Culture samples obtained from superficial wounds or sinus tracts correlate poorly with deep cultures from bone and should not be obtained.
- Antimicrobial prophylaxis for traveler's diarrhea is effective, but it is generally not recommended because of the potential for adverse effects; prophylaxis should be considered in persons with coexisting inflammatory bowel disease, immunocompromised states (including advanced HIV), and comorbidities that would be adversely affected by significant dehydration.
- Fluid replacement with aggressive oral hydration is the mainstay of treatment for travelers' diarrhea (see Item 38); antimicrobials reduce the duration of diarrhea by 1 to 2 days but are recommended only in severe disease or immunosuppressed patients.
- Antibiotic treatment of otherwise healthy patients with mild diarrheal symptoms does not hasten recovery and may lead to prolonged asymptomatic shedding of *Salmonella* bacteria.
- In most cases of bacterial gastroenteritis, infection resolves spontaneously without therapy, and further evaluation or treatment is unnecessary (see Item 91).
- Therapy for mild nontyphoidal *Salmonella* gastroenteritis should be withheld in otherwise healthy patients because treatment may increase duration of bacterial shedding (see Item 58).
- Oral metronidazole and vancomycin are equally effective in treating mild-to-moderate *Clostridium difficile* infection, with the former preferred because of its lower cost; oral vancomycin is recommended for severe disease.
- Patients with hospital-acquired diarrhea who test negative for *Clostridium difficile* infection should be treated with antimotility agents to suppress symptoms and not undergo additional testing or treatment for *C. difficile* (see Item 7).
- Documenting clearance of *C. difficile* through testing serial stool samples after an initial positive test result has no role in management.
- Testing for parasites is not recommended for diarrhea lasting less than 7 days or for patients who develop diarrhea more than 3 days into a hospital stay because it is both expensive and unlikely to be helpful.
- Approximately 65% to 70% of catheter-associated bloodstream infections and urinary tract infections and 55% of ventilator-associated pneumonia cases and surgical site infections may be preventable.
- Preventing catheter-associated urinary tract infection relies on using urinary catheters only if they are essential to the patient's care and only for as short a period of time as possible (see Item 28).
- Routine urinalysis and culture should not be performed for patients with indwelling urinary catheters without symptoms or signs of urinary tract infection.

- When culture data are available, therapy for catheter-associated urinary tract infections should be adjusted to the narrowest coverage spectrum possible.
- Continuing prophylactic antimicrobial agents postoperatively has not shown benefit in preventing surgical site infections.
- Hospitalized patients with central lines should be assessed daily to determine whether the line can be removed.
- No evidence indicates that hospital-acquired pneumonia or ventilator-associated pneumonia caused by *Pseudomonas* species requires combination therapy or that a synergistic combination improves outcomes.
- Avoiding intubation (if possible) and using noninvasive positive-pressure ventilation as an alternative (when feasible) can significantly decrease the risk for hospital-acquired pneumonia.
- Limiting transmission of antimicrobial-resistant organisms in health care settings is best accomplished by full compliance with hand hygiene protocols and contact precautions, cleaning and disinfecting the environment and patient care equipment before it is used for another patient, and judicious use of antimicrobial agents.
- Annual influenza vaccination is the most effective intervention for preventing influenza and is recommended for all persons 6 months of age or older.

- Tigecycline is a broad-spectrum antibiotic that should be used only when alternative treatments are not available, because it is expensive and should be reserved for treatment of resistant organisms.
- Suboptimal use of antimicrobial agents drives the emergence of antimicrobial resistance, leads to poor outcomes, and increases adverse events and costs.
- Outpatient parenteral antimicrobial therapy provides appropriately selected patients the ability to complete antimicrobial treatment in an outpatient setting.
- Patients with selective IgA deficiency require no specific therapy except for preventive measures against known potential complications and as-needed antibiotic therapy for those with recurrent sinopulmonary infections (see Item 84).
- Patients diagnosed with babesiosis who are asymptomatic should undergo a repeat polymerase chain reaction assay in 3 months to detect parasite clearance but do not need treatment (see Item 87).
- When a patient has been reasonably evaluated (laboratory studies, repeat blood cultures, imaging studies) for ongoing fever, a diagnosis of fever of unknown origin should be reached and the patient should be observed in case further interventions would be appropriate later (see Item 106).

# Infectious Disease

## Central Nervous System Infections

### Meningitis

#### Viral Meningitis

**Causes**

Viral meningitis is the most common cause of "aseptic" meningitis, in which cerebrospinal fluid (CSF) bacterial cultures are negative. Most patients have typical meningitis symptoms, such as fever, nuchal rigidity, headache, and photophobia.

A substantial proportion of viral meningitis is caused by enteroviruses, which commonly occur in the summer and fall in temperate climates when these organisms circulate in the environment. Enteroviral meningitis can also occur in winter and spring months; seasonal enteroviral infections are typically caused by coxsackievirus, echovirus, or other nonpolio enteroviruses.

Herpes simplex virus (HSV) can also cause meningitis. These meningitis syndromes can be related to primary infections, with central nervous system (CNS) involvement as a secondary consequence, or reactivation of latent infection presenting as aseptic meningitis. Most patients with HSV meningitis associated with primary infection will have genital lesions. HSV type 2 (HSV-2) is more commonly associated with meningitis, whereas HSV type 1 (HSV-1) is associated with encephalitis. An association exists between Mollaret meningitis, a benign recurring form of lymphocytic meningitis, and HSV-2; at least 84% of patients have evidence of HSV-2 in CSF.

Primary HIV infection can present with an aseptic meningitis syndrome, which may occur in isolation from the other symptoms. Meningitis due to acute HIV infection is typically self-limited and may be clinically indistinguishable from other viral meningitis syndromes.

Mumps virus can cause meningitis, with typical symptoms of fever, headache, and neck stiffness. Since the advent of universal childhood vaccination for measles, mumps, and rubella, the incidence of mumps-related meningitis has dramatically decreased. Meningitis from mumps virus can occur at any point during the course of clinical mumps infection. Parotitis or orchitis may be present.

Infections with arboviruses, such as West Nile virus or St. Louis encephalitis virus, can cause meningitis, although these infections more typically produce encephalitis. Cytomegalovirus, Epstein-Barr virus, adenovirus, and varicella virus infections can also cause meningitis.

**Diagnosis**

Symptoms of viral meningitis include fever, headache, neck stiffness, photophobia, and change in mental status and may be indistinguishable from symptoms of bacterial meningitis. Characteristics of the CSF profile are outlined in **Table 1**. Additional physical examination findings (rash and pharyngitis in acute HIV infection; parotitis or orchitis in mumps-related meningitis) can support the presumptive diagnosis. Polymerase chain reaction (PCR) and other molecular tests are available for diagnosis of numerous viral causes. CSF PCR studies may be used for diagnosing HSV and enterovirus meningitis; antibody detection in CSF is preferred for West Nile virus meningitis. Viral cultures of CSF are not clinically useful because of poor sensitivity and long turn-around times. Serologic testing may be an adjunctive diagnostic tool in meningitis caused by mumps.

**TABLE 1.** Typical CSF Findings in Patients with Viral and Bacterial Meningitis

| CSF Parameter | Viral Meningitis[a] | Bacterial Meningitis |
|---|---|---|
| Opening pressure | ≤250 mm H$_2$O | 200-500[b] mm H$_2$O |
| Leukocyte count | 50-1000/µL (50-1000 × 10$^6$/L) | 1000-5000/µL (1000-5000 × 10$^6$/L)[c] |
| Leukocyte predominance | Lymphocytes[d] | Neutrophils |
| Glucose | >45 mg/dL (2.5 mmol/L) | <40 mg/dL (2.2 mmol/L)[e] |
| Protein | <200 mg/dL (2000 mg/L) | 100-500 mg/dL (1000-5000 mg/L) |
| Gram stain | Negative | Positive in 60%-90%[f,g] |
| Culture | Negative | Positive in 70%-85%[g] |

CSF = cerebrospinal fluid.

[a]Primarily nonpolio enteroviruses (echoviruses and coxsackieviruses).

[b]Values exceeding 600 mm H$_2$O suggest the presence of cerebral edema, intracranial suppurative foci, or communicating hydrocephalus.

[c]Range may be <100/µL (100 × 10$^6$/L) to >10,000/µL (10,000 × 10$^6$/L).

[d]May have neutrophil predominance early in infection, but lymphocyte predominance occurs after the first 6 to 48 hours.

[e]The CSF-to-plasma glucose ratio is ≤0.40 in most patients.

[f]The likelihood of a positive Gram stain correlates with number of bacteria in the CSF.

[g]The yield of positive results is significantly reduced by previous administration of antimicrobial therapy.

**CONT.**

Meningitis can also result from medications; autoimmune diseases; malignancy; and other nonviral infectious causes, including spirochetes, fungi, or mycobacteria. Serology may be helpful to diagnose aseptic meningitis caused by syphilis, *Borrelia burgdorferi* (Lyme disease), or certain fungal organisms.

## Treatment

Anti-infective treatments are not available for viral meningitis with the exception of underlying herpes viruses. The primary focus of management in viral meningitis is to distinguish it from other causes of infectious meningitis, particularly bacterial meningitis. Symptomatic and supportive management for viral meningitis and rigorous evaluation to exclude bacterial meningitis are the cornerstones of management. Empiric antimicrobial agents may be initiated until full CSF profiles and cultures are finalized and bacterial meningitis can be excluded. Antibiotics can be started and continued as empiric treatment for 48 to 72 hours, after which most routine CSF cultures will show preliminary results. The increasing availability of enteroviral PCR testing can shorten the time required to exclude bacterial infection. Repeat lumbar puncture can be performed after the initial 2 to 3 days if lack of clinical response is a concern or if documenting the evolution of the CSF profile to that more characteristic of viral meningitis is desired. **H**

### KEY POINTS

- Viral meningitis is most commonly caused by enteroviruses, herpes simplex virus type 2, and arboviruses.

- Clinical signs and symptoms aiding in the diagnosis of viral meningitis include parotitis or orchitis with mumps virus, rash in enterovirus and HIV, pharyngitis with acute HIV, and genital lesions with herpes simplex virus.

**HVC**
- Viral meningitis is managed supportively, with empiric antimicrobials given only until cerebrospinal fluid cultures exclude bacterial meningitis.

## Bacterial Meningitis

### Causes

Bacterial meningitis usually results from bacteremic dissemination of meningeal pathogens that colonize the nasopharynx or from another distant focus of infection but may also occur from contiguous spread of infection to the CSF (sinusitis or otitis media), direct inoculation (traumatic injury or neurosurgical procedure), or prosthetic device infection (CSF shunts or drains, intracranial pressure monitors).

Individual host factors, such as colonization of the nasopharynx with potential meningeal pathogens, complement deficiency, anatomic or functional asplenia, glucocorticoid use, diabetes, hypogammaglobulinemia, and altered cell-mediated immunity, can also contribute to increased susceptibility to acute bacterial meningitis. Exposure to other persons with bacterial meningitis (for certain pathogens, such as

*Neisseria meningitidis*) or travel to regions of the world where certain organisms are more prevalent and endemic (such as sub-Saharan Africa, where endemic meningococcal disease is present) will also increase the risk for bacterial meningitis.

The two most common organisms causing bacterial meningitis are *Streptococcus pneumoniae* and *N. meningitidis*, which together are responsible for more than 80% of infections (**Table 2**).

### Diagnosis

Bacterial meningitis is classically described as producing fever, nuchal rigidity, and altered mental status. However, all three symptoms may not be present in many patients with confirmed disease. Other clinical manifestations that suggest bacterial meningitis include photophobia, headache (often a very severe headache distinctly different from what the patient may typically experience), and dermatologic manifestations (rash, petechiae, purpura) or neurologic abnormalities

| TABLE 2. | Causes of Bacterial Meningitis | |
|---|---|---|
| **Infecting Organism** | **Cases (%)** | **Comments** |
| *Streptococcus pneumoniae* | >70 | Many cases caused by serotypes not covered by pneumococcal vaccination; functionally and anatomically asplenic patients at greater risk |
| *Neisseria meningitidis* | 12 | Can be transmitted through droplet exposure; functionally and anatomically asplenic patients at greater risk |
| Group B streptococci | 7 | Persons with diabetes, alcoholism, malignancy, liver disease at risk |
| *Staphylococcus aureus* | <5 | Primary infection is associated with neurosurgery or CNS prosthetic device; secondary infection arises from bacteremia |
| *Haemophilus influenzae* | 6 | Decreased prevalence in the pediatric age group since type B conjugate vaccine; functionally and anatomically asplenic patients at greater risk |
| *Listeria monocytogenes* | <5 | Immunosuppressed and decreased cell-mediated immunity (because of medications or medical conditions) as well as age (very old and very young) are risk factors |
| Gram-negative bacteria | <5 | Nosocomial settings; complication of neurosurgery |

CNS = central nervous system.

(focal neurologic or cranial nerve deficits, seizures). Physical examination maneuvers, such as testing for Brudzinski and Kernig signs, lack adequate sensitivity and specificity, although the presence of one or both of these findings is consistent with bacterial meningitis.

Before proceeding with lumbar puncture, it should be determined whether CT of the head should be performed. CT of the head before lumbar puncture is indicated if signs or symptoms of increased intracranial pressure or a CNS mass lesion, such as papilledema, focal neurologic deficits, or altered mental status, are present; it is also indicated in patients who are immunocompromised or have a history of CNS disease (mass lesion, stroke, focal infection). In the absence of these findings, lumbar puncture can be undertaken without CNS imaging. Elevated CSF opening pressure is common. Characteristic CSF profiles in bacterial meningitis are outlined in Table 1. CSF Gram stain and cultures, when obtained before

antimicrobial therapy initiation, are usually diagnostic for the infecting organism. Rapid CSF tests, such as latex agglutination and molecular testing with PCR, can be supplemental diagnostic tools, although the diagnostic utility of latex agglutination testing is limited by a lack of specificity. Elevated CSF lactate levels suggest bacterial meningitis, but this is not a specific finding. Blood cultures, if obtained before antimicrobial therapy, are often positive and may be an adjunctive diagnostic tool in isolating the bacterial causative pathogen if CSF cannot be obtained before antibiotic administration.

## Management

Suspected bacterial meningitis demands prompt therapy; because of the risk for substantial morbidity and mortality with delayed treatment, empiric therapy is often initiated before CSF results are available (**Figure 1**). When a presumptive diagnosis of bacterial meningitis has been made, empiric

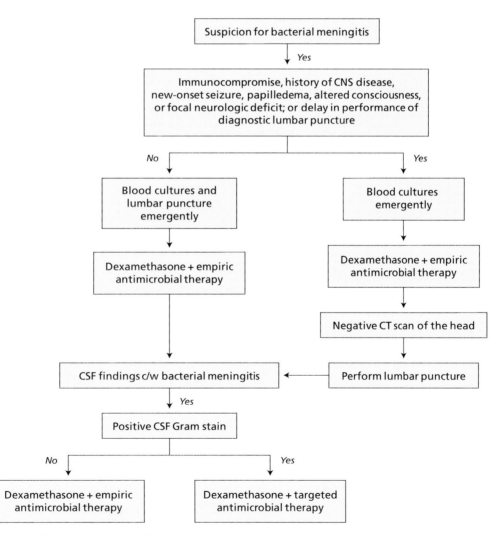

**FIGURE 1.** Management algorithm for adults suspected of having bacterial meningitis.

CNS = central nervous system; c/w = consistent with; CSF = cerebrospinal fluid.

Adapted with permission from Tunkel AR, Hartman BJ, Kaplan SL, et al. Practice guidelines for the management of bacterial meningitis. Clin Infect Dis. 2004 Nov 1;39(9):1270. [PMID: 15494903] Copyright 2004 Oxford University Press.

**H CONT.** antimicrobials directed toward the most likely causes are initiated, as outlined in **Table 3**. Because of the potential neurologic complications of bacterial meningitis, particularly pneumococcal meningitis (seizures, hearing loss, cranial nerve deficits, paresis), adjunctive dexamethasone is recommended; it should be given approximately 15 minutes before administration of antimicrobial agents and should be continued for a full course (0.15 mg/kg every 6 hours for 4 days) in patients with suspected or confirmed pneumococcal meningitis. Although benefit has been shown with dexamethasone in developed countries, the drug has not been proven beneficial in resource-poor settings. When CSF cultures have been finalized, antimicrobial therapy can be altered on the basis of the specific cause and confirmed susceptibilities. Therapy duration varies depending on the causative agent and clinical response; duration may be 7 days (*N. meningitidis*, *Haemophilus influenzae*), 10 to 14 days (*S. pneumoniae*), or up to 21 days (staphylococcal, gram-negative, or *Listeria* meningitis). **H**

**KEY POINTS**

- The most common organisms causing bacterial meningitis are *Streptococcus pneumoniae*, *Neisseria meningitidis*, group B streptococcus, *Haemophilus influenzae*, and *Listeria monocytogenes*.

- Empiric antimicrobial therapy should be initiated immediately in suspected bacterial meningitis, with more specific targeted therapy implemented after culture results are obtained.

- Dexamethasone is recommended as adjunctive therapy in all cases of bacterial meningitis in developed countries.

| TABLE 3. Antibiotic Management of Bacterial Meningitis | |
|---|---|
| **Clinical Characteristics** | **Empiric Antibiotic Regimen** |
| Immunocompetent host age <50 y with community-acquired bacterial meningitis | IV ceftriaxone *or* cefotaxime plus IV vancomycin |
| Patient age >50 y or those with altered cell-mediated immunity | IV ampicillin (*Listeria* coverage) plus IV ceftriaxone *or* cefotaxime plus IV vancomycin |
| Allergies to β-lactams | IV moxifloxacin instead of cephalosporin |
| | IV trimethoprim-sulfamethoxazole instead of ampicillin |
| Hospital-acquired bacterial meningitis | IV vancomycin plus either IV ceftazidime, cefepime, or meropenem |
| Neurosurgical procedures | IV vancomycin plus either IV ceftazidime, cefepime, or meropenem |
| IV = intravenous. | |

# Focal Central Nervous System Infections  **H**

## Brain Abscess

A brain abscess is a focal infection of the brain parenchyma that arises from hematogenous dissemination or, more commonly, direct spread of infection from contiguous anatomic structures. Multifocal brain abscesses more commonly arise from hematogenous routes of infection, whereas solitary brain abscesses most often result from extension of contiguous infections into the brain. Brain abscesses caused by contiguous infections may be a complication of otitis media, sinusitis, or odontogenic infections. Brain abscesses can also present as complications from foreign bodies that become lodged in the brain parenchyma or arise postoperatively from neurosurgical procedures. No source of infection is determined in approximately 20% to 40% of brain abscesses.

Many brain abscesses are polymicrobial, and a substantial proportion of cases involve anaerobic organisms. The microbiology and clinical characteristics of brain abscesses are outlined in **Table 4**.

Clinical presentation of brain abscess includes headache, which can be severe and unresponsive to analgesia; fever is not always present. Neck stiffness is typically present only with occipital lobe involvement. Mental status changes and vomiting indicate later-stage progression of the brain abscess and are poor prognostic signs. Physical examination may show focal neurologic signs and cranial nerve deficits. CNS imaging is the cornerstone of diagnosis; lumbar puncture is contraindicated because of the potential for increased intracranial pressure and risk for herniation. Although MRI is more sensitive than CT, contrast-enhanced CT can often be performed more rapidly. Stereotactic CT-guided aspiration can be performed to obtain microbiologic samples, but this invasive diagnostic method is often impractical before a clinical decision is made to treat a suspected brain abscess.

If brain abscess is suspected, empiric antimicrobial therapy should be started. Empiric regimens are based on predisposing conditions and suspected causative agents (see Table 4). Abscesses larger than 2.5 cm should be surgically excised or drained stereotactically. If abscesses are not drained, follow-up CNS imaging should occur within several days to assess for worsening cerebral edema. CNS imaging should be repeated urgently if any mental status or neurologic changes are noted.

Antimicrobial therapy duration is typically 4 to 8 weeks. Therapy duration should be guided by follow-up clinical evaluation and repeat neuroimaging, ideally by using the same modality as the original imaging study. Expert opinion recommends administration of glucocorticoids when substantial cerebral edema is present. A substantial portion of patients with brain abscess can have residual neurologic sequelae, particularly seizures. **H**

**TABLE 4.** Predisposing Conditions, Causative Agents, and Empiric Antimicrobial Therapy in Patients with Bacterial Brain Abscess

| Predisposing Condition | Usual Causative Agents | Empiric Antimicrobial Therapy |
|---|---|---|
| Otitis media or mastoiditis | Streptococci (aerobic or anaerobic), *Bacteroides* species, *Prevotella* species, Enterobacteriaceae | Metronidazole plus a third-generation cephalosporin[a] |
| Sinusitis | Streptococci, *Bacteroides* species, Enterobacteriaceae, *Staphylococcus aureus*, *Haemophilus* species | Metronidazole plus a third-generation cephalosporin[a,b] |
| Dental sepsis | Mixed *Fusobacterium, Prevotella,* and *Bacteroides* species; streptococci | Penicillin plus metronidazole |
| Penetrating trauma or after neurosurgery | *S. aureus*, streptococci, Enterobacteriaceae, *Clostridium* species | Vancomycin plus a third-generation cephalosporin[a,c] |
| Lung abscess, empyema, bronchiectasis | *Fusobacterium, Actinomyces, Bacteroides,* and *Prevotella* species; streptococci; *Nocardia* species | Penicillin plus metronidazole plus a sulfonamide[d] |
| Endocarditis | *S. aureus*, streptococci | Vancomycin plus gentamicin |
| Hematogenous spread from pelvic, intra-abdominal, or gynecologic infections | Enteric gram-negative bacteria, anaerobic bacteria | Metronidazole plus a third-generation cephalosporin[a,b,c] |
| Immunocompromised patients<br><br>HIV-infected patients | *Listeria* species, fungal organisms (*Cryptococcus neoformans*), or parasitic or protozoal organisms (*Toxoplasma gondii*); *Aspergillus, Coccidioides,* and *Nocardia* species | Metronidazole plus a third-generation cephalosporin[a,b,c,d,e]; antifungal or antiparasitic agent |

[a]Cefotaxime or ceftriaxone; the fourth-generation cephalosporin cefepime may also be used.

[b]Add vancomycin if infection caused by methicillin-resistant *Staphylococcus aureus* is suspected. Vancomycin can then be transitioned to antistaphylococcal β-lactam (oxacillin-nafcillin)-penicillin if methicillin-sensitive *Staphylococcus aureus* is confirmed.

[c]Use ceftazidime or cefepime if infection caused by *Pseudomonas aeruginosa* is suspected. Meropenem can also be used for antipseudomonal coverage.

[d]Use trimethoprim-sulfamethoxazole if infection caused by *Nocardia* species is suspected.

[e]Use ampicillin if infection caused by *Listeria* species is suspected.

NOTE: If predisposing condition is unknown, empiric treatment should include vancomycin plus metronidazole and third-generation cephalosporin.

---

**KEY POINT**

- Empiric antimicrobial therapy should be initiated immediately if brain abscess is suspected, and successful treatment usually combines antimicrobial therapy with surgical drainage.

## Spinal Epidural Abscess

Spinal epidural abscesses (SEAs) usually result from contiguous spread from infected vertebrae or intervertebral body disc spaces or hematogenous dissemination from a distant site. Risk factors include prolonged epidural catheter placement, paraspinal glucocorticoid or analgesic injections, diabetes mellitus, HIV infection, trauma, injection drug use, tattooing, alcoholism, and acupuncture. Most SEAs are caused by *Staphylococcus aureus*. Other, less frequent, causative organisms include gram-negative bacilli, *Streptococcus* species, anaerobic organisms, and, rarely, fungi or other unusual pathogens.

SEA can be challenging to diagnose because symptoms can be mild or nonspecific and fever may not always be present. A high index of suspicion, particularly in patients with atypical or persistent back pain, will facilitate more prompt diagnosis. Symptoms may progress from back pain to accompanying neurologic symptoms, such as bowel or bladder dysfunction, lower-extremity weakness, paresthesias, and, in the last stages, paralysis. MRI of the spine with contrast is the preferred imaging modality for diagnosis. If MRI cannot be done, CT of the spine with contrast may be an acceptable alternative. Microbiologic sampling with CT-guided needle aspiration can be attempted, and blood cultures should be obtained. At least two blood culture sets should be drawn in patients suspected of having SEA because the causative agent can be confirmed from these cultures more than 60% of the time. Empiric antibiotics can be started if the suspicion for SEA is high.

SEA is treated with a combination of antimicrobial therapy and surgical drainage. Medical therapy alone is often successful if no neurologic deficits are present at the time of diagnosis or if substantial complications from surgery are likely because of comorbid conditions. Serial clinical evaluations and follow-up MRI of the spine (at approximately 4-6 weeks into therapy or with any sign of clinical deterioration) are necessary adjuncts to management without surgery. Empiric parenteral antimicrobial therapy should include coverage for *S. aureus*, *Streptococcus* species, and gram-negative bacilli and may be narrowed on the basis of culture results, if available. Therapy typically lasts between 6 and 8 weeks (or until resolution of abscess on follow-up MRI) but may require

CONT.
modification depending on clinical and radiologic recovery. Antibiotic therapy is parenteral to ensure adequate penetration into the CNS. H

## Cranial Subdural Empyema

Subdural empyema is a focal infection or abscess that occurs between the dura mater and the arachnoid mater. This condition is a medical emergency warranting immediate neurosurgical intervention. Sinusitis, otitis media, or mastoiditis can be the inciting infection, with subdural empyema arising as a complication. Patients with subdural empyema initially have fevers and altered cognition, with deteriorating mental status as the infection progresses. Microbiologic testing of these infections reflects the source, with most subdural empyemas caused by *S. pneumoniae*, *H. influenzae*, aerobic and anaerobic *Streptococcus* species, *Staphylococcus* species (coagulase-positive and coagulase-negative), gram-negative bacilli, and anaerobic organisms (*Bacteroides* species). Diagnosis is based on clinical presentation, which often includes fever; headache;

nausea and vomiting; mental status changes; and a history of preceding sinusitis, otitis, meningitis, mastoiditis, or recent neurosurgical procedures or sinus surgeries. The diagnosis is confirmed by MRI with gadolinium; CT with contrast is an alternative. Lumbar puncture is contraindicated when increased intracranial pressure is evident. Prompt and immediate neurosurgical intervention to drain the infected collection of purulent material is necessary. Empiric antimicrobial therapy consists of intravenous vancomycin, ceftriaxone (or another cephalosporin that penetrates the CSF well), and metronidazole. Therapy duration is guided by clinical and radiologic improvement. Surgical intervention directed toward the primary source of infection may be a necessary adjunct to successful treatment. H

# Encephalitis

Encephalitis is a life-threatening condition. Select viral pathogens causing encephalitis are shown in **Table 5**. Encephalitis often exists as an overlap syndrome with meningitis or inflammation of the spinal cord (encephalomyelitis). Clinically, encephalitis is defined as alteration in mental status lasting 24 hours or more that is associated with two or more of the following: fever, focal neurologic deficit, seizure, CSF pleocytosis, and abnormal findings on electroencephalography or

**TABLE 5.** Selected Viral Causes of Acute Encephalitis

| Organism | Epidemiology and Transmission | Clinical Features | Laboratory Diagnosis | Treatment |
|---|---|---|---|---|
| Herpes simplex virus type 1 | Reactivation of latent virus | Fever, altered mental status, temporal lobe seizures | Herpes simplex virus type 1 PCR on CSF[a] | Acyclovir (IV) |
| Varicella zoster virus | Can occur at time of acute infection or reactivation, increased risk in HIV | Cutaneous lesions variably present | Varicella zoster virus PCR on CSF, CSF antibodies (if vasculitis suspected) | Acyclovir (IV) |
| Enterovirus | Typically late summer-fall | Fever, altered mental status, variable rash or oral lesions | Enterovirus PCR on CSF | Supportive care |
| West Nile virus | Mosquito-borne (summer/fall) | Fevers, altered mentation with or without muscle weakness (including acute asymmetric flaccid paralysis); seizures rare | West Nile virus IgM antibody on CSF | Supportive care |
| Rabies virus | Bite from infected animal (most commonly bat) | Paresthesia at site of inoculation, hydrophobia, progressive obtundation | Nape of neck skin biopsy for immunohistochemistry  Rabies PCR of saliva or CSF (testing coordinated with local health department) | Supportive care; prophylaxis of close contacts |

CSF = cerebrospinal fluid; IV = intravenous; PCR = polymerase chain reaction.

[a]Herpes simplex virus PCR result can be negative at the time of initial presentation; must repeat test on a second CSF sample in 3-7 days if clinical suspicion remains high.

neuroimaging. A specific cause is found in less than 50% of patients despite intensive investigation; even when a pathogen is identified, no antimicrobial therapy is available for many viral causes, and care is supportive. Nevertheless, an attempt to define the cause is indicated because establishing a diagnosis allows directed treatment, discontinuation of ineffective therapies, and determination of prognosis.

Initial management requires attention to potential comorbidities, particularly in patients with a decreased level of consciousness. All patients should undergo neuroimaging to exclude a mass lesion or cerebral edema as a contraindication to lumbar puncture. If the delay in obtaining CSF is significant (>30 minutes), empiric antimicrobial agents should be administered. Patients with evidence of cerebral edema are usually best managed in an intensive care setting with close neurologic monitoring and consideration of ventriculostomy for patients whose condition deteriorates with medical management. Electroencephalography should be considered in all patients with depressed consciousness, even without seizure activity, because nonconvulsive status epilepticus may be present in the absence of myoclonic movements.

## Herpes Simplex Encephalitis

Infection with HSV-1 is the most common cause of endemic encephalitis in the United States. Most infections result from reactivation of latent virus. Herpes simplex encephalitis (HSE) is characterized by unilateral or bilateral localized infection of the temporal lobes, but the clinical presentation is nonspecific. Cerebrospinal fluid testing typically shows lymphocytic pleocytosis and, when necrosis is extensive, abundant erythrocytes. The presence of temporal lobe abnormalities on imaging is highly suggestive of HSE, with MRI (**Figure 2**) being more sensitive than CT. Periodic lateralizing epileptiform discharges on electroencephalography suggest HSE but may not be present.

Atypical presentations of HSE may occur, and laboratory testing for HSV-1 infection is recommended for all patients with encephalitis regardless of the presence of temporal lobe lesions. HSV PCR of the CSF allows rapid diagnosis of HSE, with sensitivity greater than 95% and specificity approaching 100%; however, very early in the course of infection, the result of this test may be negative. For cases with a high suspicion based on imaging consistent with HSE, testing should be performed on a subsequent CSF sample. PCR findings remain positive for up to 1 week following initiation of acyclovir treatment. The sensitivity of viral culture of CSF for HSV is less than 5%; as a result this test is discouraged. Serologic testing has limited utility because most adults have detectable HSV-1 antibody related to previous infection.

Delay in acyclovir therapy is a negative prognostic factor, and empiric therapy should be initiated for all patients suspected of having encephalitis. Acyclovir must be administered parenterally to achieve therapeutic levels in brain parenchyma. Empiric treatment can be discontinued when an alternative cause of encephalitis is discovered or, in patients with a relatively low suspicion of HSE, when the HSV PCR has negative

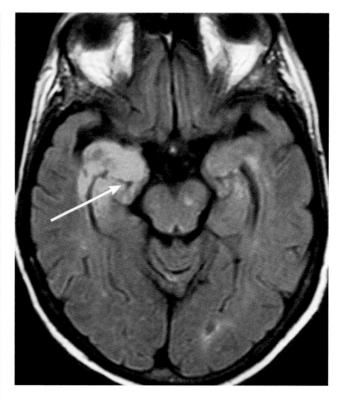

**FIGURE 2.** Brain MRI exhibiting right temporal lobe enhancement (*arrow*) in a patient with herpes simplex encephalitis.

results. When HSE is confirmed, high-dose intravenous acyclovir should be continued for 14 to 21 days.

### KEY POINTS

- Herpes simplex encephalitis is characterized by unilateral or bilateral localized infection of the temporal lobes; cerebrospinal fluid testing typically shows lymphocytic pleocytosis and, when necrosis is extensive, abundant erythrocytes; and MRI may show temporal lobe abnormalities.

- Herpes simplex virus polymerase chain reaction testing on the cerebrospinal fluid is highly sensitive and specific for herpes simplex encephalitis.

- Empiric intravenous acyclovir therapy should be initiated for all patients suspected of having encephalitis.

## Varicella-Zoster Virus Encephalitis

Varicella-zoster virus (VZV) encephalitis may occur at the time of acute varicella infection or with viral reactivation. VZV encephalitis is more common in patients with HIV/AIDS or defects in cellular immunity but also may occur in otherwise healthy persons.

Besides the characteristic skin findings, few specific features suggest VZV encephalitis. The time between the onset of zoster and the development of CNS symptoms may be prolonged, and in some cases encephalitis may predate onset of

CONT.

skin lesions. Even the presence of zoster in a patient with encephalitis is not sufficient proof of CNS infection because cutaneous reactivation may result from the physiologic stress of another infection. Most diagnostically challenging is the condition "herpes sine zoster," in which central nervous system infection occurs in the absence of skin lesions. VZV may also infect cerebral arteries, presenting as an ischemic stroke rather than encephalitis.

Confirmation of VZV encephalitis requires identification of viral infection of the CNS. Findings on VZV PCR of CSF are typically positive in cases of encephalitis associated with acute varicella or zoster. When vasculitis predominates, or when symptoms are more insidious, intrathecal VZV antibodies also should be measured because VZV PCR results can be negative in these cases. Although data on treatment are limited, parenteral acyclovir is recommended in cases of VZV encephalitis or vasculopathy. **H**

**KEY POINTS**

- Varicella-zoster virus encephalitis is more common in patients with HIV/AIDS or defects in cellular immunity.
- Varicella-zoster virus polymerase chain reaction testing of cerebrospinal fluid should be performed to identify viral infection of the central nervous system.
- Parenteral acyclovir is recommended for varicella-zoster virus encephalitis or vasculopathy.

## Neuroinvasive West Nile Virus

West Nile virus (WNV), first detected in the United States in 1999, has emerged as a national public health problem, with infections reported throughout the continental United States. Mosquitoes serve as the primary vector, and most human infections occur during the summer and early fall. Transmission through blood transfusion and organ transplantation has been reported but is much less frequent since the advent of universal screening of donor blood products. Most infected persons remain asymptomatic, with approximately 20% developing West Nile fever. The most severe clinical presentation, West Nile neuroinvasive disease (WNND), occurs in less than 1% of cases. These patients may present with meningitis, encephalitis, or myelitis, either singly or as overlap syndromes. WNND is significantly more common among adults age 50 years or older and in solid organ and bone marrow transplant recipients. HIV infection does not appear to be a significant risk factor for WNND.

Limb weakness, which may be symmetric or involve a single extremity, is a characteristic feature of WNND. Severe disease may manifest as acute asymmetric flaccid paralysis and may progress to cause respiratory failure, akin to that seen with poliomyelitis. Other clinical findings of WNND are rarely helpful in suggesting the diagnosis. Fever is almost universally present. A nonspecific viral exanthema may be found in less than 50% of patients. MRI may show focal lesions of the thalami, basal ganglia, and spinal cord in some patients.

CSF serology is the preferred test to confirm WNND. Most acutely infected patients have detectable IgM antibody to WNV in the first week of symptoms, although titers may remain detectable for more than 1 year. Detection of IgG antibody may confirm previous infection but is less sensitive for diagnosis of acute illness. Serologic cross-reactivity between WNV and other flaviviruses is significant, and caution should be used in interpreting a positive WNV IgG result in a patient with natural infection or vaccination against St. Louis encephalitis virus, Japanese encephalitis virus, yellow fever virus, or dengue virus. For these reasons, testing of CSF is preferred, and the presence of intrathecal WNV IgM antibody is considered diagnostic of acute infection. Results of WNV PCR of serum or CSF are infrequently positive except in immunocompromised patients, who may exhibit delayed viral clearance. Viral culture is insensitive and is not recommended.

No antiviral therapy is effective for WNV infection, and treatment is limited to supportive care. Patients with substantial muscle weakness should be monitored in an intensive care setting for impending respiratory failure. **H**

**KEY POINTS**

- West Nile neuroinvasive disease occurs in less than 1% of infections with West Nile virus and presents with meningitis, encephalitis, or myelitis, either singly or as overlap syndromes.
- Cerebrospinal fluid serology is the preferred diagnostic test for West Nile neuroinvasive disease, with most patients having detectable IgM antibody to West Nile virus in the first week of symptoms.

## Autoimmune Encephalitis

**H**

A newly described autoimmune condition termed anti-*N*-methyl-D-aspartate receptor (anti-NMDAR) antibody encephalitis has emerged as an increasingly common cause of encephalitis. Anti-NMDAR encephalitis is associated with ovarian teratomas in greater than 50% of patients with the disease because of production of an antibody to a tumor protein that cross-reacts with neuronal tissue. In patients without evidence of teratoma, an inciting antigenic stimulus is rarely identified. The diagnosis is suggested by the presence of choreoathetosis, psychiatric symptoms, seizures, and autonomic instability and is confirmed by detection of anti-NMDAR antibody in serum. Treatment includes removal of the teratoma to eradicate the immune stimulus and immunosuppression with glucocorticoids or intravenous immune globulin. **H**

**KEY POINTS**

- Anti-*N*-methyl-D-aspartate receptor (anti-NMDAR) antibody encephalitis presents with choreoathetosis, psychiatric symptoms, seizures, and autonomic instability; is associated with ovarian teratomas in greater than 50% of patients with the disease; and is confirmed by detection of anti-NMDAR antibody in serum.
- Treatment of anti-NMDAR encephalitis includes removal of the teratoma and immunosuppression with glucocorticoids or intravenous immune globulin.

# Prion Diseases of the Central Nervous System

## Introduction

Prion diseases (also known as transmissible spongiform encephalopathies) are a group of rare, closely related, fatal, neurodegenerative conditions that occur in humans and other mammals. They are caused by an accumulation of aggregated forms of the prion protein in the central nervous system. Human prion diseases include sporadic, infectiously transmitted, and genetic disorders. Sporadic disease accounts for most cases. Known infectious acquisition is very rare in humans and accounts for less than 1% of cases in most populations.

The infectiously transmitted forms of prion disease are kuru, variant Creutzfeldt-Jakob disease (CJD), and iatrogenic CJD. Prion disease has been transmitted to humans through dietary practices and iatrogenic exposure. Kuru was the first prion disease recognized to be transmissible and was linked to cannibalism among tribes in New Guinea.

## Creutzfeldt-Jakob Disease

CJD is the most common form of prion disease in humans, with most cases being sporadic. Iatrogenic transmission of CJD is possible and has resulted mainly from receipt of growth hormone prepared from cadaveric pituitaries and contaminated cadaveric dura mater allografts. Contaminated surgical instruments have also been documented to transmit CJD in rare instances. Sporadic CJD does not appear to be transmissible by blood. Although the age range of affected persons is wide, onset usually occurs in the seventh decade of life. The most prominent neurologic sign is disordered cognition. Typically, patients also have motor signs, such as ataxia or spasticity, vague sensory problems, or changes in visual perception. Myoclonus is common. Progressive neurologic decline resulting in death occurs rapidly, typically within 6 to 12 months.

## Variant Creutzfeldt-Jakob Disease

Variant CJD is a novel infectious human prion disease caused by the bovine spongiform encephalopathy agent. Most infections have occurred after consumption of infected beef, although transmission by blood and blood products from donors with variant CJD has been reported. Compared with sporadic CJD, variant CJD has a younger age at onset, psychiatric and sensory signs earlier in the disease process, and development of dementia and motor signs more than 6 months after disease onset; however, it typically resembles sporadic CJD, with the most common neurologic sign being impaired cognition. Motor signs, such as ataxia, spasticity, and myoclonus, are prominent.

Prion disease should be considered in the differential diagnosis of any patient who presents with rapidly progressive dementia. Elevated cerebrospinal fluid levels of the 14-3-3 protein are relatively specific for CJD. Definitive diagnosis is made by brain biopsy. No effective treatment exists.

**KEY POINTS**

- Creutzfeldt-Jakob disease is the most common form of prion disease in humans, with most cases being sporadic.
- Iatrogenic transmission of Creutzfeldt-Jakob disease (CJD) has resulted mainly from receipt of growth hormone prepared from cadaveric pituitaries and contaminated cadaveric dura mater allografts, whereas variant CJD infection has occurred after consumption of infected beef as well as reports of transmission by blood and blood products from donors with variant CJD.

# Skin and Soft Tissue Infections

## Introduction

Skin and soft tissue infections (SSTIs) usually occur when skin microbes penetrate underlying layers of the epidermis. Predisposing conditions include skin trauma, onychomycosis, tinea pedis, vascular insufficiency, lymphatic compromise, obesity, diabetes mellitus, and immune suppression. The most common organisms causing SSTIs are β-hemolytic streptococci, particularly group A β-hemolytic streptococci (GABHS), and *Staphylococcus aureus*. See **Table 6** for cellulitis risk factors and the associated causative microorganisms.

Erysipelas is a superficial infection of the epidermis that usually involves the lower extremities or face. It is typically caused by GABHS. Involved skin is erythematous (with well-demarcated borders), glistening, indurated, painful, and warm. Fever and malaise are often present. Desquamation may develop, but necrosis of the skin does not.

Cellulitis is a diffuse, spreading skin infection that involves the dermis and subcutaneous tissues. Clinical features include warmth, redness, swelling, and tenderness in addition to fever and malaise; regional lymphadenopathy also may be present. Unlike erysipelas, cellulitis is characterized by poorly defined erythema. Cellulitis is categorized as purulent or nonpurulent. Cellulitis associated with purulent drainage or exudate is typically caused by methicillin-resistant *S. aureus* (MRSA). Nonpurulent cellulitis is usually caused by β-hemolytic streptococci.

Skin infection is usually diagnosed clinically. Radiography may be helpful when the diagnosis is uncertain, when necrotizing fasciitis is suspected, or when an associated abscess is a concern. A causative agent is established in few patients. Cultures obtained directly from a purulent skin lesion may be helpful. Blood cultures are positive in less than 5% of patients. It also is estimated that the clinical diagnosis of lower-extremity cellulitis is inaccurate in up to one third of patients. Mimics include stasis dermatitis, contact dermatitis,

**TABLE 6. Cellulitis Pathogens and Associated Risk Factors and Clinical Signs**

| Pathogen | Risk Factor | Comment |
|---|---|---|
| *Aeromonas hydrophila* | Contact with or participation in recreational sports in fresh water lakes, streams, or rivers (including brackish water)<br><br>Contact with medicinal leeches | Cellulitis is nonspecific in clinical appearance; minor trauma to skin usually leads to inoculation of organism |
| *Vibrio vulnificus*, other *Vibrio* species | Contact with salt water or brackish water or contact with drippings from raw seafood | May cause cellulitis through direct inoculation into skin or may be ingested, leading to bacteremia with secondary skin infection<br><br>Hallmark is hemorrhagic bullae in area of cellulitis |
| *Erysipelothrix rhusiopathiae* | Contact with saltwater marine life (also associated with freshwater fish); contact with infected animals such as swine and poultry | Cellulitis usually involves the hand or fingers in those handling fish, shellfish, or, occasionally, poultry or meat contaminated with bacterium<br><br>Causes erysipeloid disease |
| *Pasteurella multocida* | Contact primarily with cats | Cellulitis occurs as a result of cat scratch or bite |
| *Capnocytophaga canimorsus* | Contact primarily with dogs | Cellulitis and sepsis particularly in patients with functional or anatomic asplenia |
| *Bacillus anthracis* | Contact with infected animals or animal products<br><br>Target of bioterrorism | Edematous pruritic lesion with central eschar; spore-forming organism |
| *Francisella tularensis* | Contact with or bite from infected animal (particularly cats) or arthropod bites (particularly ticks) | Ulceroglandular syndrome characterized by ulcerative lesion with central eschar and localized tender lymphadenopathy; constitutional symptoms are often present |
| *Mycobacterium marinum* | Contact with fresh water or salt water, including fish tanks and swimming pools | Lesion often trauma-associated and often involving upper extremity; papular lesions become ulcerative at site of inoculation; ascending lymphatic spread can be seen ("sporotrichoid" appearance); systemic toxicity usually absent |
| *Mycobacterium fortuitum* | Exposure to freshwater footbaths/pedicures at nail salons; infection following augmentation mammoplasty and open heart surgery | Multiple boils; razor shaving strongly associated |

eczema, lymphedema, lipodermatosclerosis, erythromelalgia, deep venous thrombosis, erythema nodosum, hypersensitivity reaction, and thrombophlebitis. **H**

**KEY POINTS**

- Cellulitis associated with purulent drainage or exudate is typically caused by methicillin-resistant *Staphylococcus aureus*, whereas nonpurulent cellulitis is usually caused by β-hemolytic streptococci.
- Skin infection is usually diagnosed clinically; radiography should be reserved for when the diagnosis is uncertain, necrotizing fasciitis is suspected, or when an associated abscess or foreign body is a concern.

## Community-Associated Methicillin-Resistant *Staphylococcus aureus*

Community-associated MRSA (CA-MRSA) infections commonly present as a purulent SSTI such as a furuncle, which is infection of the hair follicle that extends into the dermis and subcutaneous tissues. Healthy young persons can become infected, especially in conditions of crowding, suboptimal hygiene (sharing of contaminated items, including razors and towels), and frequent antibiotic use. Outbreaks have been reported on athletic teams, in correctional facilities and day care centers, and among military recruits and men who have sex with men. MRSA is responsible for almost 60% of SSTIs in patients seen in the emergency department. The increased prevalence of CA-MRSA has affected the treatment of SSTIs, and the Infectious Diseases Society of America (IDSA) has published evidence-based clinical practice guidelines to inform when empiric treatment for CA-MRSA is appropriate.

The primary treatment of a cutaneous abscess is incision and drainage. Antibiotics generally are recommended only when the response to incision and drainage is inadequate; in extensive disease or rapid progression with associated cellulitis; in immunodeficiency and other comorbidities; for very young or very old patients; with clinical signs of systemic illness; when involved areas are challenging to drain, such as the genitalia, hands, or face; and in the presence of associated

**CONT.**

septic phlebitis. Outpatients with purulent cellulitis can be treated empirically for CA-MRSA with a 5- to 10-day course of oral antibiotics, such as trimethoprim-sulfamethoxazole or doxycycline. Linezolid is another treatment option, although its expense and similar efficacy to other agents limit its use to very few clinical situations. Outpatient oral antibiotic therapy for nonpurulent cellulitis should include a β-lactam antibiotic, such as cephalexin or dicloxacillin, which is effective against β-hemolytic streptococci. When coverage of both CA-MRSA and β-hemolytic streptococci is desired, outpatient oral options include clindamycin alone or trimethoprim-sulfamethoxazole or doxycycline in combination with a β-lactam agent, such as amoxicillin; linezolid is also an option in specific patients. Patients who require hospitalization for complicated SSTIs (deep soft tissue infections and abscesses, cellulitis, necrotizing infection, trauma-associated wound infection, postsurgical wound infection, infected burn/ulcer) should receive surgical evaluation for debridement in addition to empiric broad-spectrum antibiotic coverage that includes MRSA agents, such as vancomycin, daptomycin, or, in specific patients, linezolid. Rifampin is not recommended for MRSA treatment, even in an adjunctive role. Ceftaroline is a fifth-generation cephalosporin approved for treatment of SSTIs, including those associated with MRSA. It is recommended as empiric antibiotic therapy for purulent skin infections in immunocompromised hosts or immunocompetent patients with signs of systemic infection. It costs considerably more than vancomycin but less than daptomycin, linezolid, or telavancin, all of which are recommended as empiric treatment for these patients. **H**

### KEY POINTS

**HVC**
- In community-associated methicillin-resistant *Staphylococcus aureus* infections, the primary treatment of a cutaneous abscess is incision and drainage.

**HVC**
- Antibiotic therapy generally is recommended for community-associated methicillin-resistant *Staphylococcus aureus* infections only if primary treatment is inadequate, if disease is extensive or marked by rapid progression and associated cellulitis, if immunodeficiency and other comorbidities are present, if the patient is very young or very old, if clinical signs of systemic illness are noted, if involved areas are challenging to drain, or if septic phlebitis is present.

## **H** Necrotizing Fasciitis

Necrotizing fasciitis (NF) is a potentially lethal necrotizing skin infection. Type 1 NF refers to a polymicrobial infection comprising aerobic and anaerobic gram-positive and gram-negative organisms. Type II NF is a monomicrobial infection typically caused by *Streptococcus pyogenes*, although *S. aureus*, *Vibrio vulnificus*, or *Streptococcus agalactiae* can be causative. Patients who are immunocompromised, particularly those with liver disease, are at increased risk for infection with

*V. vulnificus* in the correct clinical setting (see Table 6). Type III NF (gas gangrene or clostridial myonecrosis) usually develops after surgery or other significant trauma and is primarily caused by *Clostridium perfringens*.

Necrotizing fasciitis usually arises from skin damage or trauma, although a portal of entry is not always apparent. It is more common in patients who have comorbidities, including diabetes mellitus, cancer, injection drug use, liver disease, and immunosuppression, but may occur in healthy young patients.

Cutaneous manifestations can initially resemble less complicated cellulitis. Clues to a potential underlying necrotizing process include systemic toxicity with fever, chills, altered mental status, and hypotension. The pain may be disproportionate to the physical examination findings, and loss of sensation may later result from cutaneous nerve destruction. Skin changes can evolve rapidly and become ecchymotic, vesiculobullous, and gangrenous in appearance. "Woody" induration and crepitus on palpation of the involved areas are characteristic.

Clinical suspicion is important and laboratory evaluation, although nonspecific, may be helpful. Six independent laboratory indicators that, when added together, are associated with an increased likelihood of necrotizing fasciitis are C-reactive protein (≥15.0 mg/dL [150 mg/L]), total leukocyte count (>15,000-25,000/μL [15-25 × 10$^9$/L]), hemoglobin (<11-13.5 g/dL [110-135 g/L]), sodium (<135 mEq/L [135 mmol/L]), creatinine (>1.6 mg/dL [141 μmol/L]), and glucose (>180 mg/dL [10 mmol/L]).

Plain radiographs of the affected area may demonstrate subcutaneous gas; MRI with contrast is quite sensitive and can help determine the extent of infection. Blood cultures may be useful in identifying the causative agent, but early surgical exploration is the gold standard for diagnosis and treatment. Cultures of intraoperative tissue specimens help direct antibiotic management; repeated surgeries are often necessary for source control.

Empiric broad-spectrum antibiotics are recommended for patients suspected of having NF. Initial coverage should target aerobic and anaerobic gram-positive and gram-negative bacteria, including MRSA. Appropriate regimens include an anti-MRSA agent, such as vancomycin or daptomycin, linezolid plus imipenem (or meropenem), or piperacillin-tazobactam. In type II NF secondary to GABHS and type III NF secondary to clostridial species, penicillin and clindamycin are recommended. Clindamycin is included because it inhibits toxin production and remains effective even in the presence of a high inoculum of bacteria. Discontinuation of antimicrobials is reasonable when surgical debridement is no longer required and the patient is clinically stable. No absolute recommendations exist for the use of adjunctive intravenous immune globulin (IVIG) in streptococcal necrotizing fasciitis, although some infectious disease experts recommend its use in patients with associated toxic shock syndrome (see following). Doxycycline plus ceftazidime is recommended for *Vibrio vulnificus*-associated NF, and doxycycline plus ciprofloxacin is recommended for *Aeromonas hydrophila*-associated NF. **H**

- Clues to a potential underlying necrotizing process include systemic toxicity with fever, chills, altered mental status, and hypotension; pain may be disproportionate to physical examination findings, and loss of sensation may occur because of cutaneous nerve destruction.
- Early surgical exploration is the gold standard for diagnosis and treatment of necrotizing fasciitis.

## Toxic Shock Syndrome

*S. aureus* and *S. pyogenes* can produce toxins called super antigens that stimulate cytokine production, resulting in the systemic signs of toxic shock syndrome (TSS) (**Table 7**, **Table 8**). TSS secondary to *S. aureus* (including MRSA) may be associated with tampon use during menstruation, the presence of wounds, a history of injection drug use, burns, nasal packings, or catheters. Bacteremia is present in about 5% of cases. *S. pyogenes*–associated skin infections (particularly NF) can also produce a toxic shock–like syndrome. Bacteremia is present in about 60% of cases.

Early management consists of adequate resuscitation to maintain tissue perfusion, identification of the cause and focus of infection, and source control, which typically involves

**TABLE 7. Diagnostic Criteria for Staphylococcal Toxic Shock Syndrome**

| |
|---|
| Fever >38.9 °C (102.0 °F) |
| Systolic blood pressure <90 mm Hg |
| Diffuse macular rash with subsequent desquamation, especially on palms and soles |
| Involvement of three of the following organ systems: |
|    Gastrointestinal (nausea, vomiting, diarrhea) |
|    Muscular (severe myalgia or fivefold or greater increase in serum creatine kinase level) |
|    Mucous membrane (hyperemia of the vagina, conjunctivae, or pharynx) |
|    Kidney (blood urea nitrogen or serum creatinine level at least twice the upper limit of normal) |
|    Liver (bilirubin, aspartate aminotransferase or alanine aminotransferase concentration twice the upper limit of normal) |
|    Blood (platelet count <100,000/µL [100 × 10⁹/L]) |
|    Central nervous system (disorientation without focal neurologic signs) |
| Negative results on serologic testing for Rocky Mountain spotted fever, leptospirosis, and measles; negative cerebrospinal fluid cultures for organisms other than *Staphylococcus aureus* |

Adapted with permission from Moreillon P, Que YA, Glauser MP. *Staphylococcus aureus*. In: Mandell GL, Dolin R, Bennett JE, eds. Principles and Practice of Infectious Disease. 6th ed. Philadelphia, PA: Churchill Livingstone; 2005:2331. Copyright 2005, Elsevier.

**TABLE 8. Diagnostic Criteria for Streptococcal Toxic Shock Syndrome**

| |
|---|
| **Definite case:** |
| Isolation of GABHS from a sterile site |
| **Probable case:** |
| Isolation of GABHS from a nonsterile site |
| **Hypotension:** |
| The presence of two of the following findings: |
|    Kidney (acute kidney injury or failure) |
|    Liver (elevated aminotransferase concentrations) |
|    Skin (erythematous macular rash, soft tissue necrosis) |
|    Blood (coagulopathy, including thrombocytopenia and disseminated intravascular coagulation) |
|    Pulmonary (acute respiratory distress syndrome) |

GABHS = group A β-hemolytic streptococci.

surgical debridement. Empiric antimicrobial agents are the same as those used in NF. When identified, pathogen-directed therapy for *S. pyogenes* consists of penicillin plus clindamycin. Methicillin-sensitive *S. aureus*–associated TSS therapy consists of nafcillin or oxacillin plus clindamycin; if TSS is associated with MRSA, vancomycin plus clindamycin or linezolid can be used. Some experts recommend the use of adjunctive IVIG for TSS, although data are limited. Neutralizing antibodies to streptococcal toxins in IVIG provide the rationale for its use.

Hyperbaric oxygen treatment has also been used adjunctively. Droplet precautions are recommended until effective antibiotic therapy has been administered for 24 hours to prevent transmission of group A streptococcal infection to others; contact precautions are also recommended if the wound is draining. Antibiotic prophylaxis against invasive group A streptococcal infections among household contacts of patients with streptococcal TSS-like syndrome may be considered in older adults or in patients with comorbidities, such as diabetes mellitus, HIV infection, cancer, varicella infection, heart disease, steroid use, and injection drug use. Benzathine penicillin G plus rifampin, clindamycin, or azithromycin is recommended.

- Early management of toxic shock syndrome consists of adequate resuscitation to maintain tissue perfusion, identification of the cause and focus of infection, and source control, which typically involves surgical debridement.

## Animal Bites

Animal bites, most of which are caused by cats and dogs, account for 1% of all visits to the emergency department; up to 20% become infected. Cat bites are more likely to become infected (approximately 40%) owing to deep puncture wounds caused by sharp narrow teeth; dog bites become infected in 5% to 15% of patients. The infections result from the host's skin flora and the animal's mouth flora. This flora is a mix of aerobic and anaerobic organisms, including staphylococci, streptococci, *Bacteroides* species, *Porphyromonas* species, *Fusobacterium* species, and *Pasteurella* species. *Capnocytophaga canimorsus* is a gram-negative bacillus that can cause overwhelming sepsis in patients with functional or anatomic asplenia who have experienced a dog bite or scratch.

The type of animal involved, circumstances under which the attack occurred, timing of the bite, location of the bite, type of injury incurred, and health status of the animal and patient are important. The extremities, particularly the hands, are more likely to become infected than other areas. Physical examination should include evaluation for purulence, necrosis, erythema, edema, and extent/depth of the wound as well as careful neurovascular assessment. Prompt wound irrigation with normal saline, removal of any foreign bodies, and debridement of necrotic tissue can decrease the risk for infection. Radiography is recommended if fracture or bone penetration is possible. Surgical consultation is recommended when the hand is involved. In general, primary wound closure is not performed, particularly if infection is suspected. The need for rabies and tetanus prophylaxis should be assessed in all cases of animal bites.

A 3- to 5-day course of prophylaxis with amoxicillin-clavulanate is recommended for patients who are immunosuppressed (including those with asplenia or who have significant liver disease); have moderate-to-severe wounds, particularly on the face or hand; have wounds near a joint or bone; or have wounds associated with significant crush injury or edema. Alternatively, doxycycline alone or a combination of a fluoroquinolone (ciprofloxacin or levofloxacin) or trimethoprim-sulfamethoxazole plus an anaerobic antibiotic (such as clindamycin or metronidazole) can be used in patients allergic to β-lactam antibiotics.

Infected wounds require antibiotics. Outpatient oral treatment consisting of the same agents used for prophylaxis can be given for 5 to 10 days. Patients with sepsis; infected hand bites; nerve, tendon, or crush injuries; or severe or deep infections should be hospitalized. Recommended intravenous antibiotic options include β-lactam/β-lactamase inhibitor combinations, such as ampicillin-sulbactam or piperacillin-tazobactam; carbapenems, such as imipenem, meropenem, or ertapenem; or cefoxitin. The combination of clindamycin or metronidazole and a fluoroquinolone, such as ciprofloxacin or levofloxacin, is an alternative for patients allergic to β-lactam antibiotics. The anticipated length of therapy is usually less than 14 days unless bone or joint involvement mandates longer courses. **H**

**KEY POINTS**

- Prompt wound irrigation with normal saline, removal of any foreign bodies, and debridement of necrotic tissue can decrease the risk for infection of animal bites.
- The need for rabies and tetanus prophylaxis should be assessed in all patients with animal bites.
- Amoxicillin-clavulanate prophylaxis is recommended only for patients with animal bites who are immunosuppressed; have moderate-to-severe wounds, particularly on the face or hand; have wounds near a joint or bone; or have wounds associated with significant crush injury or edema.

**HVC**

## Human Bites

Human bite wounds usually result from occlusive injuries sustained after an intentional bite or from clenched fist injuries that develop after a punch to another's mouth. The microbiology of these wounds primarily reflects mouth flora, which is a mixture of aerobic streptococci (particularly viridans group streptococci); staphylococci; *Eikenella corrodens*; *Haemophilus* species; and β-lactamase–producing anaerobes, such as *Fusobacterium* species, peptostreptococci, *Porphyromonas* species, and *Prevotella* species.

The same general approach to management of animal bite–associated wounds is pursued. Additionally, evaluation for potential transmission of HIV, hepatitis B and C viruses, and other transmissible pathogens is recommended. Prophylactic antibiotics consisting of 3 to 5 days of amoxicillin-clavulanate should be given for all human bite wounds. Clenched-fist injuries require evaluation by a hand specialist and usually require hospitalization and intravenous ampicillin-sulbactam, a β-lactam/β-lactamase inhibitor, or a carbapenem, such as ertapenem. In patients allergic to β-lactam antibiotics, alternative regimens include fluoroquinolones, such as levofloxacin or ciprofloxacin plus metronidazole. While culture results are pending, an agent such as vancomycin can be considered in patients with risk factors for MRSA infection. **H**

**KEY POINT**

- Prophylactic amoxicillin-clavulanate should be given for all human bite wounds.

## Diabetic Foot Infections

Patients with diabetes mellitus often have associated immunodeficiency, neuropathy, and vasculopathy, which increase the risk for foot infection. Factors reported to be significantly associated with infection include persistent ulcer for more than 1 month, peripheral arterial disease in an involved limb, amputation involving a lower extremity, recurrent foot ulcers, posttraumatic foot wound, diagnosis of kidney insufficiency, walking barefoot, and the ability to palpate bone within the wound with a sterile metal probe.

CONT.

The Infectious Diseases Society of America has developed a validated system that classifies severity of foot infections as uninfected, mild, moderate, or severe. Uninfected wounds/ulcers demonstrate no clinical evidence of infection.

Mild infections are associated with at least two factors, including purulent discharge, warmth, pain/tenderness, swelling/induration, and erythema. The infection must not extend deeper than the skin and subcutaneous tissues, and any erythema must not expand more than 2 cm beyond the ulcer. The patient must not meet criteria for systemic inflammatory response syndrome (SIRS) (Table 9). The microbiology of these infections typically consists of aerobic streptococci and staphylococci. These patients can usually be treated with a short course of oral antibiotics directed against these organisms.

In moderate infections, the erythematous infection expands more than 2 cm around the ulcer or extends deeper than the skin and subcutaneous tissues as a deep tissue abscess, joint or muscle infection, fasciitis, or osteomyelitis. The patient must not meet SIRS criteria.

Infections are considered severe when SIRS criteria are met, other evidence of systemic infection is present (hypotension, confusion, vomiting, acidosis, severe hyperglycemia, acute kidney injury), or infection occurs in the presence of critical ischemia. The microbiology of severe infections is typically polymicrobial, consisting of staphylococci, streptococci, enteric gram-negative bacilli, *Pseudomonas aeruginosa*, and anaerobes. These limb-threatening infections require surgical evaluation and empiric broad-spectrum antibiotic coverage that includes MRSA. Antibiotics can be adjusted on the basis of culture results.

All patients with infection should be assessed for the possible presence of arterial insufficiency (using ankle-brachial index), sensory deficits, and biomechanical abnormalities. Wound care consisting of wound cleansing, debridement, and foot pressure off-loading is recommended. Cultures obtained should not be from superficial swab specimens but from deep tissue specimens. Foot imaging is recommended for all patients with new diabetic foot infections. A multidisciplinary team for diabetic foot infections is optimal. **H**

**TABLE 9. Definition of Systemic Inflammatory Response Syndrome**

**Presence of two or more of the following in the absence of other known causes:**

Temperature >38.0 °C (100.4 °F) or <36.0 °C (96.8 °F)

Heart rate >90/min

Respiration rate >20/min or arterial $P_{CO_2}$ <32 mm Hg (4.3 kPa)

Leukocyte count >12,000/µL ($12 \times 10^9$/L) or <4,000/µL ($4 \times 10^9$/L) or with 10% bands

**KEY POINTS**

- Wound care for diabetic foot infections consists of wound cleansing, debridement, and off-loading of foot pressure.

- Imaging of the foot is recommended for those with new diabetic foot infections.

# Community-Acquired Pneumonia

## Epidemiology

Community-acquired pneumonia (CAP) is a significant cause of morbidity and mortality in adults, ranking as the seventh most frequent cause of mortality in the United States. Certain conditions, including COPD or emphysema, alcoholism, bronchiectasis, and smoking, increase the likelihood of developing CAP and also influence the causative organisms. Older adults are particularly affected by CAP, with some estimates of U.S. case surveillance data noting that more than 900,000 adults age 65 years or older will die of this infection annually. Rates of CAP increase with age, and prevalence appears higher among blacks than whites and among men than women.

**KEY POINT**

- Community-acquired pneumonia (CAP) is more prevalent among older adult patients, and certain conditions, including COPD, emphysema, alcoholism, bronchiectasis, and smoking, increase the likelihood of developing CAP.

## Microbiology

When infection develops in the lower respiratory tract, the pulmonary and host defenses have been breached, leading to the entry of microorganisms present in the upper respiratory tract into the usually sterile lower respiratory airways. Because of this, the common microorganisms causing CAP represent the typical colonizers present in the upper respiratory tract. The most common organism causing CAP is *Streptococcus pneumoniae*; other important causes include *Mycoplasma pneumoniae*, *Haemophilus influenzae*, *Chlamydophila pneumoniae*, and respiratory viruses.

Respiratory viruses are an important contributor to CAP, particularly influenza A and B viruses. Other respiratory viral pathogens, including respiratory syncytial virus, parainfluenza virus, and adenoviruses, are a substantial source of morbidity from viral CAP. These viral infections can also lead to complications of postviral bacterial superinfection, most commonly with *S. pneumoniae*, *Staphylococcus aureus*, and *H. influenzae*. Postviral bacterial pneumonias typically occur approximately 1 to 2 weeks after viral infection symptoms start to resolve. Secondary bacterial pneumonias occurring after primary viral infection will manifest with fever, productive cough, shortness of breath, and pulmonary infiltrates. The index of suspicion for possible secondary bacterial pneumonia should be high in patients whose apparent recovery from a viral infection is complicated by clinical recrudescence.

Specific epidemiologic or geographic exposures may be associated with different and sometimes unusual pathogens causing CAP (**Table 10**).

The subcategory of "atypical" CAP pathogens refers to *M. pneumoniae*, *Legionella* species, *C. pneumoniae*, and *Chlamydophila psittaci*. Atypical CAP is often clinically indistinguishable from typical CAP syndromes. However, *M. pneumoniae* and *C. pneumoniae*, compared with many of the

bacterial pathogens causing typical CAP, can be transmitted person to person. Legionellosis is particularly notable for outbreaks where the source of exposure is traced back to equipment or devices that aerosolize the organisms, such as air conditioning towers.

Gram-negative bacteria, including *Klebsiella pneumoniae*, *Pseudomonas aeruginosa*, *Acinetobacter* species, *Escherichia coli*, and *Enterobacter* species, are rarely implicated in CAP. Most patients with CAP caused by gram-negative bacteria have a predisposing risk factor (see Table 10), such as bronchiectasis, cystic fibrosis, or COPD, and develop severe pneumonia necessitating admission and care in the ICU.

| TABLE 10. Possible Microbial Causes of Community-Acquired Pneumonia | |
|---|---|
| **Characteristics** | **Commonly Encountered Pathogens** |
| **Clinical Presentation** | |
| Aspiration | Gram-negative enteric pathogens, oral anaerobes |
| Cough >2 weeks with whoop or posttussive vomiting | *Bordetella pertussis* |
| Lung cavity infiltrates | Community-associated methicillin-resistant *Staphylococcus aureus*, oral anaerobes, endemic fungal pathogens, *Mycobacterium tuberculosis*, atypical mycobacteria |
| **Epidemiology or Risk Factor** | |
| Alcoholism | *Streptococcus pneumoniae*, oral anaerobes, *Klebsiella pneumoniae*, *Acinetobacter* species, *M. tuberculosis* |
| COPD and/or smoking | *Haemophilus influenzae*, *Pseudomonas aeruginosa*, *Legionella* species, *S. pneumoniae*, *Moraxella catarrhalis*, *Chlamydophila pneumoniae* |
| Exposure to bat or bird droppings | *Histoplasma capsulatum* |
| Exposure to birds | *Chlamydophila psittaci* (if poultry: avian influenza) |
| Exposure to rabbits | *Francisella tularensis* |
| Exposure to farm animals or parturient cats | *Coxiella burnetii* |
| Exposure to rodent excreta | Hantavirus |
| HIV infection (early) | *S. pneumoniae*, *H. influenzae*, *M. tuberculosis* |
| HIV infection (late) | *S. pneumoniae*, *H. influenzae*, *M. tuberculosis*, *Pneumocystis jirovecii*, *Cryptococcus* species, *Histoplasma* species, *Aspergillus* species, atypical mycobacteria (especially *Mycobacterium kansasii*), *P. aeruginosa* |
| Hotel or cruise ship stay in previous 2 weeks | *Legionella* species |
| Travel or residence in southwestern United States | *Coccidioides* species, hantavirus |
| Travel or residence in Southeast and East Asia | *Burkholderia pseudomallei*, avian influenza, severe acute respiratory syndrome–coronavirus (SARS-CoV) |
| Travel or residence in (or exposure to an ill traveler from) the Middle East | Middle East respiratory syndrome–coronavirus (MERS-CoV) |
| Influenza activity in community | Influenza, *S. pneumoniae*, *S. aureus*, *H. influenzae* |
| Injection drug use | *S. aureus*, anaerobes, *M. tuberculosis*, *S. pneumoniae* |
| Endobronchial obstruction | Anaerobes, *S. pneumoniae*, *H. influenzae*, *S. aureus* |
| Bronchiectasis or cystic fibrosis | *Burkholderia cepacia*, *P. aeruginosa*, *S. aureus* |
| Bioterrorism | *Bacillus anthracis*, *Yersinia pestis*, *Francisella tularensis* |

Adapted with permission from Mandell LA, Wunderink RG, Anzueto A, et al; Infectious Diseases Society of America; American Thoracic Society. Infectious Diseases Society of America/American Thoracic Society consensus guidelines on the management of community-acquired pneumonia in adults. Clin Infect Dis. 2007 Mar 1;44(suppl 2):S27-72. [PMID: 17278083] Copyright 2007, Oxford University Press.

Group A streptococcus can lead to a rapidly progressive and complicated pulmonary infection, with subsequent empyema. CAP from group A streptococcus has a substantial mortality rate.

*S. aureus* CAP can occur in a heterogeneous group of settings. A postinfluenza bacterial pneumonia syndrome is typically attributed to *S. aureus*, although *S. pneumoniae* more commonly leads to this complication. Older adult patients are also susceptible to *S. aureus* CAP. *S. aureus* pneumonia is commonly seen among injection drug users. Methicillin-resistant *S. aureus* (MRSA) as a cause of CAP more commonly occurs with nosocomial exposures and in certain patient populations, such as those undergoing hemodialysis. Recent nursing home exposure and exposure to persons with skin and soft tissue infection are also risk factors for MRSA CAP. The morbidity from MRSA causing CAP is substantial because a significant proportion of patients present with necrotizing pneumonia, in which a portion of the involved lung tissue becomes devitalized. This complication leads to pulmonary airway hemorrhage, severe respiratory failure, and fulminant clinical deterioration.

### KEY POINTS

- Community-acquired pneumonia is most commonly caused by *Streptococcus pneumoniae*.

- Influenza A and B are the most common respiratory viruses contributing to development of community-acquired pneumonia.

- Methicillin-resistant *Staphylococcus aureus* (MRSA) as a cause of community-acquired pneumonia more commonly occurs with nosocomial exposures and in certain patient populations, such as those undergoing hemodialysis; recent nursing home exposure or exposure to persons with skin and soft tissue infection are also risk factors for MRSA.

## Diagnosis

Initial evaluation of the patient suspected of having CAP starts with a comprehensive history and physical examination. Suggestive clinical symptoms include fever, cough, sputum production, and dyspnea, although these are only at most 50% sensitive for a diagnosis of CAP. Pleuritic chest pain may be present. The absence of fever does not exclude CAP, particularly in older adults. Tachypnea is often present, and tachycardia can be seen. Pulmonary examination may be positive for adventitious sounds. However, no pathognomonic findings on physical examination can indicate CAP, so a combination of suggestive and supportive symptoms and examination findings are needed to make the diagnosis.

If clinical findings suggest a CAP diagnosis, chest radiography should be performed. Chest radiography must show an infiltrate for pneumonia to be diagnosed. Radiographic findings can be characterized as interstitial infiltrates, lobar consolidation, or cavitary lesions. When clinical symptoms and examination findings otherwise support the diagnosis of CAP, a false-negative chest radiograph is a possibility; volume depletion can cause an initial negative finding on chest radiograph that, upon rehydration and repeat imaging, may become positive.

Empiric antibiotic therapy for CAP is generally not recommended without evidence of positive findings on chest radiograph. However, empiric antimicrobial treatment may be instituted for hospitalized patients with a high clinical suspicion of CAP when the chest radiograph is negative, with repeat chest radiography in 1 to 2 days to confirm or exclude the diagnosis.

Although chest CT has higher sensitivity than chest radiography for diagnosing CAP and is particularly effective for detecting interstitial infiltrates, empyema, cavitary lung lesions, or hilar lymphadenopathy, no evidence indicates clinical outcomes are improved by using CT for diagnosing CAP. It is also substantially more expensive than plain chest radiography and involves more radiation exposure. Therefore, guidelines do not recommend its use in most patients with CAP, and it is reserved for specific clinical situations in which diagnostic uncertainty will affect management.

Although an infiltrate on chest radiograph is necessary to confirm the diagnosis of CAP, microbiologic confirmation is not typically an essential diagnostic criterion. The diagnostic yield of sputum cultures varies widely, and culture data for ambulatory patients with uncomplicated CAP do not positively influence outcomes relative to empiric antibiotic therapy. Therefore, sputum cultures are not recommended for these patients. Sputum cultures (with Gram stain to ensure the adequacy of the sample) are indicated for hospitalized patients with severe disease (ICU admission), complications (pleural effusions, cavitary lesions), underlying lung disease, active alcohol abuse, asplenia, liver disease, leukopenia, or unsuccessful outpatient antimicrobial therapy.

Blood cultures are positive in few CAP cases and are not recommended for ambulatory patients. However, they should be performed in patients with an indication for sputum culture. Blood cultures should be obtained before empiric antimicrobial therapy initiation for maximal diagnostic yield. Most positive blood cultures in hospitalized patients with CAP indicate *S. pneumoniae*.

*Legionella* and pneumococcal urinary antigen testing are also recommended when confirmation of a microbiologic diagnosis is indicated, when ICU admission is being considered, and when outpatient antimicrobial therapy fails. However, *Legionella* urinary antigen testing, although specific, detects only *Legionella pneumophila* type 1 and is, therefore, less sensitive. Molecular tests for *C. pneumoniae* and *M. pneumoniae* and numerous other respiratory viruses have recently become available. These tests are useful in confirming these pathogens because they are fast (test results within hours) and accurate (high sensitivity and specificity); however, they are not always routinely used in practice because of limitations in availability or cost. Particularly in instances of

**CONT.**

CAP caused by underlying viral infection, the availability of rapid polymerase chain reaction respiratory virus panel tests can lead to reduction of unnecessary antimicrobial therapy and additional diagnostic studies. The molecular tests for *C. pneumoniae* and *M. pneumoniae*, as well as respiratory viruses, should be considered when CAP outpatient therapy fails, when ICU admission is being considered, and when risk factors are present for more severe or complicated pneumonia (such as chronic lung disease, underlying liver disease, functional or anatomic asplenia, or alcoholism). For patients who present with CAP-associated pleural effusion, diagnostic thoracentesis is an additional indicated study.

An emerging area of interest in the evaluation of CAP is the use of biologic markers, such as C-reactive protein (CRP) and procalcitonin, to help differentiate between bacterial and nonbacterial pneumonia and help exclude a bacterial CAP diagnosis in outpatients. CRP is a marker of inflammation, and levels are increased in bacterial pneumonia. Procalcitonin is produced by cells as a response to bacterial toxins, which result in serum procalcitonin elevations in bacterial infections. In viral infections, procalcitonin levels are reduced. Procalcitonin and CRP can potentially be used to help reduce unnecessary antibiotic use because they can assist in the decision to stop empirically initiated antibiotics for presumed bacterial CAP. However, the use of procalcitonin and CRP in evaluating CAP should be one of several factors in determining bacterial vs viral cause and should be considered as adjunctive diagnostic tools that will support clinical, microbiologic, and radiologic data rather than take precedence over other information. **H**

---

**KEY POINTS**

- Clinical symptoms of community-acquired pneumonia include fever, cough, sputum production, and dyspnea, with or without pleuritic chest pain.

- Pulmonary infiltrate on chest radiograph is required for a pneumonia diagnosis.

- Microbiologic testing and sputum and blood cultures are recommended in hospitalized patients with severe disease necessitating ICU admission, complications (pleural effusions, cavitary lesions), underlying lung disease, active alcohol abuse, asplenia, liver disease, leukopenia, or unsuccessful outpatient antimicrobial therapy.

---

# Management

## Site of Care

An initial step in managing CAP is to determine the appropriate site of care based on disease severity. Decision support tools have been formulated to help determine the site of care for CAP. The Pneumonia Severity Index (PSI) tabulates points based on sex; age; comorbid conditions; and physical examination, laboratory, and radiologic findings to determine a score

predicting one of five classes of mortality risk. The higher the PSI, the greater the need is for hospital admission. Although effective, the PSI encompasses multiple data points and may be challenging to use, particularly in office-based settings.

The CURB-65 tool uses five categories to predict a patient's morbidity risk, assigning 1 point for each category that is positive: confusion, blood urea nitrogen >20 mg/dL (7.14 mmol/L), respiratory rate ≥30/min, blood pressure (systolic <90 mm Hg, diastolic ≤60 mm Hg), and age 65 years or older. Those patients with a CURB-65 score of 0 or 1 are considered safe to manage in the ambulatory setting. Those with a CURB-65 score of 2 should be admitted for management. CURB-65 scores of 3 or greater warrant consideration of patient admission to the ICU. The modified CRB-65, which omits the BUN component of the original tool, can be used in office-based settings to expedite determining the need for hospitalization. A CRB-65 score of anything other than 0 warrants hospital admission.

The Infectious Diseases Society of America/American Thoracic Society (IDSA/ATS) guidelines use a combination of major and minor criteria to classify severe CAP. Patients who have one or more major criteria or at least three minor criteria for severe CAP warrant ICU admission. Major criteria include invasive mechanical ventilation and septic shock with need for vasopressors. Minor criteria are provided in **Table 11**. Recognizing severe CAP is essential to help prevent associated morbidity and mortality because those with severe disease may have a 30-day mortality rate as high as 40%. Prompt and appropriate placement of patients who warrant hospitalization

---

**TABLE 11.    IDSA/ATS Minor Criteria for Severe Community-Acquired Pneumonia**

| Clinical Criteria |
| --- |
| Confusion (new-onset disorientation to person, place, or time) |
| Hypothermia (core temperature <36.0 °C [96.8 °F]) |
| Respiration rate ≥30/min[a] |
| Hypotension necessitating aggressive fluid resuscitation |
| Multilobar pulmonary infiltrates |

| Laboratory Criteria |
| --- |
| Arterial $Po_2/Fio_2$ ratio ≤250[a] |
| Leukopenia (<4000 cells/μL [4.0 × 10⁹/L])[b] |
| Thrombocytopenia (<100,000 platelets/μL [10 × 10⁹/L]) |
| Blood urea nitrogen ≥20 mg/dL (7.1 mmol/L) |

IDSA/ATS = Infectious Diseases Society of America/American Thoracic Society; $Po_2/Fio_2$ = partial pressure of oxygen/fraction of inspired oxygen.

[a]A patient who requires noninvasive positive-pressure ventilation should be considered to meet this criterion.

[b]As a result of infection alone.

Reprinted with permission from Mandell LA, Wunderink RG, Anzueto A, et al; Infectious Diseases Society of America; American Thoracic Society. Infectious Diseases Society of America/American Thoracic Society consensus guidelines on the management of community-acquired pneumonia in adults. Clin Infect Dis. 2007 Mar 1;44(suppl 2):S27-72. [PMID: 17278083] Copyright 2007, Oxford University Press.

CONT.

or ICU management can reduce poor outcomes; use of objective criteria in accurately triaging the appropriate management setting can help standardize care and minimize practice variation. H

**KEY POINT**

HVC • One of several decision support tools (Pneumonia Severity Index, CURB-65/CRB-65, Infectious Diseases Society of America/American Thoracic Society criteria for severe pneumonia) should be used to assess the need for outpatient versus hospitalized patients care of community-acquired pneumonia.

## Antimicrobial Therapy

Empiric antimicrobial treatment for CAP is usually started before a pathogen is identified, so drug selection is based on the predicted or suspected causative organism, clinical history, radiologic findings, and epidemiologic clues. Concerns about emerging drug resistance with community-acquired *S. pneumoniae* and *S. aureus* as well as potential nosocomial resistance may influence empiric therapy. Risk factors for drug-resistant *S. pneumoniae* include age older than 65 years, recent (within the past 3-6 months) antimicrobial therapy (with a β-lactam, macrolide, or fluoroquinolone antibiotic), alcoholism, immunosuppression, and certain medical comorbidities (COPD, chronic liver or kidney disease, cancer, diabetes mellitus, functional or anatomic asplenia, chronic heart disease). Those who work or live in nursing homes and children and workers in day care centers can develop antibiotic-resistant pneumococcal infections. Guidance for empiric treatment in outpatients depends on underlying risk factors (**Table 12**).

**TABLE 12.** Antibiotic Therapy for Community-Acquired Pneumonia in Outpatients

| Risk Factors | Treatment |
|---|---|
| Previously healthy and no risk factor(s) for drug-resistant *Streptococcus pneumoniae* | Macrolide (azithromycin, clarithromycin, or erythromycin) or doxycycline |
| Risk factor(s) for drug-resistant *S. pneumoniae* or underlying comorbidities[a] | Respiratory fluoroquinolone (moxifloxacin, gemifloxacin, or levofloxacin) or β-lactam[b] plus a macrolide or doxycycline |

[a]Comorbid conditions (chronic heart, lung, liver, or kidney disease; diabetes mellitus; alcoholism; malignancies; asplenia; and immunosuppressive conditions or use of immunosuppressive drugs), recent (within 3 months) antimicrobial use, or residence in regions with a high rate (>25%) of infection with high-level (minimum inhibitory concentration ≥16 µg/mL) macrolide-resistant *S. pneumoniae*.

[b]Amoxicillin, 1 g every 8 hours, or amoxicillin-clavulanate, 2 g every 12 hours (preferred), or cefpodoxime or cefuroxime, 500 mg twice daily (alternative).

For patients who require hospitalization for CAP from an emergency department setting, the first antimicrobial dose should be given in the emergency department. The time to first antimicrobial dose has been a focus of quality-of-care evaluations, with several retrospective studies of the Medicare population showing significantly reduced mortality among patients who received antimicrobial therapy within 4 to 8 hours of presentation to the emergency department. However, IDSA/ATS guidelines do not include specific timing for antibiotic administration and only support administering the first antimicrobial dose in the emergency department (**Table 13**).

Hospitalized patients initially treated with parenteral therapy can be switched to oral agents, generally of the same antimicrobial class and with similar spectrum of activity, when clinical stability has been attained. Clinically stable

**TABLE 13.** Empiric Antibiotic Therapy for Community-Acquired Pneumonia in Inpatients

| Inpatient Setting | Treatment |
|---|---|
| Medical ward | β-lactam[a] plus a macrolide or doxycycline; *or* respiratory fluoroquinolone (moxifloxacin, gemifloxacin, or levofloxacin) |
| ICU | β-lactam[b] plus either azithromycin or a fluoroquinolone[c]; if penicillin allergic, a respiratory fluoroquinolone[d] plus aztreonam[e] |
| If risk factor(s) for *Pseudomonas aeruginosa* or gram-negative rods on sputum Gram stain | Antipseudomonal β-lactam with pneumococcal coverage (cefepime, imipenem, meropenem, or piperacillin-tazobactam) plus ciprofloxacin or levofloxacin (750 mg); *or* antipseudomonal β-lactam with pneumococcal coverage plus an aminoglycoside plus azithromycin; *or* antipseudomonal[e] β-lactam with pneumococcal coverage plus an aminoglycoside plus a respiratory fluoroquinolone |
| If risk factor(s) for CA-MRSA, cavitary infiltrates, or compatible sputum Gram stain | Add vancomycin or linezolid to β-lactam[b] plus either azithromycin or a fluoroquinolone[c] |

CA-MRSA = community-associated methicillin-resistant *Staphylococcus aureus*.

[a]Cefotaxime, ceftriaxone, or ampicillin; ertapenem is an alternative in patients with an increased risk for enteric gram-negative pathogens (not *P. aeruginosa*).

[b]Cefotaxime, ceftriaxone, or ampicillin-sulbactam.

[c]Moxifloxacin, gemifloxacin, ciprofloxacin, or levofloxacin.

[d]Moxifloxacin, gemifloxacin, or levofloxacin.

[e]Aztreonam can be used in a patient with a severe β-lactam allergy.

**CONT.**

patients are characterized as having (1) temperature of 37.8 °C (100.0 °F) or less, (2) heart rate of 100/min or less, (3) respiration rate of 24/min or less, (4) systolic blood pressure of 90 mm Hg or greater, (5) arterial oxygen saturation of 90% or more or partial pressure of oxygen of 60 mm Hg or greater breathing ambient air, (6) ability to maintain oral intake, and (7) normal mental status. Continued in-hospital monitoring of stable patients following the transition from parenteral to oral therapy has not been shown to improve outcomes.

If a specific pathogen is identified, the empiric antimicrobial regimen should be tailored to the isolated organism(s), with antimicrobial agent selection guided by in vitro susceptibility testing. ▪

**KEY POINTS**

- Empiric therapy for community-acquired pneumonia should consist of a macrolide antibiotic or doxycycline in outpatients without comorbidities or recent antimicrobial use or a respiratory fluoroquinolone or β-lactam plus a macrolide (doxycycline as an alternative) in outpatients with comorbid conditions, recent antimicrobial use, or residence in an area where macrolide-resistant *Streptococcus pneumoniae* is prevalent.

**HVC**
- Hospitalized patients with community-acquired pneumonia who have received parenteral therapy can be switched to oral agents when clinical stability has been attained.

**HVC**
- Continued in-hospital monitoring of stable patients following the transition from parenteral to oral therapy has not been shown to improve outcomes.

## ▪ Complications

Patients treated with the appropriate antimicrobial course will typically show improvement in clinical symptoms (fever, cough, dyspnea) within 2 to 3 days. Nonresponsive pneumonia is identified if patients do not show some clinical response within 72 hours of therapy initiation. Nonresponse to treatment can occur because of a pulmonary-related complication, such as a complicated parapneumonic pleural effusion, empyema, lung abscess, or postobstructive or necrotizing pneumonia. Rarely, nonresponse may occur with extrapulmonary manifestations of the infectious process, such as meningitis or endovascular infection (endocarditis). In addition to nonresponse, CAP infection may progress or deteriorate. Progressive pneumonia can lead to the need for intubation and mechanical ventilation or, in fulminant cases, result in severe sepsis. Particularly in hospitalized patients, unrelated nosocomial infections (catheter-related infection, urinary tract infection, *Clostridium difficile* infection) can contribute to clinical deterioration or progressive disease. Unsuccessful treatment, because of inadequate coverage of the empiric regimen, host factors, or delayed response to appropriate therapy, is associated with risk factors such as multilobar pneumonia; infection with MRSA, *Legionella* species, or gram-negative bacilli; PSI of

90 or more; and initial treatment with an antimicrobial regimen to which the causative pathogen was not susceptible.

Clinical nonresponse may necessitate more detailed pulmonary imaging with chest CT to exclude the possibility of such complications. These infectious or anatomic complications merit directed targeted investigations and interventions to further define the extent of disease. Antimicrobial therapy may need to be modified to adequately treat extrapulmonary infections. More invasive management is often needed to address pulmonary complications, including thoracentesis for pleural effusions, video-assisted thoracoscopy for empyema, and bronchoscopy for postobstructive/necrotizing pneumonia or lung abscess. In severe enigmatic cases, thoracoscopic or open lung biopsy may be necessary. Multiorgan involvement may result from hematogenous spread or involvement of certain organisms (MRSA); in these subsets of CAP, the antimicrobial course and management will usually require longer therapy duration and further diagnostic studies. ▪

**KEY POINTS**

- Patients with pneumonia treated with the appropriate antimicrobial course will typically show improvement in clinical symptoms within 2 to 3 days.

- Unsuccessful treatment, because of inadequate coverage of the empiric regimen, host factors, or delayed response to appropriate therapy, is associated with risk factors such as multilobar pneumonia; infection with methicillin-resistant *Staphylococcus aureus*, *Legionella* species, or gram-negative bacilli; Pneumonia Severity Index of 90 or more; and initial treatment with an antimicrobial regimen to which the causative pathogen was not susceptible.

## Follow-up ▪

Antimicrobial treatment duration for CAP is typically 5 days in outpatients. Longer treatment courses have not shown clinical benefit and should be avoided to minimize unnecessary antimicrobial use and avoid extra expense of care. Secondary symptoms of CAP, such as cough, fatigue, and other constitutional symptoms, may persist for several days after completion of antimicrobial treatment, but the ongoing presence of these symptoms, in the absence of continued fevers, does not mandate extending the course of therapy. For hospitalized patients, total course of antimicrobial therapy should continue until the patient has been afebrile at least 48 to 72 hours, does not require supplemental oxygen, and does not have more than one sign of clinical instability (defined as heart rate >100/min, respiration rate >24/min, and systolic blood pressure <90 mm Hg). Patients requiring hospitalization usually have intravenous therapy initiated, but they can be switched to oral therapy when they are hemodynamically stable, improving clinically, and able to take oral medications and their gastrointestinal tract function has normalized. Total duration of antimicrobial therapy in patients who respond clinically within the first 2 to 3 days of treatment is generally not longer than 7 days. Complications of CAP, such as lung abscess, empyema, necrotizing pneumonia, or extrapulmonary infections, will mandate longer courses of therapy. In these patients, management must be tailored to the particular circumstances and CAP complications. In the specific instance of MRSA CAP without metastatic infection, guidelines recommend between 7 and 21 days of treatment, depending on the severity and extent of infection and clinical response.

Findings on chest radiography can often linger despite clinical improvement and symptom resolution. As a result, the routine use of follow-up chest radiography after successful treatment is not generally recommended. Follow-up chest radiography may have the greatest utility in patients older than 50 years, particularly for men and smokers. In these subsets of patients, the posttreatment follow-up chest radiograph should be obtained 2 to 3 months after antimicrobial treatment.

An important aspect of treatment includes interventions to prevent future episodes of CAP. Administration of clinically indicated vaccinations, including pneumococcal and annual influenza vaccine (see MKSAP 17 General Internal Medicine), are important components of prevention of future CAP. Counseling to reduce or eliminate modifiable risk factors for CAP, such as smoking and heavy alcohol use, should be initiated. Stabilization of underlying chronic lung disease (COPD) may be an important adjunct to decreasing future CAP. **H**

### KEY POINTS

- **HVC** • Treatment courses for community-acquired pneumonia longer than 5 days have not shown clinical benefit and should be avoided to minimize unnecessary antimicrobial use and avoid extra expense of care.

- **HVC** • The routine use of follow-up chest radiography after successful treatment of community-acquired pneumonia is not recommended because findings may linger despite clinical improvement and symptom resolution.

# Tick-Borne Diseases

## Lyme Disease

Lyme disease, caused by infection with *Borrelia burgdorferi*, is the most common vector-borne infection in the United States. More than 30,000 new cases are reported each year, but the true incidence is likely several-fold higher. More than 95% of all cases occur in regions where the vector *Ixodes* tick is abundant (**Figure 3**). The *Ixodes* tick also serves as the vector for the pathogens causing anaplasmosis and babesiosis, and coinfections may occur. *Borrelia miyamotoi*, a newly described cause of fever and meningoencephalitis, is also transmitted by *Ixodes* ticks. See **Figure 4** for various tick life cycles.

Human infection occurs through inoculation of spirochetes in infected tick saliva and usually requires tick attachment for more than 36 hours. The clinical presentation and

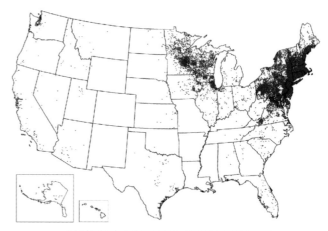

1 dot placed randomly within county of residence for each confirmed case

**FIGURE 3.** Geographic distribution of cases of Lyme disease in the United States, 2013. One dot is placed randomly within county of residence for each confirmed case.

Reproduced from Centers for Disease Control and Prevention. Reported cases of Lyme disease - United States, 2013. www.cdc.gov/lyme/stats/maps/map2013.html. Updated March 4, 2015. Accessed June 30, 2015.

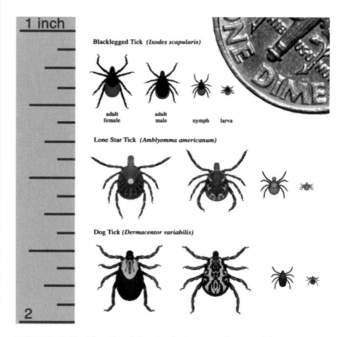

**FIGURE 4.** The life cycles of three hard tick species that spread disease.

Reproduced from Centers for Disease Control and Prevention. Life cycle of hard ticks that spread disease. www.cdc.gov/ticks/life_cycle_and_hosts.html. Updated February 3, 2014. Accessed June 30, 2015.

appropriate diagnostic strategy for Lyme disease vary according to the stage of infection (**Table 14**).

The first stage involves localized symptoms occurring 1 to 4 weeks after infection. This early stage is usually characterized by erythema migrans, a target lesion occurring at the site of tick attachment and present in 60% to 80% of localized infections (**Figure 5**). Fever and other systemic symptoms are rarely present. Results of serologic testing at this stage are frequently negative; therefore, documentation of erythema

**TABLE 14.** Clinical Manifestations and Diagnostic Testing for Lyme Disease

| Stage | Onset After Inoculation | Signs/Symptoms | Diagnosis | Treatment |
|---|---|---|---|---|
| Localized | 1-4 weeks | Single erythema migrans at site of inoculation | Clinical | Oral doxycycline[a], amoxicillin, or cefuroxime axetil |
| Early disseminated | Weeks to months | Multiple erythema migrans, often with fever, headache, myalgias | Clinical (serologic testing can support diagnosis) | Same as for localized |
| | | Heart block, myocarditis | Serologic testing | First-degree heart block: same as for localized |
| | | | | Higher-grade heart block: ceftriaxone or intravenous penicillin G |
| | | Cranial nerve palsies, meningitis | Serologic testing | Facial nerve palsy: doxycycline[a] |
| | | | | Other neurologic manifestations: ceftriaxone or intravenous penicillin G |
| Late disseminated | Months to years | Oligoarticular arthritis | Serologic testing, PCR of synovium or synovial fluid | Doxycycline[a] or amoxicillin; intravenous ceftriaxone for recurrent symptoms |
| | | Encephalopathy or encephalomyelitis | Serologic testing, intrathecal antibody, CSF PCR | Ceftriaxone or intravenous penicillin G |

CSF = cerebrospinal fluid; PCR = polymerase chain reaction.

[a]Doxycycline should not be used in pregnancy; instead, a β-lactam antibiotic should be used.

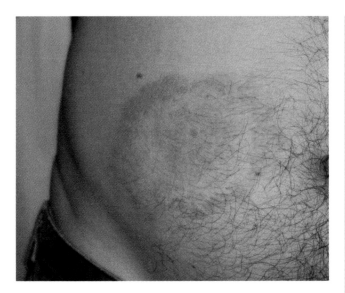

**FIGURE 5.** An erythema migrans lesion characteristic of Lyme disease. These lesions are often found near the axilla, inguinal region, popliteal fossa, or at the belt line. Lesions typically expand over time and, when large enough, often demonstrate central clearing. Some will have more complex configurations, such as a target or bull's eye, as seen in this patient.

Figure courtesy of Karen Bloch, MD

migrans with a compatible epidemiologic history is sufficient for diagnosis, and laboratory confirmation is not indicated. Atypical skin lesions, including vesicles or erythematous patches without central clearing, are more diagnostically challenging. In these cases, testing acute and convalescent sera may allow retrospective diagnosis. Results of polymerase chain reaction (PCR) on a specimen from skin biopsy of erythema migrans are usually positive, but this invasive procedure is rarely necessary.

Treatment of early localized disease prevents progression of infection. Therapy is outlined in Table 14. Doxycycline offers the advantage of treating possible coinfection with *Anaplasma phagocytophilum*. Treatment of localized Lyme disease does not protect against subsequent infection.

Untreated patients may progress to early disseminated infection. This stage typically presents as a febrile illness associated with erythema migrans at multiple sites distant from the initial tick attachment. Constitutional symptoms are common and include fever, myalgia, arthralgia, and headache. Although antibodies to *B. burgdorferi* are typically present at this stage, the diagnosis of early disseminated disease is also clinical; treatment of uncomplicated disease is the same as for localized infection.

Focal cardiac or neurologic symptoms may also occur in early disseminated disease. Cardiac involvement ranges from asymptomatic PR interval prolongation to complete heart block. Progression to complete heart block may be rapid; therefore, symptomatic patients with dyspnea or presyncope, or any patient with second-degree or greater heart block, require hospitalization for cardiac monitoring. Oral antibiotics are effective for treatment of first-degree atrioventricular block, but parenteral therapy is necessary for higher degrees of atrioventricular block. Because Lyme-associated atrioventricular block is reversible with antibiotic treatment, implantation of a permanent cardiac pacemaker is not indicated. Less

CONT.

commonly, diffuse Lyme myocarditis may occur and may be fatal with minimal prodromal symptoms.

The most common neurologic manifestation of early disseminated Lyme disease is facial nerve palsy, which may be unilateral or bilateral. Oral antibiotics are typically curative, but resolution of neurologic deficits may take weeks or even months. Meningitis or other neurologic presentations require parenteral antibiotic therapy. In addition to positive results on serologic testing for *B. burgdorferi*, intrathecal measurement of antibody production or *B. burgdorferi* PCR on cerebrospinal fluid (CSF) may help confirm the diagnosis, although the significance of a positive CSF PCR result in the absence of positive serologic findings is uncertain. **H**

Late manifestations of Lyme disease may occur months to years after infection. The most common clinical presentation is oligoarticular inflammatory arthritis involving large joints, such as the knee. The natural history is for arthritis to wax and wane, often resolving spontaneously only to recur in the same or a different joint. Results of serologic testing for *B. burgdorferi* are invariably positive at this stage and, in the absence of an alternative cause for arthritis, are diagnostic. PCR of synovial fluid or tissue may confirm the presence of infection, but

the findings should be interpreted with caution if serologic results are negative. Treatment with prolonged oral antibiotics (1-2 months) is indicated; parenteral therapy may ultimately be required if the clinical response is incomplete.

Post–Lyme disease syndrome, sometimes erroneously termed "chronic Lyme disease," occurs in some patients despite appropriate antibiotic therapy. These patients experience nonspecific but disabling symptoms, such as fatigue, poor concentration, insomnia, diffuse pain, and malaise. No evidence of latent or persistent infection is found in these patients; symptoms may result from an exuberant host inflammatory response. Management focuses on amelioration of symptoms. Because of the absence of latent *B. burgdorferi* infection in these patients, prolonged administration of antibiotics is not beneficial and is contraindicated.

In patients requiring laboratory confirmation of Lyme disease, serologic testing is the primary means of diagnosis using a two-step serologic testing strategy (**Figure 6**). The initial test is an enzyme-linked immunosorbent assay (ELISA), which is extremely sensitive and is used as a screening test. Occasionally, an indirect immunofluorescence assay may be used. For positive or equivocal results, the more specific

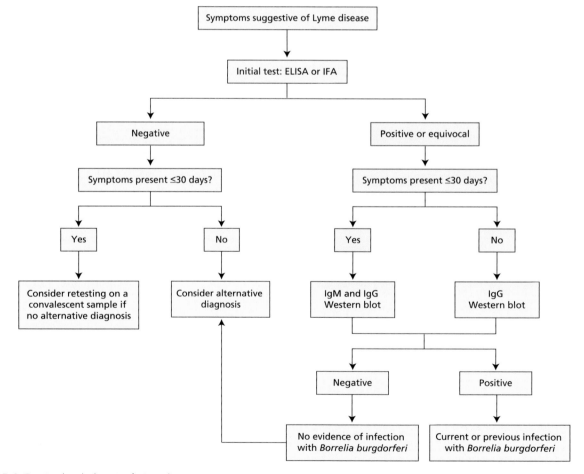

**FIGURE 6.** Two-tiered antibody testing for Lyme disease.

ELISA = enzyme-linked immunosorbent assay; IFA = immunofluorescence assay.

Western blot test is required; a positive result on this second step confirms the presence of antibodies to *B. burgdorferi*.

Early in the course of infection, antibodies may not yet be detectable, and the development of an IgM antibody predates that of IgG. However, an isolated IgM Western blot in a patient with symptoms for more than 30 days suggests a false-positive result. Antibodies remain positive indefinitely, and repeat testing or re-treatment for persistently positive antibody is not indicated. Finally, patients who have acquired infection internationally may be infected with a *Borrelia* species that does not cross-react serologically with the *B. burgdorferi* assay. In these cases, an alternative ELISA that identifies antibodies to the highly conserved C6 *Borrelia* peptide is recommended for diagnosis.

### KEY POINTS

- Lyme disease symptoms occur 1 to 4 weeks after infection and are characterized by erythema migrans, a single target lesion present in 60% to 80% of localized infections.

- **HVC** • Antibodies may not be present early in Lyme disease infection; documentation of erythema migrans with a compatible epidemiologic history is sufficient for diagnosis, and serologic testing is not indicated and may be falsely negative in localized disease.

- *Borrelia burgdorferi* antibodies will likely be present in later (disseminated) disease stages, and a two-step serologic testing strategy that uses an enzyme-linked immunosorbent assay as an initial screening test followed by a confirmatory Western blot is the best way to confirm the diagnosis of disseminated Lyme disease.

- **HVC** • Post–Lyme disease syndrome or "chronic Lyme disease" occurs in some patients despite appropriate antibiotic therapy and includes nonspecific but disabling symptoms; management focuses on amelioration of symptoms, and prolonged administration of antibiotics is not beneficial and is contraindicated.

## Southern Tick-Associated Rash Illness

Southern tick–associated rash illness (STARI) was initially recognized in patients who presented with erythema migrans (see Figure 4) but had not traveled to an area endemic for Lyme disease. Results of laboratory testing for *B. burgdorferi* are invariably negative in patients with STARI, suggesting infection with an as-yet undiscovered tick-borne pathogen. STARI cases are most prevalent in the southeastern and southcentral parts of the United States, and disseminated infection has not been documented. However, because STARI is clinically indistinguishable from localized Lyme disease, treatment with an oral antibiotic active against localized Lyme disease is indicated (see Table 14).

### KEY POINT

- Southern tick-associated rash illness is clinically indistinguishable from localized Lyme disease, so treatment with an oral antibiotic active against localized Lyme disease is indicated.

## Babesiosis

Human babesiosis is caused by protozoal infection of erythrocytes. In the United States, babesiosis is primarily caused by *Babesia microti*, although other species are increasingly recognized. *B. microti* is transmitted by the same tick vector as Lyme disease and has similar geographic distribution (see Figure 3). Transmission through transfusion of infected blood products has been reported.

In most patients, infection is asymptomatic or causes a mild illness. The onset of symptoms is typically within the first month after infection. Mild infection presents with a febrile illness variably associated with myalgias, headache, and fatigue. In cases of transfusion-associated infection, the time from exposure to symptom onset may be as long as 6 months. Physical findings may include splenomegaly, hepatomegaly, and jaundice.

Patients with asplenia or those who are older or immunocompromised typically have higher parasitic burdens, leading to more severe disease. Patients with high-level parasitemia may present with acute respiratory failure, disseminated intravascular coagulation, or kidney injury. Splenic rupture can also occur.

Laboratory findings are related to hemolysis and include anemia, elevated reticulocyte count, increased lactate dehydrogenase, and decreased haptoglobin. Elevated liver enzyme levels and thrombocytopenia are also common. Organisms may be identified on blood smears by using Giemsa or Wright staining (**Figure 7**). Trophozoites appear as ring forms inside erythrocytes and may be confused with malaria unless a thorough travel history is obtained. Less commonly, protozoa may resemble a tetrad or Maltese cross formation. The sensitivity of microscopy depends on the level of parasitemia and the number of fields reviewed; however, if results are positive, this test is diagnostic for infection. For patients with mild disease and low parasitic burden, PCR is recommended as the initial test. The utility of serologic testing in the diagnosis of acute infection is limited. Among inhabitants of endemic areas, detection of antibody may indicate previous asymptomatic infection. A positive IgM antibody or seroconversion result denotes recent infection; however, the serologic response may be delayed and findings on antibody testing may be falsely negative early in the course of infection.

When *Babesia* infection is detected in an asymptomatic patient, monitoring for resolution of parasitemia is recommended. If organisms persist for more than 3 months, with or without symptoms, treatment is indicated. All patients with symptomatic babesiosis require therapy. Atovaquone

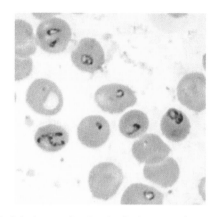

**FIGURE 7.** *Babesia* sp. trophozoites visualized as intraerythrocytic ring forms.

Reproduced from Centers for Disease Control and Prevention, DPDx. Babesiosis. www.cdc.gov/dpdx/babesiosis/gallery. html#thinblood. Updated November 29, 2013. Accessed June 30, 2015.

plus azithromycin is the treatment of choice for mild-to-moderate disease. This regimen is as effective as combination therapy with clindamycin and quinine but is associated with significantly fewer adverse effects. In severe disease, clindamycin plus quinine is preferable. Exchange transfusion should be considered in patients with 10% or greater parasitemia or multiorgan system failure. In immunocompromised patients or those with sustained parasitemia, antibiotics should be continued for at least 6 weeks. Relapse in immunosuppressed patients is common, and a repeat course of treatment is often necessary.

**KEY POINTS**

- Babesiosis is typically asymptomatic or causes a mild febrile illness variably associated with myalgias, headache, and fatigue, whereas more severe disease presents with acute respiratory failure, disseminated intravascular coagulation, kidney injury, and possibly splenic rupture.

- Polymerase chain reaction is a more sensitive test for diagnosing patients with mild babesiosis and low parasitic burdens; the sensitivity of microscopy of Giemsa- or Wright-stained blood smears depends on the level of parasitemia.

- When treatment for babesiosis is indicated, atovaquone plus azithromycin or clindamycin plus quinine are the therapies of choice, depending on disease severity.

## Ehrlichiosis and Anaplasmosis

The clinical presentations of human monocytic ehrlichiosis (HME) and human granulocytic anaplasmosis (HGA) are similar despite transmission by different ticks. The vector for HME is the Lone Star tick, endemic to the southcentral and southeastern parts of the United States. HGA is transmitted by the same vector as are Lyme disease and babesiosis (Figure 3).

The spectrum of clinical disease with HME and HGA ranges from a nonspecific febrile condition to a fulminate illness, with a mortality rate of 1% to 3%. Fever is present in more than 90% of patients, followed in frequency by headache, myalgia, arthralgia, and meningismus. Rash is rare. Life-threatening complications may include acute kidney injury, meningoencephalitis, and acute respiratory distress syndrome.

Laboratory abnormalities raise suspicion for these diagnoses. Both conditions are associated with leukopenia and thrombocytopenia. Aminotransferases are frequently elevated, with bilirubin and alkaline phosphatase usually unaffected. Patients undergoing lumbar puncture may have lymphocytic pleocytosis.

Morulae, basophilic inclusion bodies composed of clusters of bacteria, may be found in leukocyte cytoplasm (**Figure 8**). Morulae are identified in monocytes in fewer than 30% of patients with HME but are seen in neutrophils in more than 50% of patients with HGA; considering the low sensitivity, other diagnostic tests are recommended when microscopic findings are negative. Antibodies are often absent at presentation; however, the sensitivity of serologic testing on a convalescent specimen is greater than 90%, allowing retrospective diagnosis. Whole-blood PCR is the most sensitive test for diagnosis of acute infection, particularly when performed before initiation of antibiotics.

Doxycycline is effective therapy for both infections. Therapy should be given empirically when a diagnosis of HME or HGA is considered because delay in therapy has been associated with adverse outcomes. Given their limitations, a negative result on serologic testing or microscopy should not affect the decision to start or continue doxycycline. A negative PCR result, particularly if obtained before initiation of doxycycline, would suggest an alternative diagnosis. Treatment options for patients allergic to or intolerant of doxycycline are limited, and desensitization may be required.

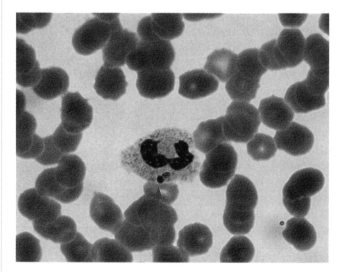

**FIGURE 8.** Morulae (*arrow*), appearing as basophilic inclusion bodies in leukocytes of a patient with ehrlichiosis.

Figure courtesy of Charles Stratton, MD

- Human monocytic ehrlichiosis and human granulocytic anaplasmosis are associated with a nonspecific febrile illness, frequently accompanied by headache, myalgia, arthralgia, and meningismus.
- Whole-blood polymerase chain reaction is extremely sensitive for diagnosing ehrlichiosis and anaplasmosis when performed before antibiotic initiation and allows rapid diagnosis at acute presentation.
- Doxycycline should be given empirically when ehrlichiosis or anaplasmosis is a diagnostic consideration because delay in therapy is associated with adverse outcomes.

## Rocky Mountain Spotted Fever

Rocky Mountain spotted fever (RMSF) has been reported throughout the United States. Infections predominate in warmer months when ticks are active. The hallmark of RMSF is a petechial rash, seen in more than 85% of patients by the end of the first week of illness (**Figure 9**). Skin lesions may lag behind other symptoms; only 50% of patients have visible rash by the third day of illness. Therefore, the diagnosis should be considered in any patient presenting with a fever and possible tick exposure regardless of the presence of a rash. Skin lesions typically start at the distal extremities and progress centrally. The rash involves the palms and soles in more than 30% of patients but usually spares the face.

Thrombocytopenia and elevated aminotransferase levels are common. The leukocyte count in RMSF may be elevated, normal, or low. When lumbar puncture is performed, CSF demonstrates a lymphocyte-predominant pleocytosis.

Development of rickettsial antibodies takes several weeks; therefore, serologic testing is of limited utility during the acute illness. Testing paired acute and convalescent serum may demonstrate seroconversion or a fourfold rise in antibody titer, both of which are diagnostic of acute infection. Serologic cross-reactivity is common, and a positive test result may represent infection with another spotted fever group *Rickettsia* species. Immunohistochemistry or PCR of a skin biopsy specimen allows diagnosis at the time of acute infection.

Doxycycline is effective against all spotted fever group rickettsioses. Symptoms typically improve within 72 hours, and continued fevers or progressive constitutional symptoms after this time period strongly suggest an alternative diagnosis. Doxycycline is contraindicated in pregnancy; chloramphenicol is an alternative option.

- The diagnosis of Rocky Mountain spotted fever should be considered in any patient presenting with a fever and possible tick exposure regardless of the presence of a rash.
- Serologic testing is of limited utility during acute illness with Rocky Mountain spotted fever.
- Doxycycline is the therapy of choice for all spotted fever group rickettsioses; chloramphenicol is an alternative option in pregnancy.

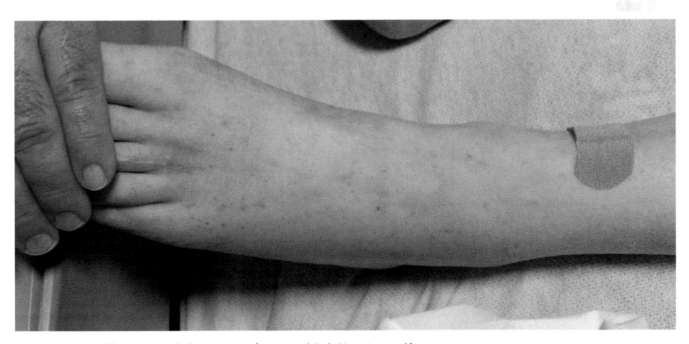

**FIGURE 9.** Petechial skin eruption on the lower extremity of a patient with Rocky Mountain spotted fever.

# Urinary Tract Infections
## Epidemiology and Microbiology

Urinary tract infection (UTI) is broadly defined as infection anywhere in the urinary tract, including the urethra, the bladder, the ureters, and the kidneys. UTI accounts for more than eight million office visits and one million emergency department visits and results in approximately 100,000 hospital admissions each year in the United States. UTIs are common among hospitalized patients, with the predominant risk factor being bladder catheterization. Other risk factors for UTIs include female sex; postmenopausal status; previous UTI; sexual activity; genital trauma or surgery; diabetes; condom, diaphragm, or spermicide use in women; vaginal infection; obesity; genital tract abnormalities or obstructions; and host susceptibility, including genetic factors and immunosuppression. Bacteria that cause UTI generally have special virulence factors that enable them to survive in the urinary tract. Most of the research in bacterial uropathogenesis has been done with *Escherichia coli*. Uropathogenic *E. coli* expresses such traits as fimbrial and nonfimbrial adhesins for attachment, flagellae for motility, enterobactin that inactivates host defenses, metal acquisition systems that enhance survival in urine, toxins, and fimbrial phase variation mechanisms that change antigens before the host can respond.

*E. coli* is the most common organism associated with asymptomatic bacteriuria, cystitis, pyelonephritis, and catheter-associated UTI. The urinary tract is the most common source of bacteremia caused by gram-negative organisms. Other common urinary pathogens include *Klebsiella* species, *Proteus* species, *Pseudomonas aeruginosa*, and *Staphylococcus saprophyticus*, the latter being a frequent cause of acute uncomplicated cystitis. Infections with non–*E. coli* organisms are more likely to occur in men, in patients with recurrent UTIs, in those with obstruction, or in the presence of a urinary catheter. Multiple urinary pathogens may be isolated when structural abnormalities of the urinary tract or calculi are present. *Candida* species cause UTI in patients with diabetes mellitus or indwelling urinary catheters; however, in most patients, candiduria represents colonization and does not require treatment.

Antimicrobial resistance among urinary pathogens is increasing in frequency in the community and hospital settings because of antibiotic overuse, inappropriate treatment of asymptomatic bacteriuria, and local differences in antibiotic use. The frequency of resistant organisms varies by patient population and geographic location. Risk factors for multidrug-resistant organisms are current or recent hospitalization, immunocompromise, presence of underlying structural abnormalities of the urinary tract, previous UTI, kidney transplantation, and recent antimicrobial therapy.

**KEY POINTS**

- Risk factors for urinary tract infection (UTI) with multidrug-resistant organisms are current or recent hospitalization, immunocompromise, presence of underlying structural abnormalities of the urinary tract, previous UTI, kidney transplantation, and recent antimicrobial therapy.

- Antimicrobial resistance among urinary pathogens is increasing in frequency in the community and hospital settings because of antibiotic overuse, inappropriate treatment of asymptomatic bacteriuria, and local differences in antibiotic use.

HVC

## Diagnosis

UTIs are classified as uncomplicated or complicated. Acute cystitis and pyelonephritis occurring in healthy, premenopausal, nonpregnant women with no history of urinary tract abnormalities are classified as uncomplicated. Complicated UTI is defined as infection occurring in a patient with comorbid conditions or anatomic abnormalities of the urinary tract that increase the risk for adverse outcomes, including poor response to therapy, a need for hospitalization, presence of resistant organisms, and morbidity. Common complicating factors are diabetes, pregnancy, male sex, advanced age, kidney transplantation, anatomic or functional abnormalities of the urinary tract, urinary catheterization or manipulation, recent antibiotic exposure, and recent hospitalization.

Urine dipsticks are used to assess for pyuria and bacteriuria by detecting leukocyte esterase and nitrites, respectively, which are markers of infection in the urine. They are easy to use and fairly reliable in confirming infection if results are positive and the patient has signs or symptoms consistent with UTI. Sensitivity of both tests together (with results of one or both being positive) is between 68% and 88%, depending on patient group. When both results of tests are positive, specificity and predictive value increase. Negative results for both tests, however, strongly predict the absence of UTI when the pretest probability is low. Reasons for a false-negative nitrite test result include inability of some organisms, such as *Enterococcus faecalis*, to convert nitrate to nitrite; low urinary excretion of nitrate; low urine pH; and insufficient bladder incubation time. On urine microscopy, the presence of at least 10 leukocytes/μL of unspun urine from a midstream, clean-catch specimen indicates significant pyuria; 5-10 leukocytes/hpf on a centrifuged specimen of urine is also significant. Pyuria is a nonspecific finding and may or may not indicate infection.

A urine culture is used to confirm the presence of bacteriuria and yield the causative organism for antimicrobial susceptibility testing. A urine culture should be obtained in patients with suspected pyelonephritis, complicated UTI, recurrent UTI, and multiple antimicrobial allergies and in

**CONT.** those in whom the presence of a resistant organism is suspected. It is also recommended that urine cultures be obtained in pregnant women during the first trimester of pregnancy to screen for asymptomatic bacteriuria and for patients undergoing urologic procedures so that appropriate therapy can be instituted. Urine cultures are not indicated for the diagnosis of uncomplicated cystitis because patient history is reliable in establishing the diagnosis and treatment is completed before the availability of culture results. Because contamination of urine from bacteria that normally colonize the urethra and periurethral areas is frequent, quantitating bacteria in midstream, clean-void urine allows for differentiation of contamination and infection. Patients with infection usually have at least 105 colony-forming units (CFU)/mL on culture. In symptomatic patients with pyuria, a colony count between 102 and 105 CFU/mL may still indicate a UTI. Standard criteria are insensitive for cystitis because up to half of women with cystitis have colony counts of 102 to 104 CFU/mL. Reasons for this are unclear but may represent an earlier stage of infection or bladder washout during urination. Similarly, low colony counts may still indicate infection in patients receiving antimicrobial therapy, in men, and in those with organisms other than *E. coli* and *Proteus* species. Diagnosis is complicated in patients with indwelling catheters. Most patients with catheter-associated UTI have colony counts of $10^5$ CFU/mL or greater. Symptoms may be nonspecific. Although pyuria is frequently found in asymptomatic patients who are catheterized, the absence of pyuria in a symptomatic patient should prompt consideration of an alternative diagnosis.

**KEY POINT**

**HVC**
- A culture of midstream, clean-void urine should be reserved for patients with suspected pyelonephritis, complicated urinary tract infection, recurrent urinary tract infection, or multiple antimicrobial allergies and in those in whom the presence of a resistant organism is suspected.

## Management

### Asymptomatic Bacteriuria

Asymptomatic bacteriuria is defined by the presence of bacteria (two consecutive voided specimens with isolation of the same strain in counts ≥$10^5$ CFU/mL in women, a single voided specimen with one bacterial species in counts ≥$10^5$ CFU/mL in men, or a single catheterized specimen with isolation of one species in a count ≥$10^2$ CFU/mL in women or men) in an uncontaminated urine specimen collected from a patient without signs or symptoms. It is important to recognize that screening for and possibly treating asymptomatic bacteriuria are supported by only two indications: pregnancy and medical clearance before an invasive urologic procedure. In actual practice, treatment decisions are usually based on a single voided specimen without a repeat culture. Urinalysis and urine culture are not indicated as part of routine health surveillance in asymptomatic patients and should not be performed.

### Cystitis in Women

The most common symptoms of cystitis in premenopausal women are dysuria, frequency, urgency, and suprapubic discomfort. Postmenopausal women with cystitis may present with incontinence or gross hematuria. Fever is unusual. Progression to pyelonephritis is rare. Recommended first-line antimicrobial agents for acute uncomplicated cystitis in women include nitrofurantoin and trimethoprim-sulfamethoxazole; fosfomycin has lower efficacy and is more expensive than the first two options. Trimethoprim-sulfamethoxazole should not be used if it was taken in the preceding 3 months or if the prevalence of resistance is known to exceed 20%. Resistance rates for nitrofurantoin and fosfomycin are low. Short-course regimens (single dose to 5 days, depending on the agent used) are recommended. They are as effective in achieving cures as longer regimens and have fewer adverse effects. Fluoroquinolones (ciprofloxacin, levofloxacin, ofloxacin) and β-lactams are considered second-line therapy. Oral β-lactams are less effective than fluoroquinolones. Increasing resistance of urinary isolates of *E. coli* to fluoroquinolones has been reported. Strains that produce extended-spectrum β-lactamases have increased in frequency.

**KEY POINTS**

- Urinalysis and urine culture are not indicated as part of routine health surveillance in asymptomatic patients and should not be performed.

- Fosfomycin has lower efficacy and is more expensive than nitrofurantoin or trimethoprim-sulfamethoxazole in first-line antimicrobial therapy for women with acute uncomplicated cystitis. **HVC**

## Acute Pyelonephritis

Clinical manifestations of acute pyelonephritis include fever, chills, back/flank pain, nausea, and vomiting. Antecedent or concurrent symptoms of cystitis may or may not be present. Most episodes of acute uncomplicated pyelonephritis are treated in the ambulatory setting. This is appropriate for patients who are otherwise healthy and have mild to moderate uncomplicated illness, but close supervision is essential. Empiric therapy should be initiated after a urine culture is obtained. Fluoroquinolones (ciprofloxacin, levofloxacin, or ofloxacin) are recommended for outpatient empiric therapy. Indications for hospitalization include hemodynamic instability, inability to tolerate oral medications, host factors such as pregnancy or presence of kidney stones or other obstructions, presence of comorbidities, and an unstable social situation that may compromise adherence or follow-up. Inpatient antimicrobial regimens include intravenous fluoroquinolones, aminoglycosides with or without ampicillin,

CONT.

extended-spectrum cephalosporins or extended-spectrum penicillins with or without an aminoglycoside, and carbapenems. Ceftolozane-tazobactam was recently approved for treatment of complicated UTI caused by resistant organisms, including those producing extended-spectrum β-lactamases. Imaging with CT (preferred) or ultrasonography should be performed if symptoms and fever persist longer than 72 hours to rule out perinephric or intrarenal abscess. In patients who have symptoms suggesting a stone or obstruction, a urologic evaluation should be performed emergently.

The duration of therapy for acute uncomplicated pyelonephritis treated with fluoroquinolones is 5 to 7 days; complicated infections should be treated for 14 days. Hospitalized patients who are treated initially with parenteral antibiotics can be switched to oral agents after clinical improvement is noted and they are able to tolerate oral therapy. Oral therapy can be chosen on the basis of susceptibility results from urine culture; however, oral cephalosporins generally should be avoided. Trimethoprim-sulfamethoxazole or fluoroquinolones are preferred. Bacteremia is not uncommon in patients who require hospitalization for pyelonephritis; although these patients may take longer to reach clinical stability, more prolonged courses of parenteral antibiotics are not required.

**KEY POINTS**

HVC
- Acute uncomplicated pyelonephritis should be treated with fluoroquinolones for 5 to 7 days, complicated infections should be treated for 14 days, and hospitalized patients treated initially with parenteral antibiotics can be switched to oral agents after clinical improvement is noted and oral therapy can be tolerated.

- Trimethoprim-sulfamethoxazole or fluoroquinolones are preferred for oral therapy in acute pyelonephritis, and oral cephalosporins should generally be avoided.

## Recurrent Urinary Tract Infections in Women

Recurrent UTI is defined as three episodes of UTI in the preceding 12 months or two episodes in the preceding 6 months. Recurrent UTI is common in women. A recurrent UTI may be a relapse or reinfection. Relapse is defined as an infection caused by the same strain (by repeat culture) as the initial UTI and occurs within 2 weeks of the completion of initial therapy. Reinfection is diagnosed if the UTI is caused by a different strain than that causing the initial infection or if a sterile urine culture was documented between the episodes. Most recurrences are reinfections. For relapsed UTI, therapy can be given with the same antibiotic for a longer period; 7 to 10 days is reasonable.

Prevention includes considering an alternate method of contraception in patients using condoms, diaphragms, and spermicides. Low-dose antimicrobial prophylaxis with a daily or every-other-day dose of nitrofurantoin or trimethoprim-sulfamethoxazole, usually taken at bedtime, is an effective method to prevent frequent UTIs but does not alter the long-term risk for recurrence after prophylaxis is discontinued. This strategy may aid women who desire a respite from recurrent UTI. Antimicrobial prophylaxis, consisting of a single dose of an agent (such as nitrofurantoin or trimethoprim-sulfamethoxazole), can be administered after sexual intercourse and reduces the rate of recurrent cystitis. This strategy is useful when recurrent UTI is clearly linked to sexual intercourse. An additional, nonpreventive strategy is for patients with previously diagnosed cystitis to self-diagnose and self-treat at the onset of symptoms. In postmenopausal women, two small studies have shown the use of topical vaginal estrogens reduces the number of UTIs compared with placebo. Some cranberry products decrease the frequency of recurrent UTIs by about one third but are less effective compared with low-dose antimicrobial prophylaxis.

A urologic evaluation is indicated if a structural or physiologic abnormality is suspected, if multiple relapses occur caused by the same strain, and when renal calculi as a nidus for infection are a concern.

**KEY POINTS**

- Continuous antimicrobial prophylaxis with a daily bedtime dose of nitrofurantoin or trimethoprim-sulfamethoxazole reduces recurrences of cystitis, but adverse effects are common.

- Antimicrobial prophylaxis, consisting of a single dose of an agent (such as nitrofurantoin or trimethoprim-sulfamethoxazole), can be administered after sexual intercourse and reduces the rate of recurrent cystitis when it has been linked to sexual activity.

## Acute Bacterial Prostatitis

Acute bacterial prostatitis is a common and important infection. Patient groups at high risk include those with diabetes, immunosuppression, and cirrhosis. Risk factors include unprotected sexual intercourse, the presence of indwelling urinary catheters, urinary tract manipulation, urinary stasis (obstruction), and benign prostatic hyperplasia. Most cases result from ascending urethral infection and intraprostatic reflux, although bacterial cystitis, epididymo-orchitis, and seeding during a transrectal prostate biopsy can also lead to acute bacterial prostatitis. Rarely, prostatitis can develop from spread from the rectum by the lymphatic system or hematogenously during bacterial sepsis. Common symptoms include fever, chills, malaise, nausea and vomiting, dysuria, urgency, frequency, and pain in the lower abdomen, perineum, and rectum. Patients may be quite ill. On rectal examination, the prostate is very tender and tense. Excessive palpation of the prostate should be avoided due to lack of diagnostic or therapeutic benefit and because bacteremia may result. The causative organisms are the same as those that cause most UTIs, including *E. coli* and other gram-negative organisms and *Enterococcus* species. *Neisseria gonorrhoeae* may cause acute prostatitis in sexually active men. The diagnosis is established in most cases by a urine Gram stain and culture. Blood cultures should be obtained in patients who require hospitalization and in outpatients who have systemic symptoms. The therapy of choice for uncomplicated cases in patients with low risk for a sexually transmitted infection is an oral fluoroquinolone (levofloxacin or ciprofloxacin) for 4 to 6 weeks; trimethoprim-sulfamethoxazole is an alternative. Follow-up evaluation with repeat culture is necessary to ensure response to treatment.

Complications include development of prostatic abscess, infarction, chronic bacterial prostatitis, and granulomatous prostatitis. Imaging studies are not necessary unless a prostatic abscess is suspected. Chronic prostatitis is discussed in MKSAP 17 General Internal Medicine. **H**

> **KEY POINT**
> - The therapy of choice for uncomplicated acute prostatitis is an oral fluoroquinolone (levofloxacin or ciprofloxacin) for 4 to 6 weeks, with repeat culture needed to ensure response to treatment.

# *Mycobacterium tuberculosis* Infection

## Epidemiology

One third of the world (approximately 2 billion people) is infected with *Mycobacterium tuberculosis*. In 2012, almost 9 million people worldwide developed active tuberculosis, and 1.3 million people died as a result of tuberculosis. The greatest number of new cases reported was in Asia (60% of all new cases worldwide), but the largest tuberculosis case rate was reported in sub-Saharan Africa. More than one third of persons with HIV worldwide are also infected with tuberculosis, a concern because active disease is 25 times more likely in this population than in those without HIV. More than 1 million new HIV-associated tuberculosis cases were reported in 2012, and 20% of HIV-associated deaths occur because of tuberculosis.

In 2013, the total number of tuberculosis cases in the United States was 9582, the lowest since reporting began in 1953. The incidence rate of infection in foreign-born persons is 13 times higher than that of persons born in the United States. The percentage of cases in foreign-born persons was 65% of all cases in the United States and has continued to increase since 1993, when the percentage was 29%. Eighty percent of all cases of tuberculosis in foreign-born persons living in the United States occurred in those of Hispanic and Asian descent.

Ninety-five cases of primary multidrug-resistant (MDR) tuberculosis were reported in the United States in 2013, and 89.5% of these infections occurred in foreign-born persons. Extensively drug-resistant (XDR) tuberculosis remains rare in the United States.

> **KEY POINTS**
> - The percentage of tuberculosis cases in foreign-born persons was 65% of all cases in the United States in 2013; this rate has continued to increase since 1993, when the percentage was 29%.
> - More than one third of persons with HIV worldwide are infected with tuberculosis, which is 25 times more likely in this population than in those without HIV; 20% of HIV-associated deaths occur because of tuberculosis.

## Pathophysiology

Actively infected patients transmit tuberculous mycobacteria by aerosolized droplets. Even patients whose sputum specimens are negative on an acid-fast bacilli (AFB) smear but positive on AFB culture can infect others. Approximately 90% of patients who become infected after inhaling viable mycobacteria remain asymptomatic with latent infection. The risk for active tuberculosis after initial infection is approximately 5% within the first 24 months and then approximately 5% for the remainder of the person's lifetime. Active disease that occurs early after infection is known as primary progressive tuberculosis. Reactivation tuberculosis, which represents at least two thirds of all recognized cases, refers to active disease that develops remotely after infection. Patients who are most likely to develop active disease are those with impaired host defenses from immunocompromising conditions, such as HIV infection; malignancy; diabetes mellitus; chronic kidney disease; injection drug use; tobacco smoking; and malnutrition; or those receiving such medications as cytotoxic chemotherapy, glucocorticoids, and tumor necrosis factor α inhibitors.

> **KEY POINT**
> - Patients most likely to develop active tuberculosis are those with impaired host defenses from immunocompromising conditions, such as HIV infection, malignancy, diabetes mellitus, chronic kidney disease, injection drug use, tobacco smoking, and malnutrition or from medications.

## Clinical Manifestations

Latent infection with tuberculosis is asymptomatic. In patients with active disease, pulmonary tuberculosis accounts for 70% of cases. Patients typically present with an indolent syndrome characterized by fever, chronic cough, purulent or blood-streaked sputum, chest pain, malaise, weight loss, night sweats, anorexia, and fatigue. Physical examination findings of pulmonary crackles, rhonchi, or evidence of pleural effusion are nonspecific, resulting in a delay of diagnosis. This is particularly true in patients with HIV and low CD4 cell counts (<200/μL), who can present with subtle and atypical features. *M. tuberculosis* can also disseminate through the lymphatic system and blood stream, resulting in miliary tuberculosis, which can present fulminantly with sepsis and acute lung injury. Extrapulmonary tuberculosis, more commonly seen in immunocompromised patients, can involve any organ, including the pleura, lymph nodes, central nervous system, skeletal system, pericardium, larynx, peritoneum, and genitourinary system.

**KEY POINT**

- Pulmonary tuberculosis, which accounts for 70% of active disease, is characterized by fever, chronic cough, purulent or blood-streaked sputum, chest pain, malaise, weight loss, night sweats, anorexia, and fatigue.

# Diagnostic Testing

Diagnostic testing is used to detect latent tuberculosis infection (LTBI) or confirm tuberculosis infection in those with clinical findings suggesting active disease. The tuberculin skin test (TST) and interferon γ release assay (IGRA) are the initial diagnostic studies used to evaluate for tuberculosis infection. However, neither test can distinguish between latent and active tuberculosis, nor should they be administered to persons who are at low risk for infection with *M. tuberculosis* (targeted testing is reserved for those at high risk). The exception includes persons who will be at increased future risk, such as those beginning employment in a hospital setting.

LTBI is diagnosed when an asymptomatic patient has a positive TST or IGRA result without clinical evidence of active tuberculosis infection by history, physical examination, or chest imaging. In patients suspected of having active disease, additional microbiologic testing, including AFB staining and culture and nucleic acid–based testing, is indicated to confirm the diagnosis.

**KEY POINT**

- Latent tuberculosis infection is diagnosed when an asymptomatic patient has a positive tuberculin skin test or interferon-γ release assay result without clinical evidence of active tuberculosis infection.

## Tuberculin Skin Test

The Mantoux TST requires intradermal injection of 5 tuberculin units into the volar aspect of the forearm. Forty-eight to 72 hours later, the transverse width of induration (not erythema) is measured in millimeters, serving as a marker of a delayed hypersensitivity cell-mediated immunity response. Skin test reactivity develops 2 to 12 weeks after infection. The criteria for a positive reaction have been established by the Centers for Disease Control and Prevention (CDC) based on the patient's risks for tuberculosis (**Table 15**). An increase in induration of 10 mm or more within 2 years is also considered a positive TST reaction in persons without a history of reactive TST. False-negative TST results can occur in patients who are immunosuppressed, are very young or old, or have active overwhelming tuberculosis. Conversely, false-positive TST reactions can result from infection with nontuberculous mycobacteria or in patients who have received bacillus Calmette-Guérin (BCG) as a vaccine or chemotherapy. In adults who received BCG vaccine as a child, TST results should be interpreted in the same way as in those who have not received BCG. Patients with a remote history of tuberculosis infection who have an initially negative skin test result may receive a second "booster" TST up to 4 weeks later that causes a true-positive skin test result. This two-step testing is also administered as a baseline assessment for persons who will need to undergo serial testing in the future.

| TABLE 15. | Interpretation of Tuberculin Skin Test Results | |
|---|---|---|
| **Criteria for Tuberculin Positivity by Risk Group** | | |
| **≥5 mm Induration** | **≥10 mm Induration** | **≥15 mm Induration** |
| HIV-positive persons | Recent (<5 years) arrivals from high-prevalence countries | All others with no risk factors for TB |
| Recent contacts of persons with active TB | Injection drug users | |
| Persons with fibrotic changes on chest radiograph consistent with old TB | Residents or employees of high-risk congregate settings: prisons and jails, nursing homes and other long-term facilities for the elderly, hospitals and other health care facilities, residential facilities for patients with AIDS, homeless shelters | |
| Patients with organ transplants and other immunosuppressive conditions (receiving the equivalent of ≥15 mg/d of prednisone for >4 weeks) | Mycobacteriology laboratory personnel; persons with clinical conditions that put them at high risk for active disease; children aged <4 years or exposed to adults in high-risk categories | |
| TB = tuberculosis infection. | | |

### Interferon-γ Release Assays

IGRAs are in vitro blood tests that measure T-cell–mediated interferon-γ release in response to specific *M. tuberculosis* antigens. These assays are felt to be more specific (no *Mycobacterium bovis*–associated BCG strain antigens are included) than the TST while attaining similar sensitivity in diagnosing tuberculosis infection. Like the TST, IGRAs should not be used to assess persons who have low risk for tuberculosis infection or active disease unless they will be at increased future risk (such as employment in a health care setting). According to the CDC, an IGRA can be used instead of a TST in all cases in which TST is recommended. However, the IGRA is preferred for those who have received BCG previously or are members of groups that are unlikely to return to have their TST interpreted (homeless population or drug users). A TST is preferred for evaluation of children younger than 5 years.

Two IGRAs are commercially available that have been approved by the FDA. The QuantiFERON-TB Gold In-Tube test measures the interferon-γ concentration, with possible results listed as positive, negative, or indeterminate. The T-SPOT TB test measures the number of cells that secrete interferon-γ, with results listed as positive, negative, indeterminate, or borderline. When results are reported, both of these standard qualitative test interpretations and the quantitative assay measurements should be included so that the best-informed decision can be reached.

A TST or repeat IGRA can be considered when the result from the initial IGRA reflects an uncertain likelihood of tuberculosis infection, that is, a borderline or indeterminate result, and a reason for ongoing assessment persists. Routine use of both a TST and IGRA is not recommended. In certain circumstances, however, using both tests when the result of the initial test is negative might be helpful when the risk for infection or progression is increased or risk for poor outcome exists, such as in children younger than 5 years who have been exposed to a patient with active tuberculosis or in patients with HIV infection. Use of a second test for diagnosing infection when the result of the first test is negative can also be considered when the suspicion of tuberculosis is strong based on clinical presentation or radiographic imaging. Conversely, using both tests when the result of the initial test is positive might be helpful when additional evidence to enhance patient adherence with treatment is needed or to evaluate a suspected false-positive result in a person at low risk for infection and progression to active disease.

IGRAs have several advantages in addition to the need for only a single visit to perform the test. These include availability of test results within 1 day, the lack of a booster response with subsequent tests, and fewer false-positive results in patients infected with nontuberculous mycobacteria (including those vaccinated with BCG). Disadvantages of IGRA testing include increased expense compared with TST, need for specialized personnel and equipment, and the need to process blood samples within 8 to 30 hours.

## Imaging

Lung imaging, although nonspecific, is recommended for all patients being evaluated for tuberculosis. Primary pulmonary tuberculosis may present with mid- to lower-zone unilateral infiltrates, hilar lymphadenopathy, and pleural effusions. Reactivation tuberculosis classically presents with fibrocavitary disease in the apical-posterior segments of the upper lobes or superior segments of the lower lobes (**Figure 10**). Chest radiographs may be normal, particularly in primary tuberculosis. CT is more sensitive for detecting abnormalities in the lung (particularly lymphadenopathy) or at other sites of involvement, although it is not typically used for initial screening for active disease. When pericardial disease is suspected, echocardiography can provide information about the amount of pericardial fluid present and any potential hemodynamic effects, including cardiac tamponade.

### Culture and Additional Microbiologic Testing

Confirmatory diagnostic testing requires growth of *M. tuberculosis* from culture or detection by nucleic acid–based testing. Initial screening of sputum specimens with

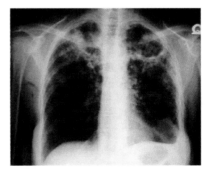

**FIGURE 10.** Chest radiograph demonstrating upper-lobe infiltrates and cavitation consistent with reactivation pulmonary tuberculosis.

**H**
**CONT.**

AFB staining is followed by culture in a liquid medium, which allows for faster growth and detection (approximately 2 weeks) than a solid medium (approximately 3-4 weeks). A positive AFB test result is helpful but not diagnostic because nontuberculous mycobacteria will stain similarly. Because culture recovery can be slow, faster molecular tests have been developed that can identify *M. tuberculosis* in culture media within 1 to 2 days, which speeds the diagnostic process significantly. Additionally, nucleic acid amplification testing (NAAT) is available that can target *M. tuberculosis* in sputum from patients suspected of having pulmonary tuberculosis and can expedite initiation of treatment, although this form of testing is expensive. The positive predictive value of a positive NAAT result in a patient with AFB smear–positive sputum is greater than 95%. In patients in whom tuberculosis is strongly suspected, the NAAT result is positive in approximately 65% of patients whose sputum is negative on AFB smear but eventually positive on culture. NAATs are not recommended for patients in whom the suspicion for tuberculosis is low. One FDA-approved NAAT that can detect *M. tuberculosis* infection and rifampin resistance (sensitivity of 95%; specificity of 99%) within 2 hours, the Xpert MTB/RIF test, has the potential to make a significant public health impact on the control of tuberculosis in endemic areas; however, its cost may be prohibitive. Because rifampin resistance often coexists with isoniazid resistance, this test can more rapidly identify MDR tuberculosis. Although results are available quickly with this NAAT, conventional mycobacterial cultures are still recommended for performance of drug susceptibility testing and genotyping.

Pleural tuberculosis may be difficult to diagnose from pleural fluid cultures, which typically are positive in less than half of infection cases. Pleural biopsies demonstrating caseating granulomatous inflammation may be needed to confirm the diagnosis. Adenosine deaminase levels in pleural fluid may also be helpful in the evaluation of suspected pleural tuberculosis, particularly in patients with a high clinical suspicion but negative results on culture and pleural biopsy. Tuberculous meningitis should be considered when the cerebrospinal fluid (CSF) profile demonstrates a lymphocytic pleocytosis with elevated protein and decreased glucose levels. Serial CSF sampling is recommended to increase the yield of AFB smears and cultures in the diagnosis of CSF tuberculosis. NAAT of the CSF is highly specific, but a negative test result does not rule out the diagnosis (sensitivity of approximately 50%). Pericardial fluid usually reveals an elevated protein level and leukocyte count that is lymphocytic predominant in tuberculosis pericarditis. AFB smears and cultures are recommended but often are not positive (approximately 50% of the time). Adenosine deaminase levels in pericardial fluid may be helpful, particularly in endemic areas. If findings on pericardial fluid analysis are negative, a pericardial biopsy may be considered for pathologic and microbiologic evaluation. **H**

**KEY POINT**

- Nucleic acid amplification testing targeting *Mycobacterium tuberculosis* in sputum from patients with high clinical suspicion of having tuberculosis (AFB smear–positive sputum) can expedite initiation of treatment, although it is more expensive and does not provide drug susceptibility and genotyping information necessary to guide long term treatment.

**HVC**

## Treatment

**H**

If active tuberculosis is excluded in a patient with positive results on TST or IGRA, treatment for LTBI is indicated. Several treatment options exist, and the regimen chosen should be based on comorbidities, knowledge of the drug-susceptibility data from the source patient, and possible drug interactions (**Table 16**). If isoniazid is chosen, the addition of pyridoxine is recommended for patients with diabetes, uremia, alcoholism, HIV infection, malnutrition, seizure disorder, and pregnancy because of an increased risk **for** isoniazid-associated peripheral neuropathy.

The 12-week regimen of once-weekly isoniazid and rifapentine must be administered as directly observed therapy (that is, a health care worker directly observes the ingestion of a medication) and can be used instead of 9 months of isoniazid alone for healthy adult patients, including those with HIV coinfection who are not taking antiretroviral agents. It is not recommended for patients suspected of having rifampin- or isoniazid-resistant tuberculosis strains or patients who are pregnant or plan to become pregnant while taking these agents. Four months of rifampin is acceptable for patients in whom infection with isoniazid-resistant tuberculosis is suspected or who cannot take isoniazid. A 9-month regimen of isoniazid is usually recommended for patients with HIV receiving antiretroviral medications. In pregnant patients, isoniazid is recommended for treatment of LTBI if the patient has been recently exposed to a person with known tuberculosis or if she has HIV. If not, many experts would recommend that treatment of LTBI be deferred until after delivery. Isoniazid treatment is not a contraindication for breastfeeding.

Treatment of active tuberculosis usually consists of multiple drugs for 6 to 9 months administered in two phases: initial and continuation (**Table 17**). The core first-line antituberculous agents include isoniazid, rifampin, pyrazinamide, and ethambutol (**Table 18**). These agents are administered for 8 weeks as part of the initiation phase, and then isoniazid and rifampin are continued for 4 or 7 months as part of the continuation phase. The longer course is recommended in patients who have cavitary pulmonary disease at diagnosis and positive sputum cultures after completing initial therapy, patients who did not receive pyrazinamide as part of the initial therapy, and patients who are receiving once-weekly rifapentine and

**TABLE 16.  Treatment Regimens for Latent Tuberculosis Infection**

| Drugs | Duration | Dose[a] | Frequency | Total Doses |
|---|---|---|---|---|
| Isoniazid | 9 months | 5 mg/kg<br>Maximum dose: 300 mg | Daily | 270 |
| | | 15 mg/kg<br>Maximum dose: 900 mg | Twice weekly[b] | 76 |
| | 6 months | 5 mg/kg<br>Maximum dose: 300 mg | Daily | 180 |
| | | 15 mg/kg<br>Maximum dose: 900 mg | Twice weekly[b] | 52 |
| Isoniazid and rifapentine | 3 months | Isoniazid[c,d]: 15 mg/kg rounded up to the nearest 50 or 100 mg; 900 mg maximum<br><br>Rifapentine[c,d]:<br>10.0–14.0 kg: 300 mg<br>14.1–25.0 kg: 450 mg<br>25.1–32.0 kg: 600 mg<br>32.1–49.9 kg: 750 mg<br>≥50.0 kg: 900 mg maximum | Once weekly[b] | 12 |
| Rifampin | 4 months | 10 mg/kg<br>Maximum dose: 600 mg | Daily | 120 |

[a]Doses listed are for adults.

[b]Intermittent regimens must be provided by directly observed therapy in which a health care worker observes the ingestion of medication.

[c]Isoniazid is formulated in 100-mg and 300-mg tablets. Rifapentine is formulated in 150-mg tablets in blister packs that should be kept sealed until use.

[d]For isoniazid and rifapentine, doses listed are for anyone older than 12 years.

Adapted from Centers for Disease Control and Prevention. Latent Tuberculosis Infection: A Guide for Primary Health Care Providers. Treatment of Latent TB Infection. Table 2. Choosing the Most Effective LTBI Treatment Regimen. www.cdc.gov/tb/publications/ltbi/treatment.htm#2. Accessed June 30, 2015.

**TABLE 17.  Tuberculosis Treatment Regimens**

| Treatment Phase | Preferred Regimen | Alternative Regimens |
|---|---|---|
| Initial | Daily INH, RIF, PZA, and EMB[a] for 56 doses (8 weeks) | Daily INH, RIF, PZA, and EMB[a] for 14 doses (2 weeks), then twice weekly for 12 doses (6 weeks)<br><br>Thrice-weekly INH, RIF, PZA, and EMB[a] for 24 doses (8 weeks) |
| Continuation | Daily INH and RIF for 126 doses (18 weeks)<br><br>or<br><br>Twice-weekly INH and RIF for 36 doses (18 weeks) | Twice-weekly INH and RIF for 36 doses (18 weeks)<br><br>Thrice-weekly INH and RIF for 54 doses (18 weeks) |

EMB = ethambutol; INH = isoniazid; PZA = pyrazinamide; RIF = rifampin.

[a]EMB can be discontinued if drug susceptibility studies demonstrate susceptibility to first-line drugs.

NOTE: A continuation phase of once-weekly INH/rifapentine can be used for patients who are HIV negative who do not have cavitary lesions on the chest film and who have negative acid-fast bacilli smears at the completion of the initial phase of treatment.

Source: Tuberculosis. Treatment for TB Disease. Table 1. Basic TB Disease Treatment Regimens. www.cdc.gov/tb/topic/treatment/tbdisease.htm. Accessed August 27, 2014.

CONT.

isoniazid whose sputum cultures remain positive after the initial 2-month phase.

Completion of treatment is dictated by how many doses are taken over a specified duration. When treatment interruptions of 2 weeks or more occur during the initial 2-month phase, the treatment regimen should be restarted from the beginning. In general, treatment recommendations are the same for patients with HIV with tuberculosis, with careful consideration given to the potential for drug interactions in patients receiving antiretroviral therapy.

**TABLE 18.** Antituberculous Drugs

| Agent | Adverse Effects | Notes |
|---|---|---|
| **First-Line Medications** | | |
| Isoniazid | Rash; liver enzyme elevation; hepatitis; peripheral neuropathy; lupus-like syndrome | Hepatitis risk increases with age and alcohol consumption. Pyridoxine may prevent peripheral neuropathy. Adjust for kidney injury. |
| Pyrazinamide | Hepatitis; rash; GI upset; hyperuricemia | May make glucose control more difficult in patients with diabetes. Adjust for kidney injury. |
| Rifampin | Hepatitis; rash; GI upset | Contraindicated or should be used with caution when administered with protease inhibitors and nonnucleoside reverse transcriptase inhibitors. Do not administer to patients also taking saquinavir/ritonavir. Colors body fluids orange. |
| Rifabutin | Rash; hepatitis; thrombocytopenia; severe arthralgia; uveitis; leukopenia | Dose adjustment required if taken with protease inhibitors or nonnucleoside reverse transcriptase inhibitors. Monitor for decreased antiretroviral activity and for rifabutin toxicity. |
| Rifapentine | Similar to rifampin | Contraindicated in patients who are HIV positive (unacceptable rate of failure/relapse). |
| Ethambutol | Optic neuritis; rash | Baseline and periodic tests of visual acuity and color vision. Patients are advised to call immediately if visual acuity or color vision changes. Adjust for kidney injury. |
| **Second-Line Medications**[a] | | |
| Streptomycin | Auditory, vestibular, and kidney toxicity | Avoid or reduce dose in adults age >59 years. Monitor hearing and kidney function test results. Adjust for kidney injury. |
| Cycloserine | Psychosis; convulsions; depression; headaches; rash; drug interactions | Pyridoxine may decrease CNS adverse effects. Measure drug serum levels. |
| Capreomycin | Kidney, vestibular, and auditory toxicity | Monitor hearing and kidney function test results. Adjust for kidney injury. |
| Ethionamide | GI upset; hepatotoxicity; hypersensitivity | May cause hypothyroidism. |
| Kanamycin and amikacin | Auditory, vestibular, and kidney toxicity | Not approved by the FDA for TB treatment. Monitor vestibular, hearing, and kidney function. |
| Levofloxacin, moxifloxacin | GI upset; dizziness; hypersensitivity; drug interactions | Not approved by the FDA for TB treatment. Should not be used in children. |
| Para-aminosalicylic acid | GI upset; hypersensitivity; hepatotoxicity | May cause hypothyroidism, especially if used with ethionamide. Measure liver enzymes. |
| Bedaquiline | Nausea, joint pain, headache, elevated aminotransferases, hemoptysis, prolonged QT interval | FDA-approved oral agent for MDR pulmonary TB treatment indicated for combination therapy when other alternatives are not available. Novel mechanism of action inhibits mycobacterial adenosine triphosphate synthase. Should be given as directly observed therapy. |

CNS = central nervous system; GI = gastrointestinal; MDR = multidrug resistant; TB = tuberculosis.

[a]Use these drugs in consultation with a clinician experienced in the management of drug-resistant TB.

**CONT.**

Similar to pulmonary tuberculosis, extrapulmonary tuberculosis is usually treated with a 6-month treatment course. However, a 9- to 12-month regimen is recommended for tuberculous meningitis. Adjunctive glucocorticoids are also recommended for patients with tuberculosis-associated meningitis and pericarditis.

Drug susceptibility testing should be performed on the initial isolate in all patients. Patient education about the adverse effects associated with antituberculous therapy is important. Before therapy begins, serum creatinine level, liver function tests, a complete blood count, and hepatitis B and C serologic testing (for patients at risk for these diseases) should be obtained. If pyrazinamide or ethambutol is to be used, uric acid levels or visual acuity and color vision testing are recommended, respectively. At least monthly clinical evaluations are recommended during treatment (see Table 18). Routine laboratory monitoring is recommended for patients with baseline abnormalities or increased risk for adverse effects; otherwise, laboratory studies are reserved for those who develop potential drug-associated toxicities.

- Several treatment options exist for latent tuberculosis infection, including a 12-week regimen of once-weekly isoniazid and rifapentine, which can be used instead of 9 months of isoniazid alone for healthy adult patients.

- The core, first-line, antituberculous agents for active tuberculosis include isoniazid, rifampin, pyrazinamide, and ethambutol, which are administered for an 8-week initiation phase followed by 4 to 7 months of continuation-phase therapy with rifampin and isoniazid.

HVC • At least monthly clinical evaluations are recommended during tuberculosis treatment, and routine laboratory monitoring is recommended for patients with baseline abnormalities or increased risk for adverse effects; otherwise, laboratory studies are reserved for those who develop potential drug-associated toxicities.

## Multidrug-Resistant and Extensively Drug-Resistant Tuberculosis

Resistance can develop because of suboptimal treatment regimens, medication nonadherence, drug malabsorption, or drug interactions resulting in subtherapeutic drug levels. By definition, MDR tuberculosis strains are resistant to at least rifampin and isoniazid. Extensively drug-resistant tuberculosis strains are resistant to rifampin and isoniazid, any fluoroquinolone, and at least one injectable second-line drug (kanamycin, amikacin, or capreomycin). Multiple drugs, including second-line agents (five or six agents usually), and extended courses (at least 18-24 months) are required to treat these resistant strains of tuberculosis and should be guided by expert consultation. Recently, bedaquiline, the first antituberculous drug with a novel mechanism of action approved by the FDA since 1971, became available for treatment of MDR tuberculosis. To ensure optimal outcomes, it is essential to give as directly observed therapy. ☐

## Prevention

In health care settings in which tuberculosis is encountered, effective infection control to prevent transmission includes quick identification of infected patients, initiation of airborne isolation (including use of negative-pressure rooms) and prompt treatment of suspected and proven cases. The CDC has established three criteria that must be met to establish a patient as no longer infectious: adequate treatment for tuberculosis for greater than 2 weeks; improvement of symptoms; and three consecutive negative sputum smears (collected at 8- to 24-hour intervals, including one early-morning collection). ☐

Although not routinely administered in the United States, *Mycobacterium bovis*-associated BCG vaccine is used in countries in which tuberculosis is endemic to prevent disseminated disease and meningitis in children. It has not been shown to prevent primary infection or reactivation of pulmonary tuberculosis. In nonendemic countries, such as the United States, BCG vaccination can be considered for children who have a negative TST result and are consistently exposed to adults who have untreated tuberculosis or tuberculosis caused by MDR strains. Vaccination of TST-negative adult health care workers who will be traveling to areas with a high prevalence of MDR tuberculosis can also be considered. BCG is a live attenuated vaccine, so it is contraindicated in patients who are pregnant or immunosuppressed.

- In countries where tuberculosis is endemic, *Mycobacterium bovis*-associated bacillus Calmette-Guérin vaccine is used to prevent disseminated disease and meningitis in children.

# Nontuberculous Mycobacterial Infections

Nontuberculous mycobacteria (NTM) are ubiquitous environmental acid-fast bacilli belonging to species other than *Mycobacterium leprae* or *Mycobacterium tuberculosis* complex. These opportunistic organisms most frequently cause infection in the lungs, lymph nodes, skin or soft tissue, and blood stream (disseminated disease) (**Table 19**). NTM are classified into general groups based on colony-associated morphologic features, pigmentation, and growth rate; rapidly growing mycobacteria (RGM) are a form of NTM that are unique because of their rapid growth rate in culture and different antibiotic susceptibilities relative to more slowly growing species.

Although infection may occur in normal hosts, the risk for disseminated disease is increased with immunologic abnormalities, including low CD4 lymphocyte counts and abnormalities in the interleukin-12, interferon-γ, and signal transducer and activator of transcription 1 (STAT1) pathways. Lung disease is associated with underlying structural abnormalities, such as COPD and bronchiectasis.

Isolation of NTM from clinical specimens may result from colonization, environmental contamination, or active infection. When NTM are isolated from a sterile site, pathogenic infection is more likely. With documented infection, identification to the species level is recommended. Specific DNA probes exist to rapidly identify *Mycobacterium avium* complex (MAC) and *Mycobacterium kansasii*, and high-performance liquid chromatography can be used to identify other mycobacterial species. Identification of RGM may require additional testing, including biochemical studies, ribosomal DNA sequencing, antimicrobial susceptibility testing, and

**TABLE 19. Clinical Syndromes Caused by Selected Nontuberculous Mycobacteria**

| NTM Species | Disseminated | Lymphadenitis | Lung | Skin and Soft Tissue |
|---|---|---|---|---|
| M. abscessus | X | | X | X |
| M. avium complex | X | X | X | X |
| M. chelonae | X | | | X |
| M. fortuitum | X | | | X |
| M. genavense | X | | | |
| M. haemophilum | X | X | | X |
| M. kansasii | X | | X | |
| M. malmoense | | X | X | |
| M. marinum | | | | X |
| M. mucogenicum | X | | | |
| M. scrofulaceum | | X | | |
| M. simiae | X | X | | |
| M. ulcerans | | | | X |
| M. xenopi | X | | X | |

NTM = nontuberculous mycobacteria. Genus for all organisms is *Mycobacterium*.

polymerase chain reaction restriction fragment-length polymorphism analysis.

Guidelines for diagnosing infection and initiating treatment based on clinical, microbiologic, and radiographic criteria have been developed by the American Thoracic Society and Infectious Diseases Society of America (**Table 20**). Isolation of persons with NTM infections is not required. **H**

**KEY POINT**

- With documented mycobacterial infection, species-level identification is recommended; specific DNA probes exist to rapidly identify *Mycobacterium avium* complex and *Mycobacterium kansasii*, and high-performance liquid chromatography can be used to identify other mycobacterial species.

**TABLE 20. Diagnostic Criteria for Nontuberculous Mycobacterial Lung Disease**

| Criteria | Findings |
|---|---|
| Clinical and imaging criteria | Evidence of pulmonary symptoms and abnormal findings on chest imaging studies (nodular or cavitary lung lesions on radiographs or high-resolution CT scans), with exclusion of other possible causes |
| Laboratory (microbiologic) criteria | Positive isolation of NTM from at least two separate sputum samples *or* |
| | Positive isolation of NTM from at least one bronchoalveolar lavage sample *or* |
| | Histopathologic demonstration of AFB and/or granulomatous disease with a positive culture for NTM from lung tissue specimen; or histopathologic demonstration of AFB and/or granulomatous disease on lung tissue specimen with a positive culture for NTM from one or more sputum samples or bronchoalveolar lavage sample |
| Other considerations | The isolation of an unusual NTM species or of an NTM species that is usually a contaminant should prompt consultation with an infectious diseases or pulmonary specialist |
| | The suspicion of NTM lung disease that does not fulfill the above diagnostic criteria should prompt follow-up until a definitive diagnosis is made or excluded |
| | Whether to treat pulmonary infections due to NTM should be based on the potential benefits and risks for individual patients |

AFB = acid-fast bacilli; NTM = nontuberculous mycobacteria.

## 🄷 *Mycobacterium avium* Complex Infection

Pulmonary disease is the most common manifestation of NTM infection, and MAC is the most common causative species. Pulmonary disease, a classic presentation of MAC infection, is seen in middle-aged to older adult male smokers with underlying lung disease who clinically and radiographically resemble patients with tuberculosis. Nonsmoking postmenopausal women with pectus excavatum, mitral valve prolapse, scoliosis, and joint abnormalities are another characteristic group. A chronic cough and purulent sputum production without constitutional symptoms are often noted. Radiographs reveal nodular bronchiectatic disease.

MAC is responsible for most cases of NTM lymphadenitis. Disseminated MAC infection develops in patients with HIV who have CD4 counts less than 50/µL and are not receiving MAC prophylaxis. The clinical presentation often consists of fever, night sweats, weight loss, and gastrointestinal symptoms.

Clarithromycin susceptibility testing is routinely recommended for all MAC isolates. Treatment of MAC infection usually consists of clarithromycin or azithromycin with ethambutol and either rifampin or rifabutin. 🄷

### KEY POINTS

- Pulmonary disease is the most common manifestation of nontuberculous mycobacterial infection, and *Mycobacterium avium* complex (MAC) is the most common causative species.
- Disseminated MAC infection develops in patients with HIV who have CD4 counts less than 50/µL and are not receiving MAC prophylaxis.

## 🄷 *Mycobacterium kansasii*

*M. kansasii* most commonly causes a lung infection that mimics tuberculosis, with cough, fever, weight loss, and cavitary lung disease. Risk factors for infection include COPD, cancer, HIV, alcohol abuse, and drug-associated immunosuppression. Treatment of *M. kansasii* pulmonary disease consists of isoniazid, rifampin, and ethambutol. 🄷

### KEY POINT

- *Mycobacterium kansasii* most commonly causes a lung infection that mimics tuberculosis, with cough, fever, weight loss, and cavitary lung disease.

## 🄷 Rapidly Growing Mycobacteria

*Mycobacterium abscessus* is the most common RGM-associated cause of pulmonary infection, even in patients without underlying lung disease. *M. abscessus* and *Mycobacterium fortuitum* have been associated with lymphadenitis. Disseminated *M. abscessus*, *M. fortuitum*, and *Mycobacterium*

*chelonae* infections are seen in immunosuppressed patients and appear to be increasing in incidence as a cause of localized skin and soft tissue infections, usually after trauma, surgery (often associated with implanted prosthetic material), catheter insertion, or cosmetic procedures (including pedicures, tattooing, and body piercing). Contaminated, nonsterile water is the source of these infections.

RGM are usually not susceptible to antituberculous agents. Susceptibility testing of amikacin, doxycycline, fluoroquinolones, sulfonamides, cefoxitin, clarithromycin, linezolid, imipenem (*M. fortuitum* only), and tobramycin (*M. chelonae* only) is routinely recommended for RGM. At least two to three drugs are recommended for a prolonged course depending on the type of infection, the NTM species, and the antimicrobial susceptibility profile. Consultation with infectious diseases or pulmonary experts is recommended. 🄷

### KEY POINT

- Disseminated *Mycobacterium abscessus*, *Mycobacterium fortuitum*, and *Mycobacterium chelonae* infections are seen in immunosuppressed patients and appear to be increasing in incidence as a cause of localized skin and soft tissue infections, usually after trauma, surgery (often associated with implanted prosthetic material), catheter insertion, or cosmetic procedures (including pedicures, tattooing, and body piercing).

# Fungal Infections
## Systemic Candidiasis 🄷

Systemic or invasive candidiasis includes candidemia, focal organ involvement, and disseminated candidiasis, with candidemia being the most common. Candidemia occurs most frequently in the presence of an intravascular catheter and may lead to focal organ involvement or disseminated infection as a consequence of hematogenous spread. Risk factors for candidemia and other forms of systemic candidiasis include neutropenia, malignancies, organ transplantation, broad-spectrum antimicrobial agents, immunosuppressive agents, chemotherapeutic agents, intravascular catheters, hemodialysis, parenteral nutrition, and major abdominal surgery.

### Clinical Manifestations and Diagnosis

Clinical manifestations, signs, and symptoms in focal organ involvement may be specific to that organ. Focal infections include urinary tract infections (UTIs) (catheter-related or non-catheter-related), peritonitis, bone and joint infections, and central nervous system infections. Pneumonia occurs rarely and generally only in severely immunosuppressed patients. When *Candida* is isolated from the sputum, it usually reflects contamination from the oral mucosa. With disseminated disease, microabscesses have been described in all organs.

**CONT.**

Systemic candidiasis is usually diagnosed by a positive culture from blood or a normally sterile body site, although a negative culture does not exclude the diagnosis. In the case of organ involvement, tissue biopsy specimens should be obtained for culture and histopathology. In suspected disseminated disease, white exudates may be seen in the retina on ophthalmoscopic examination (**Figure 11**), and painless skin papules or pustules on an erythematous base may be present on the skin; a biopsy of a characteristic skin lesion can aid in rapid diagnosis. When *Candida* is isolated from the blood or a normally sterile body site, identification of species should be performed to guide appropriate antifungal therapy. Antifungal susceptibility testing is indicated against the triazoles and echinocandins for *Candida glabrata* isolates from blood and sterile sites and for other *Candida* species that have failed to respond to antifungal therapy. **H**

**KEY POINT**

- Common focal infections in systemic candidiasis include urinary tract infections (catheter-related or non-catheter-related), peritonitis, bone and joint infections, and central nervous system infections.

**H** **Treatment**

Systemic candidiasis has a high mortality, so therapy should be initiated promptly when it is suspected or diagnosed. An echinocandin (anidulafungin, caspofungin, or micafungin) is recommended as initial therapy for most patients with candidemia (**Table 21**) but not for those with meningitis, UTI, or endophthalmitis because of poor organ penetration. Step-down therapy from an echinocandin to an azole (fluconazole or voriconazole) is appropriate if the *Candida* isolate is known to be susceptible and the patient is clinically stable. In patients with *Candida glabrata* infection, susceptibility testing is necessary before switching to an azole. Fluconazole is recommended for *Candida parapsilosis* complex infection because

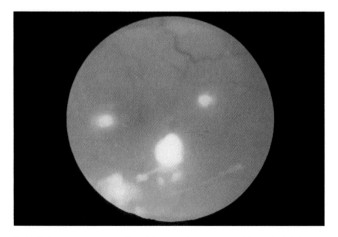

**FIGURE 11.** Disseminated candidiasis to the retina. *Candida* endophthalmitis is characterized by focal, white, infiltrative, often mound-like lesions on the retina. Endophthalmitis is a bacterial or fungal infection within the eye not caused by viruses or parasites.

*C. parapsilosis* may have reduced susceptibility to echinocandins. Treatment duration for uncomplicated candidemia is 14 days after clearance of the organism from the bloodstream and resolution of symptoms. Treatment duration for focal organ involvement is based on resolution of signs and symptoms of infection and usually extends for several weeks to months.

Removal of an intravascular catheter in addition to antifungal therapy has been associated with a shorter duration of infection and improved outcomes in nonneutropenic patients with candidemia. *C. parapsilosis* candidemia is almost always catheter related. The role of catheter removal is less clear in neutropenic patients because they may develop candidemia from translocation across the gastrointestinal tract mucosa. If candidemia persists for more than a few days in a neutropenic patient with an intravascular catheter, the catheter should be removed.

*Candida* can cause UTI by direct entry into the urinary tract or hematogenously. Most cases of *Candida* pyelonephritis occur hematogenously. It may be difficult to ascertain whether candiduria represents a contaminated specimen, colonization of the bladder or urinary catheter, or an actual infection of the bladder or kidney. Most patients with candiduria are asymptomatic and rarely develop candidemia. Treatment of asymptomatic candiduria is indicated only in neutropenic patients and those undergoing urologic procedures. The treatment of choice is oral fluconazole. **H**

**KEY POINTS**

- Therapy with an echinocandin is indicated for most patients with candidemia; however, an echinocandin should not be used to treat those with meningitis or endophthalmitis because of poor organ penetration.

- Intravascular catheter removal, in addition to antifungal therapy, is indicated for nonneutropenic patients with candidemia.

- Treatment of asymptomatic candiduria is indicated only in neutropenic patients and those undergoing urologic procedures. **HVC**

## Aspergillosis and Aspergilloma

*Aspergillus* is a ubiquitous environmental mold, and *Aspergillus fumigatus* is the most common human pathogen. The main route of acquisition is inhalation of aerosolized spores, with the lung being the principal site of clinical infection, followed by the paranasal sinuses. *Aspergillus* pulmonary disease may manifest as colonization, allergic bronchopulmonary aspergillosis, aspergilloma (fungus ball), or invasive aspergillosis.

Allergic bronchopulmonary aspergillosis, a hypersensitivity reaction that occurs with colonization of the larger airways by *Aspergillus*, is typically seen in the setting of chronic asthma or cystic fibrosis. Cardinal features include asthma-like symptoms, fleeting pulmonary infiltrates on chest

| TABLE 21. Therapy for Common Systemic Fungal Infections | | |
|---|---|---|
| **Infection** | **Therapy of Choice** | **Alternatives** |
| Candidemia | Echinocandin[a] | Fluconazole, voriconazole, lipid formulation of amphotericin B |
| Invasive aspergillosis | Voriconazole | Lipid formulation of amphotericin B, echinocandins, posaconazole, itraconazole, isavuconazonium |
| Allergic bronchopulmonary aspergillosis | Itraconazole or voriconazole | |
| Aspergilloma (fungus ball) | Itraconazole, voriconazole, posaconazole | |
| Mucormycosis | Liposomal amphotericin B, high-dose amphotericin B deoxycholate | Posaconazole, isavuconazonium |
| Cryptococcal meningitis | | |
|    Patients with AIDS | Induction period: amphotericin B and flucytosine for 2 weeks | Induction period: amphotericin B and fluconazole, fluconazole and flucytosine, or fluconazole monotherapy |
| | Consolidation period: oral fluconazole for 8 weeks | |
| | Maintenance period: oral fluconazole for ≥1 year | |
|    Transplant recipients | Induction period: lipid formulation of amphotericin B and flucytosine for 2 weeks | Induction period: lipid formulation of amphotericin B or amphotericin B deoxycholate for 4-6 weeks |
| | Consolidation period: oral fluconazole for 8 weeks | |
| | Maintenance period: oral fluconazole for 6 months to 1 year | |
|    Patients without HIV/AIDS or transplantation | Induction period: amphotericin B and flucytosine for ≥4 weeks | Induction period: amphotericin B for ≥6 weeks |
| | Consolidation period: oral fluconazole for 8 weeks | |
| | Maintenance period: oral fluconazole for 6-12 months | |
| Nonmeningeal cryptococcosis | Fluconazole | Itraconazole, amphotericin B plus flucytosine |
| Blastomycosis | | |
|    Cutaneous/pulmonary/ extrapulmonary | Lipid formulation of amphotericin B followed by itraconazole | Itraconazole, fluconazole |
|    CNS | Lipid formulation of amphotericin B followed by fluconazole | Itraconazole, voriconazole |
| Histoplasmosis | | |
|    Mild to moderate acute pulmonary[b] | Itraconazole | |
|    Moderately severe to severe pulmonary | Lipid formulation of amphotericin B followed by itraconazole | |
|    Acute progressive disseminated | Lipid formulation of amphotericin B followed by itraconazole | Conventional amphotericin B |
| Coccidioidomycosis | | |
|    Pulmonary (patient at low risk) | No treatment indicated | |
|    Primary pulmonary (patient at high risk)[c] | Itraconazole, fluconazole | |
| Severe coccidioidal pneumonia or disseminated disease | Conventional or lipid formulation of amphotericin B until improved, then itraconazole or fluconazole | |
| Coccidioidal meningitis | Fluconazole | Conventional or lipid formulation of amphotericin B plus intrathecal amphotericin B or itraconazole, or voriconazole |
| Cutaneous sporotrichosis | Itraconazole | |

CNS = central nervous system.

[a]Anidulafungin, caspofungin, or micafungin; no preference among the three available agents.

[b]Not sufficiently ill to require hospitalization.

[c]Factors include HIV/AIDS, solid organ transplantation, high-dose glucocorticoids, anti–tumor necrosis factor therapy, lymphoma, chemotherapy, pregnancy, diabetes mellitus, and African or Philippine ancestry.

imaging, peripheral eosinophilia, elevated serum IgE levels, serum *Aspergillus*-precipitating antibodies, and cutaneous reactivity to *Aspergillus* antigens. In addition to standard therapy (see Table 21), acute or recurrent exacerbations should include glucocorticoids to control acute inflammation and to limit lung damage.

Aspergilloma is generally a consequence of colonization of a preexisting pulmonary cavity or cyst or in areas of devitalized lung. Symptoms include cough, hemoptysis, dyspnea, weight loss, fever, fatigue, and chest pain. Radiographic images show a round mass within a pulmonary cavity or cyst. Sputum cultures are usually positive. Patients who are asymptomatic and have stable radiographs do not require therapy. Surgical resection is indicated for hemoptysis and is considered definitive therapy. Antifungal therapy (see Table 21) is indicated for those who are symptomatic but unable to undergo surgery; it can be administered perioperatively to reduce the risk for pleural aspergillosis.

Risk factors for invasive or disseminated aspergillosis include profound and prolonged neutropenia and immunosuppression often associated with organ transplantation. The disorder is also increasingly reported in patients who are critically ill and in intensive care units, especially with exposure to glucocorticoids.

*Aspergillus* invades pulmonary blood vessels and causes distal infarction of lung tissue. Patients present with fever, cough, chest pain, and hemoptysis; pulmonary infiltrates, nodules, or wedge-shaped densities resembling infarcts may be seen on chest radiographs. CT scans may show a target lesion with a necrotic center surrounded by ring of hemorrhage (halo sign) (**Figure 12**). Central nervous system (CNS) involvement may manifest as a brain abscess or infarction. Other sites of involvement include blood vessels in the heart, gastrointestinal tract, or skin.

Invasive aspergillosis can be difficult to diagnose with certainty. It is definitively established by tissue biopsy. Although *Aspergillus* can spread hematogenously, blood cultures are rarely positive. The galactomannan antigen

immunoassay is increasingly used for diagnosis. Galactomannan is a polysaccharide contained in the cell wall of *Aspergillus*, and its presence in serum or other body fluids suggests invasive infection. The sensitivity of the assay can be impaired by antifungal prophylaxis or specific antifungal therapy. The β-D-glucan assay, although not specific for *Aspergillus* species, can also be used to detect early infection. **H**

### KEY POINTS

- *Aspergillus* pulmonary disease may manifest as colonization, allergic bronchopulmonary aspergillosis, aspergilloma (fungus ball), or invasive aspergillosis.

- Invasive aspergillosis is definitively diagnosed by tissue biopsy; the galactomannan antigen immunoassay is increasingly used for diagnosis.

## Mucormycosis

Mucormycosis (formerly zygomycosis) is an increasingly common fungal infection that can present as acute and rapidly progressive with a high mortality rate. Various organisms are responsible for causing mucormycosis; *Rhizopus* and *Mucor* species are most common. Risk factors include immunocompromise from hematologic malignancies, organ transplantation, and cancer chemotherapy; patients with uncontrolled diabetes or ketoacidosis have a unique susceptibility. Patients treated with deferoxamine for iron-overload states also are at risk. Patients with severe burns or trauma can contract mucormycosis through contamination of wounds. Outbreaks have also been reported during natural disasters.

The most common presentation is rhinocerebral. This is a rapidly fatal infection that spreads from the sinuses retroorbitally to the CNS. Symptoms and signs include headache, epistaxis, and ocular findings, including proptosis, periorbital edema, and decreased vision. A pathognomonic finding on physical examination of the nose or palate is the presence of a black eschar. Other sites of involvement include the lungs, gastrointestinal tract, and skin. Pulmonary mucormycosis with thrombosis and infarction most frequently develops in patients with hematologic malignancies. Cutaneous involvement is rare, developing most often in burn or trauma patients or resulting from dissemination from another site. Isolated CNS mucormycosis may result from hematogenous spread or dissemination in injection drug users.

Mucormycosis is diagnosed by tissue biopsy and culture. Histologically, the organism appears as broad, irregular, and ribbon-like aseptate hyphae that have right-angle branching. Blood cultures are usually negative. A combined medical (see Table 21) and surgical approach is required for effective therapy. **H**

### KEY POINT

- The most common presentation of mucormycosis is a rapidly fatal rhinocerebral infection, with headache, epistaxis, and ocular findings (proptosis, periorbital edema, and decreased vision).

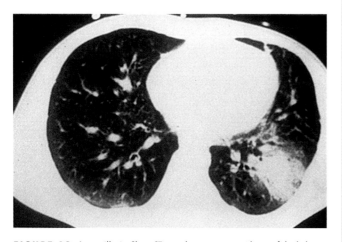

**FIGURE 12.** Aspergillosis. Chest CT scan demonstrates evidence of the halo sign, which is an area of low attenuation surrounding a nodule, reflecting hemorrhage into the tissues surrounding the fungus.

# Cryptococcosis

Two cryptococcal species exist, *Cryptococcus neoformans* and *C. gattii*, but *C. neoformans* is the predominant species causing human infection. In the United States, most infections with *C. gattii* occur in California. Cryptococcus is inhaled and causes an initial pulmonary infection. Healthy persons generally contain the initial infection owing to intact cell-mediated immunity; however, immunocompromised persons are at risk for dissemination. Pulmonary cryptococcosis found incidentally in an asymptomatic immunocompetent person may resolve without treatment; however, if the person becomes immunosuppressed, the organism can reactivate and disseminate. Therefore, treatment (typically fluconazole for 6-12 months) is given to patients with mild to moderately severe pulmonary cryptococcosis to prevent progressive or disseminated disease.

Risk factors for dissemination include AIDS, organ transplantation, glucocorticoid treatment, diabetes mellitus, liver dysfunction, and kidney injury. The CNS is the most common site of disseminated cryptococcosis, which manifests as a subacute or chronic meningoencephalitis. Common symptoms include headache, alternations in mental status, and fever. Visual abnormalities, including diplopia, decreased visual acuity, and extraocular nerve palsies, may also occur. Dissemination can occur to the skin (**Figure 13**), prostate, bone, eye, and urinary tract. When cryptococcosis is found outside of the CNS, a lumbar puncture should be done to determine whether CNS infection is present. Skin lesions (papules, nodules, ulcers, plaques, cellulitis) imply disseminated disease.

Cryptococcosis can initially be diagnosed by suggestive histopathology or by the detection of cryptococcal antigen in serum or cerebrospinal fluid (CSF). Diagnosis is confirmed by culture. The latex agglutination assay for cryptococcal antigen is highly sensitive and specific for the diagnosis of meningitis. The serum assay has been used successfully to screen febrile patients with AIDS who are at high risk, especially those with headache. However, the sensitivity of the serum assay is lower in patients without HIV infection; therefore, a negative test result in these persons cannot be used to exclude meningitis. In cryptococcal meningitis, lumbar puncture may show a high opening pressure, and the CSF typically shows a lymphocytic pleocytosis. Patients with AIDS often have normal or mildly abnormal CSF findings and may have minimal pleocytosis.

The treatment of cryptococcal meningitis differs in those with AIDS and those without AIDS (see Table 21). Maintenance therapy is indicated for patients with AIDS until they have responded to antiretroviral therapy (CD4 cell count ≥100/µL for ≥3 months) and have been receiving antifungal therapy for at least 1 year. Maintenance therapy is administered for 6 to 12 months in patients who are not infected with HIV. If a patient is receiving appropriate antifungal therapy and other measures to reduce elevated intracranial pressure have failed, management by frequent lumbar punctures and removal of CSF or placement of a ventriculoperitoneal shunt is required. Organ transplant recipients who must continue taking high-dose immunosuppressive therapy may require life-long antifungal therapy.

### KEY POINTS

- The central nervous system is the most common site of disseminated cryptococcosis.
- The latex agglutination assay for cryptococcal antigen is highly sensitive and specific for the diagnosis of meningitis in symptomatic patients with AIDS.
- Maintenance therapy is indicated for patients with AIDS and cryptococcal meningitis until they have responded to antiretroviral therapy (CD4 cell count ≥100/µL for ≥3 months) and have been receiving antifungal therapy for at least 1 year.

# Blastomycosis

*Blastomyces dermatitidis* is endemic to the Ohio and Mississippi river valleys, the Great Lakes, and the St. Lawrence River. Infection occurs by inhalation of spores and primarily involves the lungs. The second most frequent site of infection is the skin, followed by the bones, joints, and prostate. Most patients with acute pulmonary blastomycosis are asymptomatic. Those with acute pneumonia have nonspecific systemic symptoms, a nonproductive cough, and nonspecific pulmonary infiltrates on chest radiographs. Skin lesions are the most common manifestation of disseminated disease and may vary in appearance, including papules, nodules, verrucous lesions, or draining lesions. Presumptive diagnosis is based on finding characteristic yeast forms with broad-based buds on histopathologic samples. Definitive diagnosis is established by culture.

Acute pulmonary blastomycosis may be mild and self-limited in otherwise healthy persons and may not require therapy, although therapy may prevent extrapulmonary

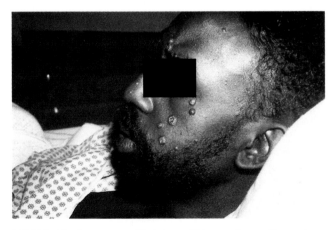

**FIGURE 13.** Cryptococcosis. Skin lesions, which are molluscum-like, are characteristic of disseminated cryptococcosis.

**H**
CONT.

dissemination. All immunocompromised patients and patients with moderate to severe pneumonia or disseminated infection require therapy (see Table 21). All patients with disseminated blastomycosis should have a bone scan to detect occult osteoarticular involvement. Genitourinary infection may be asymptomatic or associated with symptoms of prostatism. A urine culture should be obtained to document involvement because the prostate may serve as a nidus for infection and lead to relapses. Current serologic assays serve no role. Extrapulmonary blastomycosis can occur in the absence of lung disease. **H**

**KEY POINT**

- Blastomycosis infection primarily involves the lungs, followed by skin; other sites of infection include bones, joints, and prostate.

## **H** Histoplasmosis

*Histoplasma capsulatum* is the most common endemic mycosis in the United States and is found in the Ohio and Mississippi river valleys. Although infection usually is asymptomatic, acute and chronic pulmonary disease, granulomatous mediastinitis, fibrosing mediastinitis, broncholithiasis, pulmonary nodules (histoplasmomas), and acute and chronic disseminated disease may occur. Acute progressive disseminated histoplasmosis presents with nonspecific symptoms, including high fever and weight loss, hepatosplenomegaly, and pancytopenia. Small yeast forms within neutrophils may be seen on peripheral blood smear. The definitive diagnosis requires culture, which may take up to 6 weeks. Additional diagnostic modalities include histopathologic studies and antigen (primarily from the urine) determination. Because the sensitivity of these studies differs, depending on the extent of infection and the time following exposure, several different tests are usually required to confirm the diagnosis.

In most immunocompetent, symptomatic patients, pulmonary disease is mild and resolves without therapy. Therapy is indicated in those with moderately severe or severe infection, acute diffuse pulmonary infection, and chronic cavitary pulmonary disease (see Table 21). Therapy should also be considered for patients with mild infection who are immunocompromised or have had symptoms for 4 or more weeks. **H**

**KEY POINT**

- Although histoplasmosis infection is usually asymptomatic, acute and chronic pulmonary disease, granulomatous mediastinitis, fibrosing mediastinitis, broncholithiasis, pulmonary nodules (histoplasmomas), and acute and chronic disseminated disease may occur.

## **H** Coccidioidomycosis

*Coccidioides immitis* and *Coccidioides posadasii* are endemic to desert areas of the southwestern United States, including Arizona, New Mexico, Texas, and the central valley of California,

and to parts of Central and South America. Rates of infection in endemic areas are highest during dry months and increase when the soil is disturbed. Most infections are caused by inhalation of spores and are asymptomatic. Primary pulmonary infection most frequently presents as community-acquired pneumonia occurring 1 to 3 weeks after exposure. In endemic areas, up to one third of cases of community-acquired pneumonia are caused by *Coccidioides* species. Valley fever is a subacute infection with respiratory symptoms, fever, and erythema nodosum. Arthralgia of multiple joints, termed "desert rheumatism," is frequent. Risk factors for dissemination include immunosuppression, AIDS, or pregnancy. However, disseminated infection may occur in patients who have no underlying disease. The most common sites for disseminated infection include skin, bones (including vertebrae), joints, and the meninges.

Coccidioidomycosis is definitively diagnosed by isolation of the organism in culture. Serologic tests are useful for diagnosis and for monitoring the course of therapy, and they are the preferred method for diagnosing primary coccidioidal infections. Serologic studies are more helpful than cultures in diagnosing chronic coccidioidal meningitis because cultures of CSF are frequently negative. A negative serologic test result does not exclude infection; therefore, repeat tests are needed to improve sensitivity.

Treatment is indicated for patients with severe disease or those with an increased risk for disseminated infection (see Table 21). For those with meningitis, therapy should be lifelong because relapses are common after medication is discontinued. Azoles should be avoided in women during the first trimester of pregnancy because of their teratogenic potential. **H**

**KEY POINTS**

- Primary coccidioidomycosis infection most frequently presents as community-acquired pneumonia occurring 1 to 3 weeks after exposure.

- Serologic tests are useful for diagnosis and for monitoring the course of therapy and are the preferred method for diagnosing primary coccidioidal infections; however, repeat tests may be needed to improve sensitivity.

## Sporotrichosis

*Sporothrix schenckii* is found in soil, moss, and other vegetation and occurs almost exclusively in persons who encounter the organism through an occupation or hobby, such as landscaping or gardening. Infection is almost always acquired through inoculation of the organism into the skin or subcutaneous tissue. A papule appears days to weeks later at the inoculation site and usually ulcerates. Similar lesions then occur along lymphatic channels proximal to the inoculation site. Risk factors for pulmonary and osteoarticular infection include diabetes mellitus, alcoholism, and COPD. Those with HIV infection are at risk for disseminated infection. The diagnosis is established by culture. Itraconazole is the therapy of choice for cutaneous and osteoarticular sporotrichosis.

- Itraconazole is the therapy of choice for cutaneous and osteoarticular sporotrichosis.

## Exserohilum

*Exserohilum rostratum* is a mold that has rarely been described as a human pathogen. Since the fall of 2012, it has been the predominant pathogen in an outbreak of meningitis and other infections in patients who received epidural, paraspinal, or joint injections with contaminated lots of methylprednisolone acetate from a single compounding pharmacy. In addition to meningitis, epidural abscesses, arachnoiditis, and infection involving the sacroiliac and peripheral joints have occurred. Most patients infected with *Exserohilum rostratum* have been treated with voriconazole (with or without liposomal amphotericin B) for CNS and paraspinal infections and with voriconazole for bone and joint infections.

# Sexually Transmitted Infections

## Introduction

The Centers for Disease Control and Prevention (CDC) estimates that 20 million sexually transmitted infections (STIs) occur annually in the United States, accounting for an estimated $16 billion in health care expenditures. Half of these infections occur in persons aged 15 to 24 years. The appropriate evaluation and management of STIs affect the health of the patient and can help decrease the transmission of infections in the community.

## *Chlamydia trachomatis* Infection

*C. trachomatis* is the most commonly reported STI in the United States. It may cause several clinical syndromes but also may be asymptomatic or subclinical and lead to potentially significant complications, including ectopic pregnancy, tubal infertility, and chronic pelvic pain syndromes. Because of this, screening is recommended for women at risk for infection. The U.S. Preventive Services Task Force (USPSTF) recommends at least annual screening for all sexually active women aged 24 years and younger; older women should be screened if they have risk factors, including a previous STI, new or multiple partners, inconsistent condom use, or a history of exchanging sex for money or drugs. The CDC recommends screening for all pregnant women. Routine screening is not recommended for most men, although heterosexual men can be screened if they report risk factors for STIs; men who have sex with men should be screened at least annually.

Nucleic acid amplification testing (NAAT) is the preferred diagnostic test for chlamydia. NAAT can be performed on first voided urine samples or urethral swabs from men and on vaginal or endocervical swabs from women. NAAT is not FDA approved for the detection of chlamydia from rectal swabs; however, some laboratories have met the Clinical Laboratory Improvement Amendments standards for NAAT on these samples, so physicians should confer with the director of the laboratory they use to understand what testing is available. Repeat testing to document cure of infection (at 3-4 weeks) is recommended only for pregnant women. Repeat testing is recommended for all patients 3 months after a diagnosis of *C. trachomatis* infection because of the high risk for reinfection. Sexual partners who had contact during the 60 days before the onset of a patient's symptoms or diagnosis should be referred for evaluation; if the last sexual contact occurred more than 60 days before diagnosis, the most recent sexual partner should be referred.

- The U.S. Preventive Services Task Force recommends at least annual screening for *Chlamydia trachomatis* in all sexually active women age 24 years and younger and in older women if they have risk factors; men who have sex with men should be screened at least annually.
- Nucleic acid amplification testing is the preferred diagnostic test for *Chlamydia trachomatis* infection and can be performed on first voided urine samples or urethral swabs from men and on vaginal or endocervical swabs from women.

## *Neisseria gonorrhoeae* Infection

*N. gonorrhoeae* is the second most common bacterial STI in the United States, and infection rates are highest among young women aged 15 to 19 years. Many infected women are asymptomatic. The USPSTF recommends screening for gonorrhea in sexually active women with a history of infection, another STI, new or multiple partners, inconsistent condom use, or a history of exchanging sex for money or drugs. The USPSTF does not recommend screening of men; however, the CDC recommends annual screening for men who have sex with men.

In addition to causing cervicitis, pelvic inflammatory disease, urethritis, and epididymitis, *N. gonorrhoeae* can cause pharyngeal infection (usually asymptomatic) and anorectal infections. Disseminated gonococcal infection (DGI) may cause two syndromes: an arthritis-dermatitis syndrome (in which patients have the triad of migratory polyarthralgia, subsequent tenosynovitis, and, eventually, frank arthritis without purulent joint infection) or purulent arthritis alone without skin findings. The classic skin lesion of DGI is a vesiculopustular lesion on an erythematous base; however, petechial, macular, and papular lesions can also occur.

NAAT is the preferred diagnostic test for *N. gonorrhoeae* infections. NAAT can be performed on first voided urine or urethral swabs from men and on vaginal or endocervical swabs from women. NAAT is not FDA approved for pharyngeal or anorectal samples; however, some laboratories have established performance standards for testing of these specimens, and results can be used for clinical management. If available, a Gram stain of urethral discharge is highly sensitive and specific for the diagnosis of urethritis due to *N. gonorrhoeae* in men who are symptomatic; Gram stain of endocervical or vaginal specimens is inadequately sensitive to exclude infection. Blood and joint fluid cultures should be obtained if DGI is suspected but they may be negative; a presumptive diagnosis can be made by demonstrating the organism at a mucosal site (cervix/urethra, pharynx, or rectum) with NAAT or by culture.

A disadvantage of non–culture-based testing for *N. gonorrhoeae* is the lack of availability of antimicrobial susceptibility data. Because of increasing drug resistance among *N. gonorrhoeae*, culture is recommended, if possible, to provide antimicrobial susceptibility results to guide additional therapy for patients in whom treatment fails. Test of cure is not recommended; however, patients should be retested at 3 months because the risk for reinfection is high even when sexual partners have been referred for treatment. Sexual partners should be referred for evaluation as described for *C. trachomatis* infections. Patients should be advised to avoid sexual contact until therapy is completed and symptoms have resolved.

### KEY POINTS

- The U.S. Preventive Services Task Force recommends screening for gonorrhea in sexually active women with a history of infection, another sexually transmitted infection, new or multiple partners, inconsistent condom use, or a history of exchanging sex for money or drugs.
- The U.S. Preventive Services Task Force does not recommend screening men for gonorrhea; however, the CDC recommends annual screening for men who have sex with men.
- Nucleic acid amplification testing is the preferred diagnostic test for *Neisseria gonorrhoeae* infection.

# Specific Syndromes

## Cervicitis

Women with cervicitis present with vaginal discharge and intermenstrual bleeding, especially after intercourse, although infections may be asymptomatic. In addition to *N. gonorrhoeae* and *C. trachomatis*, cervicitis can be caused by herpes simplex virus (HSV), particularly primary infection; *Mycoplasma genitalium* infection and bacterial vaginosis presenting as cervicitis have also been reported. Purulent or mucopurulent discharge can be visualized from the cervical os, and passage of a cotton-tipped swab through the os elicits bleeding owing to inflamed, friable mucosa. Gram staining in women is less useful in differentiating *N. gonorrhoeae* because

other gram-negative flora may be present in the vagina. Cervicitis can also result from chemical irritation, for example from douching, so a careful history of any potential chemical exposures should be obtained.

## Pelvic Inflammatory Disease

Pelvic inflammatory disease (PID) is an ascending infection of the genital tract that is polymicrobial. *C. trachomatis* and *N. gonorrhoeae* are implicated in approximately two thirds of cases. Because the sequelae of untreated infection of the upper genital tract are significant, a diagnostic strategy that maximizes the sensitivity of the diagnosis is recommended. Sexually active women with lower genital tract symptoms who have cervical motion tenderness, uterine tenderness, or adnexal tenderness should be evaluated and treated for PID. Clinical manifestations of PID may include right upper quadrant pain and tenderness due to perihepatitis (Fitz-Hugh-Curtis syndrome). Fever, mucopurulent cervical discharge, numerous leukocytes on microscopic examination of a wet mount of vaginal fluid, and elevated inflammatory markers (C-reactive protein, erythrocyte sedimentation rate) increase the specificity of the diagnosis. NAAT for *C. trachomatis* and *N. gonorrhoeae* should be obtained, and women should be screened for other STIs, including HIV infection. Outpatient management is appropriate for most women with PID. Indications for hospitalization include inability to tolerate an oral regimen, severe signs of systemic toxicity, pregnancy, inability to exclude a surgical emergency (ectopic pregnancy, appendicitis), and suspected tubo-ovarian abscess. Women who do not respond to outpatient therapy within 72 hours should also be hospitalized. If the presence of *C. trachomatis* or *N. gonorrhoeae* is confirmed, repeat testing in 3 to 6 months is recommended because the incidence of reinfection is substantial. The risk for PID is increased in the first 3 weeks after intrauterine device insertion, but removal of the intrauterine device because of a PID diagnosis is not recommended as long as the patient responds to treatment. Sexual partners of women diagnosed with PID should be referred for evaluation.

## Urethritis

Men with urethritis usually have symptoms of urethral discharge, dysuria, and pruritus, although infections can be asymptomatic. Causative agents of urethritis include *C. trachomatis*, *N. gonorrhoeae*, and *M. genitalium*. Nongonococcal urethritis can also be caused by HSV, *Trichomonas* species, and adenovirus. Purulent urethral discharge may be visualized at the urethral meatus or expressed by applying gentle pressure with the thumb on the ventral surface and the forefinger on the dorsum of the base of the penis and moving toward the meatus. A positive result on a leukocyte esterase test on a first voided urine sample or leukocytes (≥10/hpf) on microscopic examination of urine sediment supports the diagnosis.

## Epididymitis

In sexually active young men, epididymitis is usually caused by *C. trachomatis* or *N. gonorrhoeae;* men who have insertive anal intercourse can have infections due to enteric gram-negative organisms, such as *Escherichia coli.* In older men, epididymitis can occur as a complication of urinary tract infection, often in the presence of benign prostatic hyperplasia unrelated to STI (see MKSAP 17 General Internal Medicine). Patients typically have pain and swelling of the ipsilateral testis and the spermatic cord (epididymo-orchitis) on presentation. The differential diagnosis includes testicular torsion; abrupt onset of symptoms and the absence of signs of urethral inflammation should raise concern about the possibility of this diagnosis. A Gram stain of urethral discharge with leukocytes (>5/hpf) or positive leukocyte esterase result or a first voided urine sample with leukocytes (≥10/hpf) supports the diagnosis. Patients should have NAAT for *C. trachomatis* and *N. gonorrhoeae,* and the urine should be cultured. Men with epididymitis who are at risk for STIs should be screened for other STIs and encouraged to refer sexual partners for evaluation.

## Anorectal Infections

Men and women who engage in receptive anal intercourse can develop proctitis because of sexually transmitted pathogens, including *N. gonorrhoeae*, *C. trachomatis*, syphilis, and HSV. Anorectal infection can also occur in women with cervicitis because of autoinoculation, which occurs when infected secretions from the vagina come in contact with the anal region. Persons with proctitis present with anal pain or pruritus, discharge (which may be bloody), constipation, and tenesmus.

### KEY POINTS

- Nucleic acid amplification testing for *Chlamydia trachomatis* and *Neisseria gonorrhoeae* should be obtained when pelvic inflammatory disease and epididymitis are diagnosed.
- Signs and symptoms of pelvic inflammatory disease include cervical motion, uterine, or adnexal tenderness; fever, mucopurulent cervical discharge, leukocytes on microscopic examination of a wet mount of vaginal fluid, and elevated inflammatory markers increase the specificity of the diagnosis.
- Men with epididymitis present with pain and swelling of the ipsilateral testis and the spermatic cord.

## Treatment

Recommended treatment of cervicitis, urethritis, proctitis, and their associated complications is outlined in **Table 22**. The emergence of drug resistance among isolates of *N. gonorrhoeae* has had a major impact on the antimicrobial regimens recommended for the treatment of clinical syndromes caused by this pathogen. Fluoroquinolone-resistant strains have been reported throughout the United States, so fluoroquinolones are no longer recommended for the treatment of infections due to *N. gonorrhoeae*. Additionally, cephalosporin minimal inhibitory concentrations among *N. gonorrhoeae* isolates have increased in the past several years, and cephalosporin-resistant strains of *N. gonorrhoeae* have been reported. As a result, the recommended dose of ceftriaxone has been increased from 125 mg to 250 mg, and the use of cefixime, an oral third-generation cephalosporin, is recommended only if parenteral ceftriaxone is unavailable. If cefixime is used for treatment, a test of cure using NAAT should be performed 1 week after completion of therapy; however, if results on repeat testing are positive, a culture should be obtained so that antimicrobial susceptibility testing is available to guide further treatment.

Treatment of possible concomitant *C. trachomatis* infection in persons diagnosed with gonococcal infection is recommended, and the addition of azithromycin or doxycycline to treatment regimens for *N. gonorrhoeae* may increase the chances of eradication of this pathogen. Patients with cervicitis, urethritis, and proctitis can be treated empirically at the time of presentation or on the basis of diagnostic test results. Persons seen in emergency departments, urgent care centers, or any other setting where likelihood of follow-up is a concern should receive empiric therapy. Diagnostic testing for the presence of *C. trachomatis* and *N. gonorrhoeae* should be performed even if empiric therapy is given because these infections are reportable, and the results of diagnostic testing may be helpful if the patient returns with persistent symptoms. If a *Trichomonas* species is determined as the cause of urethritis, treatment with metronidazole (500 mg twice daily for 7 days) is recommended; HSV treatment is discussed later. Patients should be offered testing for other STIs, including HIV infection, and encouraged to refer their sexual partners for evaluation.

Patients treated for chlamydial, gonococcal, or trichomonal infection should be retested 3 months after treatment.

### KEY POINTS

- Fluoroquinolones are no longer recommended for the treatment of gonorrhea, the recommended ceftriaxone dose has been increased to 250 mg, and oral cefixime is recommended only if parenteral ceftriaxone is not available.
- The addition of azithromycin or doxycycline to treatment regimens for *Neisseria gonorrhoeae* may increase the chances of eradication of this pathogen.

## Genital Ulcers

### Herpes Simplex Virus

HSV is the most common cause of genital ulcer disease in the United States. The epidemiology of primary genital HSV infections has shifted, and up to half are now caused by HSV-1 rather than HSV-2. However, HSV-1 is less able to

**TABLE 22.** Treatment of *Chlamydia trachomatis* and *Neisseria gonorrhoeae* Infections and Their Complications

| Clinical Syndrome | Preferred Regimen | Alternative Regimen |
|---|---|---|
| Cervicitis and urethritis (empiric therapy) | Ceftriaxone, 250 mg IM single dose, plus azithromycin, 1 g PO single dose (preferred), *or* doxycycline 100 mg PO twice daily for 7 days | Cefixime, 400 mg PO single dose, plus doxycycline,[a] 100 mg PO twice daily for 7 days |
| *Chlamydia* cervicitis, urethritis, or proctitis | Azithromycin, 1 g PO single dose, *or* doxycycline, 100 mg PO twice daily for 7 days | Erythromycin base, 500 mg PO four times daily, *or* erythromycin ethylsuccinate, 800 mg PO four times daily, *or* levofloxacin, 500 mg PO daily, *or* ofloxacin, 300 mg PO twice daily for 7 days |
| Gonococcal cervicitis, urethritis, or proctitis and pharyngeal infection[b] | Ceftriaxone, 250 mg IM single dose, plus azithromycin, 1 g PO single dose (preferred), *or* doxycycline, 100 mg PO twice daily for 7 days | Cefixime, 400 mg PO single dose, plus azithromycin, 1 g PO single dose (preferred), *or* doxycycline, 100 mg PO twice daily for 7 days<br><br>Test of cure of *Neisseria gonorrhoeae* 1 week after treatment |
| Disseminated gonococcal infection[c] | Ceftriaxone, 1 g IM or IV every 24 h | Cefotaxime, 1 g IV every 8 h, *or* ceftizoxime, 1 g IV every 8 h |
| Pelvic inflammatory disease | | |
|   Parenteral therapy[d] | Cefotetan, 2 g every 12 h, or cefoxitin, 2 g every 6 h, plus doxycycline, 100 mg PO or IV every 12 h, *or* clindamycin, 900 mg every 8 h, plus gentamicin, 2 mg/kg loading dose followed by 1.5 mg/kg every 8 hours or a single daily dose of 3-5 mg/kg/d | Ampicillin-sulbactam, 3 g every 6 h, plus doxycycline, 100 mg PO or IV every 12 h |
|   Oral/IM therapy | Ceftriaxone, 250 mg IM single dose, plus doxycycline, 100 mg PO twice daily for 14 days with or without metronidazole, 500 mg PO twice daily for 14 days, *or* cefoxitin, 2 g IM single dose, with probenecid, 1 g PO, plus doxycycline, 100 mg PO every 12 h for 14 days, with or without metronidazole, 500 mg PO twice daily for 14 days | |
| Epididymitis[e] | Ceftriaxone, 250 mg IM single dose, plus doxycycline, 100 mg PO twice daily for 10 days | |

IM = intramuscularly; IV = intravenously; PO = orally.

[a]Doxycyline should be avoided/used with caution in pregnant patients. Cefixime should be used only if ceftriaxone is unavailable.

[b]Treatment for possible chlamydial infection is recommended for all patients diagnosed with gonorrhea.

[c]Parenteral therapy should be used until clinical improvement. Uncomplicated infections can then be treated with cefixime, 400 mg twice daily, to complete a total of 7 to 10 days of treatment. Septic arthritis should be treated for 7 days with parenteral therapy.

[d]Patients can be switched to oral therapy within 24 to 48 hours of clinical improvement using doxycycline, 100 mg PO twice daily, with or without metronidazole, 500 mg PO twice daily, to complete a total of 14 days of therapy

[e]The recommended regimen for acute epididymitis likely due to enteric gram-negative organisms is levofloxacin, 500 mg PO daily, or ofloxacin, 300 mg PO twice daily, for 10 days.

establish latency in the genital region, so most recurrent genital infections are due to HSV-2. Most patients with serologic evidence of HSV-2 infection have never had a recognized episode of genital ulcers. Patients with genital HSV infection initially have painful lesions that begin as vesicles and progress to ulcers on an erythematous base (**Figure 14**). In immunocompromised patients, HSV may appear as extensive, painful, shallow ulcers. Those with primary infection often have multiple genital lesions accompanied by regional lymphadenopathy and systemic symptoms, such as fever, myalgia, and malaise. Recurrent episodes are often heralded by prodromal symptoms, such as tingling, burning, pruritus, or pain, and are generally much less severe and without systemic symptoms.

The initial episode of HSV genital infection should be microbiologically confirmed. In primary infections, it is

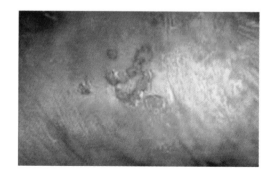

**FIGURE 14.** Penile lesions seen in herpes simplex virus type 2.

particularly important to distinguish between HSV-1 and HSV-2 because the former is much less likely to cause recurrent disease. Polymerase chain reaction testing of clinical specimens obtained from ulcers and mucocutaneous sites is the most sensitive diagnostic modality available. The use of type-specific serum antibody testing is not preferred for the diagnosis of symptomatic ulcer disease.

Antiviral therapy can reduce the severity and duration of symptoms of primary and secondary infections. Patients with frequent or severe recurrences should be offered long-term suppressive therapy. Because the frequency of recurrence decreases over time, the need for continued suppressive therapy should be reassessed periodically. Daily therapy with valacyclovir also decreases the risk for transmission to uninfected sexual partners. Treatment of HSV-associated genital ulcers is outlined in **Table 23**.

An important aspect of managing HSV-associated genital ulcer disease is counseling and education of the patient regarding the chronic nature of the infection and risks for transmission. Infected persons should understand the importance of informing sexual partners and should be counseled to abstain from sexual intercourse or oral-genital contact when prodromal symptoms or ulcers are present. It is also important that infected persons understand that asymptomatic viral shedding can occur and result in transmission of infection. Suppressive therapy does not eliminate the risk for transmission. Condoms, however, can reduce this risk. Men and women should be educated about the risk for neonatal HSV. Women should be encouraged to inform their obstetric providers and pediatricians of their history or the history of their male partner during pregnancy. Type-specific serologic antibody testing of an asymptomatic sexual partner can be useful in determining whether they are already infected and, therefore, not at risk for transmission.

**TABLE 23. Treatment of Herpes Simplex Virus Genital Infections**

| Clinical Syndrome | Recommended Regimen[a] |
|---|---|
| Primary infection[b] | Acyclovir, 400 mg three times daily, *or* acyclovir, 200 mg five times daily, *or* famciclovir, 250 mg three times daily, *or* valacyclovir, 1 g twice daily; all regimens for 7-10 days |
| Recurrent infection | Acyclovir, 400 mg three times daily for 5 days, *or* acyclovir, 800 mg twice daily for 5 days, *or* acyclovir, 800 mg three times daily for 2 days, *or* famciclovir, 125 mg twice daily for 5 days, *or* famciclovir, 1 g twice daily for 1 day, *or* famciclovir, 500 mg once followed by 250 mg twice daily for 2 days, *or* valacyclovir, 500 mg twice daily for 3 days, *or* valacyclovir, 1 g once daily for 5 days |
| Suppressive therapy | Acyclovir, 400 mg twice daily, *or* famciclovir, 250 mg twice daily, *or* valacyclovir, 500 mg daily, *or* valacyclovir, 1 g daily[c] |

[a]All regimens are given orally.

[b]Therapy can be extended if healing is incomplete after 10 days of treatment.

[c]The 500-mg dose of valacyclovir may be less effective than the 1-g dose in patients who have very frequent recurrences (≥10 episodes per year).

- Patients with genital herpes simplex virus infection present with painful lesions that begin as vesicles and progress to ulcers on an erythematous base; those with primary infection often have multiple genital lesions, regional lymphadenopathy, fever, myalgia, and malaise.

- Polymerase chain reaction is the most sensitive modality available for diagnosing herpes simplex virus.

## Syphilis

The incidence of infection with *Treponema pallidum* reached historic low levels in the United States in 2000 and then began to rise. Outbreaks among men who have sex with men are well described; however, the incidence of infection among women also has risen, as has the incidence of congenital syphilis.

Primary syphilis presents as a painless ulcer (chancre) at the site of inoculation (**Figure 15**). Chancres begin as papular lesions, which then ulcerate; the ulcer has a firm, raised border and the ulcer bed is clean. Up to one quarter of patients have multiple lesions. Regional lymphadenopathy is common. Chancres heal in 3 to 6 weeks. Secondary syphilis is a systemic illness characterized by a generalized macular and papular rash that normally involves the trunk and extremities, including the palms and soles. Lesions can coalesce in intertriginous

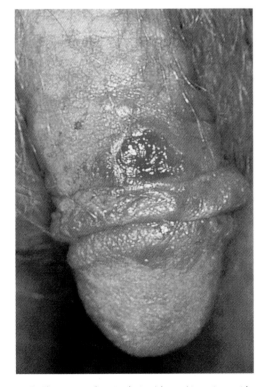

**FIGURE 15.** The primary ulcerative lesion (chancre) in patients with syphilis develops approximately 3 weeks after infection occurs, has a clean appearance with heaped-up borders, and is usually painless. It is often unrecognized. The primary chancre resolves spontaneously, and the infection progresses to a more advanced stage.

**CONT.**

areas to form plaques (condyloma lata), and superficial erosions may occur on mucosal surfaces (mucous patches). Fever, malaise, and generalized lymphadenopathy are common. Complications of tertiary syphilis (cardiovascular disease, gumma) are now rarely seen. Neurosyphilis can be asymptomatic or present as meningovascular, parenchymatous, or ocular disease.

Cerebrospinal fluid examination should be performed in patients with neurologic symptoms or signs and those who do not have an appropriate serologic response to treatment. Latent syphilis is the presence of serologic evidence of infection in the absence of clinical signs. Latent syphilis is divided into early-latent (infection ≤1 year in duration) or late-latent (infection >1 year) categories. In the absence of previous serologic results, asymptomatic patients with positive serologic findings are classified as having syphilis of unknown duration.

Primary syphilis can be diagnosed by dark field examination of scrapings from the ulcer base; however, this is not available in many clinical settings, so patients may need to be treated empirically. Serologic testing is the mainstay of syphilis diagnosis. Results of nonspecific tests (rapid plasma reagin [RPR] test, VDRL test) may be negative in primary infection but will be positive, generally at high titers, in secondary syphilis. Titers are lower in latent and tertiary infection. Positive findings on nonspecific tests should always be confirmed with a specific treponemal test (*T. pallidum* particle agglutination assay or fluorescent treponemal antibody absorption test) because biologic false-positive results can occur. Many commercial laboratories are now using a "reverse serology" testing algorithm that entails a specific treponemal test, most commonly an enzyme immunoassay (EIA), as the initial screening test followed by a nonspecific test (RPR or VDRL) for patients with a positive result on a specific test. These treponemal-specific assays allow automation of testing in the laboratory and increase the sensitivity of diagnosis

because patients with longstanding untreated syphilis may have negative results on nonspecific tests. Although the specificity of the EIA is excellent, persons with a positive EIA and a negative VDRL or RPR finding should have a second specific treponemal test to confirm the positive result. Persons with a positive (confirmed) EIA and a negative RPR or VDRL result should be offered treatment for late latent syphilis if they have no history of treatment.

Penicillin remains the treatment of choice at all stages of syphilis, and treatment recommendations are outlined in **Table 24**. Patients with primary and secondary syphilis should have repeat serologic testing at 6 and 12 months with the same testing method used for initial diagnosis; a fourfold decrease in the RPR or VDRL titer is considered significant. Patients should be offered screening for HIV infection, and sexual partners should be referred for evaluation. Partners exposed within the preceding 90 days to persons diagnosed with primary, secondary, or early latent syphilis should receive treatment regardless of serologic results.

**KEY POINTS**

- Primary syphilis presents as a painless ulcer at the site of inoculation, with a firm, raised border and clean bed; secondary syphilis is characterized by a generalized macular and papular rash that normally involves the trunk and extremities, including the palms and soles; and tertiary syphilis includes symptoms of cardiovascular disease and gumma.

- Penicillin is the treatment of choice for all stages of syphilis.

- Sexual partners should be referred for evaluation, and those exposed within the preceding 90 days of diagnosis should receive treatment regardless of serologic results.

| TABLE 24. | Treatment of Syphilis | |
|-----------|-----------------------|---|
| **Stage** | **Recommended Regimen**[a] | **Alternative Regimen for Penicillin-Allergic Patients** |
| Primary and secondary | Benzathine penicillin G, 2.4 million units IM single dose | Doxycycline, 100 mg PO twice daily, *or* tetracycline, 500 mg PO four times daily, for 14 days |
| Early latent | Benzathine penicillin G, 2.4 million units IM single dose | Doxycycline, 100 mg PO twice daily, *or* tetracycline, 500 mg PO four times daily, for 14 days |
| Late latent or syphilis of unknown duration | Benzathine penicillin G, 2.4 million units IM at 1-week intervals for 3 doses | Doxycycline, 100 mg PO twice daily, *or* tetracycline, 500 mg PO four times daily, for 28 days |
| Neurosyphilis | Aqueous crystalline penicillin G, 18-24 million units daily given as 3-4 million units IV every 4 h or by continuous infusion for 10-14 days, *or* procaine penicillin, 2.4 million units IM daily, plus probenecid, 500 mg PO four times daily, both for 10-14 days | Ceftriaxone, 2 g IM or IV daily for 10-14 days[b] |

IM = intramuscularly; IV = intravenously; PO = orally.

[a]Penicillin is the only effective antimicrobial agent for treatment of syphilis at any stage in pregnancy; therefore, pregnant penicillin-allergic patients should be desensitized and treated with the appropriate penicillin regimen as outlined above.

[b]Limited data are available to support the use of this alternative regimen, and the possibility of cross-reaction in penicillin-allergic patients must be considered.

## Chancroid

Chancroid, caused by *Haemophilus ducreyi*, is a common cause of genital ulcer disease worldwide but is uncommon in the United States. On presentation, patients have a painful genital ulcer and tender inguinal lymphadenopathy, which often suppurates. Culture of the organism is difficult. The CDC recommends consideration of this diagnosis if all of the following criteria are met: (1) presence of one or more painful genital ulcers, (2) no evidence of syphilis by dark field examination and serologic testing, (3) negative test result for HSV from the ulcer, and (4) clinical presentation consistent with chancroid. Treatment is outlined in **Table 25**. Patients who do not respond should be referred to a physician with expertise in the management of genital ulcer disease.

> **KEY POINT**
> - Patients with chancroid present with a painful genital ulcer and tender inguinal lymphadenopathy, which often suppurates.

## Lymphogranuloma Venereum

Lymphogranuloma venereum (LGV) is caused by three specific serovars of *C. trachomatis* (L1, L2, and L3). Infection presents with a genital papule or ulcer followed by tender unilateral inguinal lymphadenopathy. LGV is reported as a cause of proctocolitis, especially among men who have sex with men. Results of NAAT and most serologic tests will be positive for evidence of infection with *C. trachomatis* but cannot distinguish the LGV serovars, so the diagnosis must be made on clinical and epidemiologic grounds. Treatment is outlined in Table 25.

> **KEY POINT**
> - Lymphogranuloma venereum infection presents with a genital papule or ulcer followed by tender unilateral inguinal lymphadenopathy.

## Genital Warts

Genital warts are most commonly caused by human papillomavirus (HPV) types 6 and 11. They are typically painless lesions, although they can present with pain or pruritus. The lesions are flesh colored and exophytic (**Figure 16**); pedunculated lesions often occur. Diagnosis is generally based on clinical appearance; biopsy is indicated if the diagnosis is uncertain or lesions progress or do not respond to therapy. Pigmented or ulcerated lesions should also be biopsied. Treatment is indicated for symptomatic lesions and can be offered to patients concerned about the cosmetic appearance of the warts, although up to 80% of patients will clear the infection spontaneously. Treatment does not prevent HPV transmission. Patient-applied and provider-administered treatments are available. Patient-applied agents include podofilox (podophyllotoxin), imiquimod, and sinecatechins. Provider-administered treatments include podophyllin resin, trichloroacetic acid, cryotherapy, and surgical removal. See MKSAP 17 General Internal Medicine for discussion of HPV vaccination. Only the quadrivalent vaccine (HPV4) protects against genital warts.

> **KEY POINTS**
> - Genital warts are typically painless, flesh-colored, and exophytic lesions.
> - Treatment of genital warts does not prevent human papillomavirus transmission.

# Osteomyelitis

## Pathophysiology and Classification H

Osteomyelitis occurs by hematogenous spread, by direct introduction secondary to surgery or trauma, or contiguously from infected or colonized adjacent soft tissues. Osteomyelitis can be acute or chronic, depending on time of onset and histologic changes.

Hematogenous seeding of bone accounts for approximately 20% of adult cases, and the vertebral column is the most common location. Bloodborne pathogens are more likely

| TABLE 25. | Treatment of Chancroid and Lymphogranuloma Venereum |
| --- | --- |
| **Clinical Entity** | **Recommended Regimen** |
| Chancroid | Azithromycin, 1 g PO single dose, *or* ceftriaxone, 250 mg IM single dose, *or* ciprofloxacin, 500 mg PO twice daily for 3 days, *or* erythromycin base, 500 mg PO three times daily for 7 days |
| Lymphogranuloma venereum | Doxycycline,[a] 100 mg PO twice daily for 21 days (preferred), *or* erythromycin base, 500 mg PO four times daily for 21 days (alternative) |

IM = intramuscularly; PO = orally.

[a]Doxycyline should be avoided/used with caution in pregnant patients.

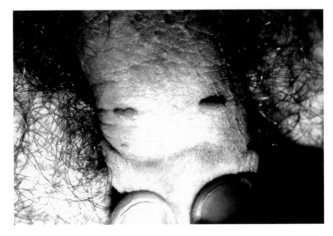

**FIGURE 16.** Genital warts due to human papillomavirus infection.

**CONT.**

to infect the sternoclavicular and sacroiliac bones, particularly in injection drug users. Frequent sources of hematogenous osteomyelitis are distant foci of infection (for example, skin and soft tissue, genitourinary, gastrointestinal), intravascular catheters, and infective endocarditis. Hematogenous osteomyelitis is typically monomicrobial, and *Staphylococcus aureus* is the most commonly isolated pathogen; however, aerobic, gram-negative bacilli cause disease in many patients. Certain patient-specific conditions are associated with less common bacterial organisms, including *Salmonella* osteomyelitis in persons with sickle cell disease and *Pseudomonas aeruginosa* bone infection in injection drug users.

Osteomyelitis associated with contiguous foci of infection, decubitus ulcers, and vascular insufficiency is often polymicrobial, although monomicrobial disease also occurs, with *S. aureus* as the most commonly involved organism. Osteomyelitis resulting from contaminated open or postsurgical closed traumatic fractures may involve soil organisms, skin flora, or hospital-acquired pathogens. The presence of a foreign body and diminished host defenses can predispose patients to infection from less pathogenic organisms. **H**

### KEY POINT

- *Staphylococcus aureus* is the most commonly isolated pathogen causing hematogenous osteomyelitis; however, aerobic, gram-negative bacilli such as *Salmonella* and *Pseudomonas aeruginosa* can cause disease in patients with sickle cell disease and in injection drug users, respectively.

## **H** Clinical Manifestations

In acute osteomyelitis, signs and symptoms typically present gradually. Often, patients report a dull pain that may intensify at the site of the infected bone, followed by local erythema, warmth, edema, and tenderness. Constitutional symptoms rarely occur. Although the clinical features of chronic osteomyelitis resemble those of acute disease, the presence of a draining sinus tract is pathognomonic of chronic infection in the bone. **H**

### KEY POINT

- The presence of a draining sinus tract is pathognomonic of chronic osteomyelitis infection in the bone.

## **H** Diagnosis

Bone biopsy is the definitive diagnostic study for osteomyelitis. However, other diagnostic studies are usually obtained for patients with suspected osteomyelitis before bone biopsy is pursued.

### Imaging Studies

Conventional plain radiographs lack sensitivity and specificity when used for diagnosing osteomyelitis because bony abnormalities can take up to 2 weeks to be detectable.

Three-phase bone scanning, gallium scanning, and tagged leukocyte scanning are potentially useful nuclear imaging modalities, especially in the setting of acute disease. Three-phase bone scans involve injection of a radionuclide with imaging of the suspected infection site at three time points: immediately after injection, 15 minutes later, and 4 hours after injection. In patients with osteomyelitis, enhancement occurs in all three phases. Gallium-67 has an affinity for acute-phase reactants and will accumulate at sites of infection following injection. Tagged leukocyte scans use a radiotracer to label autologous leukocytes, which accumulate at sites of infection or inflammation after injection. The sensitivity of these nuclear scanning modalities is high (>90%) for osteomyelitis, but specificity is more variable because patients may have alternative causes of bone inflammation or turnover, such as degenerative joint disease, surgery, trauma, or cancer. The specificity of these tests is significantly heightened if plain radiographs fail to demonstrate evidence of another osseous process. A normal result on a radionuclide imaging test has excellent negative predictive value for ruling out bone infection.

MRI is the best imaging technique for diagnosing osteomyelitis. Because of its high sensitivity for bone infection, a negative scan can reliably exclude disease in the area imaged. Additionally, it is more effective than nuclear imaging in detecting osteomyelitis in certain anatomic locations, such as the feet and vertebrae. However, bone marrow edema changes seen on MRI may be from other causes (such as fracture, surgery, contusion, and Charcot arthropathy). Gadolinium contrast-enhanced MRI is helpful in identifying abscesses and sinus tracts. Because MRI changes persist for an extended duration following effective therapy, follow-up MRI may be misleading and result in additional unwarranted treatment; thus, it should be limited to verifying equivocal clinical improvement.

CT is useful for assessing bone anatomy and delineating adjacent soft tissue and is a reasonable alternative in situations when MRI is contraindicated. Ultrasonography has limited utility in the diagnosis of osteomyelitis. PET scans are currently considered investigational. **H**

### KEY POINTS

- Conventional plain radiography lacks sensitivity and specificity for diagnosing osteomyelitis. **HVC**
- MRI is the best imaging technique for diagnosing osteomyelitis because of its high sensitivity for bone infection and superiority at delineating bone anatomy and providing excellent resolution of surrounding soft tissues; the role for follow-up MRI is limited to patients who do not clinically improve with therapy. **HVC**

### Laboratory Studies

**H**

Generally, inflammatory markers, erythrocyte sedimentation rate, and C-reactive protein are increased, but normal values do not exclude osteomyelitis. Blood cultures identify bacteremia in few cases (almost all are acute osteomyelitis), but when

CONT.

present, the organism isolated is likely the same as the bone pathogen. Accordingly, blood cultures should be obtained in all suspected cases of osteomyelitis because a positive culture may avert more invasive testing. **H**

> **KEY POINT**
>
> HVC • Blood cultures should be obtained in all suspected cases of osteomyelitis because a positive culture may avert more invasive testing.

## Bone Biopsy

The demonstration of a microorganism(s) coupled with characteristic histologic features makes bone biopsy the gold standard for diagnosing osteomyelitis. Biopsies can be accomplished by open surgical procedure or percutaneously. It is best to obtain specimens before the initiation of empiric antimicrobial agents.

With the exception of *S. aureus*, microorganisms isolated from culture samples obtained from superficial wounds or sinus tracts correlate poorly with deep cultures from bone; therefore, this practice is of limited value. **H**

> **KEY POINTS**
>
> • Bone biopsy is the gold standard for diagnosing osteomyelitis.
>
> HVC • Culture samples obtained from superficial wounds or sinus tracts correlate poorly with deep cultures from bone.

## Treatment

Identification of the inciting pathogen, administration of adequate antimicrobials for a prolonged duration (usually 6 weeks), surgical debridement (if warranted), and removal of orthopedic prosthetic devices (if feasible) influence the success of osteomyelitis treatment. Parenteral antimicrobials are used to treat osteomyelitis, except in certain circumstances in which oral therapy may be appropriate, such as using oral fluoroquinolones for infections with certain gram-negative bacilli. Long-term suppressive oral antimicrobial treatment may be indicated in patients for whom cure is not possible. Negative pressure is an adjunctive therapy used to manage open wounds that applies subatmospheric pressure to the wound surface and may benefit select patients. Hyperbaric oxygen therapy has been advocated as an adjunctive therapy for refractory osteomyelitis. However, few randomized, controlled clinical trials support its use in this setting. **H**

> **KEY POINTS**
>
> • Successful osteomyelitis treatment involves antimicrobial administration for a prolonged period, surgical debridement, and removal of orthopedic hardware.
>
> • Parenteral antimicrobials are used to treat osteomyelitis except in certain circumstances; however, chronic osteomyelitis can be treated with oral agents alone.

## Evaluation and Management of Diabetes Mellitus–Associated Osteomyelitis

Patients with diabetes mellitus are prone to frequent skin and soft tissue infections of the feet with subsequent ulcer formation, which, if left unrecognized, eventually result in contiguous osteomyelitis.

Patients with diabetes and complex foot infections often lack classic signs of infection, including fever. Characteristic findings that predict contiguous osteomyelitis are ulcers that have been present for 2 weeks or longer, ulcer size greater than 2 cm, grossly visible bone or the ability to probe to bone, and an erythrocyte sedimentation rate greater than 70 mm/h.

The same imaging and laboratory studies are used for patients with diabetes-associated osteomyelitis as in those without diabetes. However, these tests may not be necessary when bone is visualized or probable using a sterile instrument in the depth of a foot ulcer.

A combined medical and surgical approach incorporating meticulous attention to wound management, glycemic control, assessment of vascular supply, and adequate antimicrobial administration are imperative to maximize chances for a successful outcome. Curetted samples from the ulcer base following debridement, or preferably bone biopsy specimens obtained before antimicrobial initiation, provide the best method for identifying the likely pathogen(s). Early surgical intervention for debridement and drainage decreases the risk for subsequent amputations. If indicated, revascularization procedures improve the arterial blood supply, promoting healing and preventing further ischemic necrosis.

Broad-spectrum antimicrobial therapy is usually required considering the polymicrobial nature of diabetic foot infections. Parenteral administration is necessary in patients with severe infections or those suspected of having osteomyelitis. Oral agents with reliable bioavailability may be adequate in the setting of milder infections. Standard antimicrobial regimens use monotherapy or combinations of agents against staphylococci, streptococci, aerobic gram-negative bacilli, and anaerobes. Acceptable choices include advanced-generation cephalosporins (ceftriaxone and cefepime) and fluoroquinolones (ciprofloxacin or levofloxacin) combined with an agent with anaerobic activity, such as metronidazole or clindamycin. Similarly, β-lactam/β-lactamase inhibitor combinations or carbapenems would provide appropriate coverage. The increasing prevalence of methicillin-resistant *S. aureus* underscores the importance of making an accurate microbiologic diagnosis and may require the use of agents active against this pathogen (vancomycin, daptomycin, linezolid, and ceftaroline) until its presence is excluded. After culture and sensitivity information becomes available, modifications to narrow the initial empiric antimicrobial regimen should be undertaken, keeping in mind that not every isolate from these polymicrobial infections requires treatment. Generally, antimicrobials are continued until the wound adequately heals and

**CONT.**

the signs of infection have resolved (usually 2-4 weeks). In patients with osteomyelitis, 6 weeks of antimicrobial therapy after surgical debridement is the preferred treatment course, unless all infected bone and soft tissue has been removed, in which case antimicrobial agents can be stopped when the wound has adequately healed.

The use of vacuum-assisted wound closure is advantageous in achieving complete closure in diabetic foot ulcers. The benefit of hyperbaric oxygen therapy is less clear. **H**

**KEY POINTS**

- Findings that predict contiguous osteomyelitis are ulcers that have been present for 2 weeks or longer, ulcer size greater than 2 cm, grossly visible bone or the ability to probe to bone, and an erythrocyte sedimentation rate greater than 70 mm/h.
- Debridement and culturing of samples before antimicrobial initiation are the best methods for identifying the offending pathogen(s).
- In patients with diabetes-associated osteomyelitis, 6 weeks of antimicrobial therapy after surgical debridement is the norm.

## Evaluation and Management of Vertebral Osteomyelitis

The term *spondylodiskitis* refers to infection of the vertebrae and contiguous disk space. Most infections are hematogenous in origin. Less commonly, infection results from the direct introduction of bacteria or other microorganisms at the time of spinal surgery, is a rare complication from local injection or catheter placement, or is caused by contiguous spread from organs adjacent to the spine. The lumbar spine is involved most frequently, followed by the thoracic and cervical vertebrae. Most patients are men older than 50 years. *S. aureus* (including methicillin-resistant strains) is the pathogen most often isolated. Gram-negative bacilli, streptococci, *Candida* species, and unusual organisms (*Brucella* species) may be involved.

A diagnosis of vertebral osteomyelitis should be considered in patients reporting worsening back or neck pain without an alternative explanation. Local tenderness over the site of spinal infection is frequently detected. Radicular pain, motor weakness, and sensory changes may be present. If infection spreads posteriorly into the epidural space, more severe neurologic deficits may develop. Fever is present in approximately half of infected patients.

Blood cultures should be obtained before administration of empiric antimicrobials because cultures will be positive in more than 50% of patients and help guide appropriate therapy and limit unnecessary testing. Increased erythrocyte sedimentation rate (often >100 mm/h) and C-reactive protein level are noted in more than 80% of patients. Leukocyte counts are often normal, so they are less helpful.

Early in the course of disease, the utility of plain radiography is limited because of its lack of sensitivity. MRI is the most sensitive imaging modality to detect vertebral osteomyelitis, but results can be falsely positive in cases of uninfected fractures. With the exception of gallium scanning, other radionuclide scanning is less reliable in diagnosing vertebral osteomyelitis. When blood cultures are negative, CT-guided percutaneous needle aspiration biopsy and culture are required to confirm the microbiologic diagnosis. A second biopsy attempt is strongly recommended to help determine the microbial cause if the first sample is nondiagnostic.

Lengthy parenteral antimicrobial therapy is the mainstay of treatment. When no pathogen is successfully isolated, empiric antimicrobial therapy must include a reliable agent aimed at gram-positive cocci, such as vancomycin or daptomycin, together with a broad-spectrum antimicrobial against gram-negative bacilli, such as ceftriaxone, ceftazidime, cefepime, or a fluoroquinolone. Because anaerobic bacteria are uncommon pathogens in this setting (except when the pathogenesis is secondary to contiguous infection), the inclusion of empiric antimicrobial agents with specific anaerobic activity is not necessary.

Oral antimicrobial agents are generally used only to treat vertebral osteomyelitis in specific situations, such as when a fluoroquinolone-sensitive, gram-negative bacillus proves to be the infecting pathogen or, possibly, when long term-term chronic antimicrobial suppression is warranted, such as in patients with retained orthopedic prosthetic devices.

Antimicrobial therapy is given for 6 to 8 weeks, but longer treatment courses may be necessary in patients with extensive or advanced disease. Surgical intervention is indicated in few patients, except when required to stabilize the spine, drain an abscess, or pursue the diagnosis when empiric treatment is ineffective.

Follow-up MRIs should be performed in patients without expected improvement, when complications develop, or when inflammatory markers remain elevated without explanation. **H**

**KEY POINTS**

- Worsening back or neck pain without an alternative explanation, local tenderness, radicular pain, motor weakness, sensory changes, or more severe neurologic deficits should prompt evaluation for vertebral osteomyelitis; fever is present in approximately half of infected patients.
- Blood cultures will be positive in more than 50% of patients and help guide therapy and limit unnecessary testing. **HVC**
- Antimicrobial therapy is generally given for 6 to 8 weeks.

# Fever of Unknown Origin
## Introduction

Fever is a common problem, although it is usually self-limited or the cause is promptly diagnosed. Fever of unknown origin (FUO) is a sustained, unexplained fever despite a comprehensive diagnostic evaluation. FUO can be classified into classic, nosocomial, neutropenic, and HIV-associated categories based on the clinical setting and the patient's underlying immune status (**Table 26**).

# Causes

The spectrum of diseases causing classic FUO changed considerably in recent decades with improved diagnostic modalities for infections, malignancies, and connective tissue diseases. Better methods of diagnosing bacterial and viral infections have become available; with the development of serologic studies to detect connective tissue diseases and improved imaging techniques to detect malignancies, the proportion of patients with classic FUO that remains undiagnosed following evaluation has decreased from half to one third of all cases. The most recently available data show classic FUO is caused by infection (25%-50%; most commonly tuberculosis, abscesses, system fungal infections, infective endocarditis, cytomegalovirus infection), malignancy (20%-30%, leukemia, lymphoma, solid tumors, carcinomatosis), and connective tissue disease (15%-30%; systemic lupus erythematosus, temporal arteritis, Still disease, polyarteritis nodosa, rheumatoid arthritis). Miscellaneous causes include thromboembolic disorders, pancreatitis, medications, inflammatory bowel disease, and granulomatous hepatitis.

**KEY POINT**

- Fever of unknown origin is primarily caused by infections, malignancies, and connective tissue diseases.

# Evaluation

The longer a fever persists without a diagnosis, the less likely it is to have an infectious origin. Most patients with undiagnosed FUO recover spontaneously. The diagnostic evaluation should be based on a detailed history and physical examination, with further evaluation based on the most likely cause in a given patient. Initial studies in most patients typically include a complete blood count with differential, complete metabolic profile with kidney and liver studies, at least three blood culture sets (preferably obtained over 24 hours) and cultures of other bodily fluids (such as urine or from other sources based on clinical suspicion), an erythrocyte sedimentation rate, tuberculosis testing (skin testing or interferon-γ release assay), and serology for HIV. It is reasonable to perform chest imaging (radiography or CT) and a CT of the abdomen as initial diagnostic imaging. CT of the chest showing patchy or nodular infiltration (especially if cavitary) in the lung apices suggests pulmonary tuberculosis, which can occur in those with normal chest radiographs; however, culture is the gold standard for diagnosis. Miliary tuberculosis has nonspecific symptoms, but anemia and pancytopenia are common. The diagnosis is most often established by culture and histopathology of tissue from enlarged lymph nodes, liver biopsy if aminotransferases and alkaline phosphatase are elevated, or bone marrow biopsy if pancytopenia is present. Mycobacterial blood cultures may also be positive. Blood cultures are the most important test for the diagnosis of infective endocarditis. Echocardiography should also be performed if endocarditis is suspected. In cases

| TABLE 26. Categories and Common Causes of Fever of Unknown Origin | | |
|---|---|---|
| **Category** | **Definition** | **Common Causes** |
| Classic | Temperature >38.3 °C (100.9 °F) for at least 3 weeks with at least 1 week of in-hospital investigation[a] *or* Temperature >38.3 °C (100.9 °F) for at least 3 weeks that remains undiagnosed after 2 visits in the ambulatory setting[b] or 3 days in hospital | Infection (endocarditis, tuberculosis, abscesses, complicated urinary tract infection), neoplasm, connective tissue disease |
| Health care associated | Temperature >38.3 °C (100.9 °F) in patients hospitalized ≥72 hours but no fever or evidence of potential infection at the time of admission, and negative evaluation of at least 3 days | Drug fever, septic, thrombophlebitis, pulmonary embolism, sinusitis, postoperative complications (occult abscesses), *Clostridium difficile* enterocolitis, device- or procedure-related endocarditis |
| Neutropenic (immune deficient) | Temperature >38.3 °C (100.9 °F) and neutrophil count <500/μL for >3 days and negative evaluation after 48 hours | Occult bacterial and opportunistic fungal infections (aspergillosis, candidiasis), drug fever, pulmonary emboli, underlying malignancy; cause not documented in 40%-60% of cases |
| HIV associated | Temperature >38.3 °C (100.9 °F) for >3 weeks (outpatients) or >3 days (inpatients) in patients with confirmed HIV infection | Primary HIV infection, opportunistic infections (cytomegalovirus, cryptococcosis, typical and atypical mycobacteria, toxoplasmosis), lymphoma, IRIS |

IRIS = immune reconstitution inflammatory syndrome.

[a]First definition of fever of unknown origin.

[b]The ambulatory setting is the preferred venue for evaluation and treatment.

**CONT.**

of culture-negative endocarditis, serologic tests for Q fever, psittacosis, and *Bartonella* species may yield a causative organism. Brain imaging and cultures and histopathology of biopsy specimens of lung, bone marrow, and liver may establish a diagnosis in HIV-associated FUO. Imaging and bacterial cultures are potentially useful in diagnosing hospital-acquired and neutropenic FUO. **H**

**KEY POINT**

- The longer a fever persists without a diagnosis, the less likely it is to have an infectious origin.

# Primary Immunodeficiencies

## Introduction

Diseases of primary immunodeficiency are relatively uncommon, and many, including X-linked agammaglobulinemia and severe combined immunodeficiency, are initially diagnosed in infancy or early childhood. This discussion focuses on immunodeficiencies most likely to be encountered in adults. Immunodeficiencies are classified as B-cell antibody immunodeficiencies, T-cell or cellular immunodeficiencies, and immunodeficiencies associated with the phagocytic or complement system. Most primary immunodeficiencies manifest with infection at certain sites (sinopulmonary, gastrointestinal) and with recurrent infection. The most frequent B-cell immunodeficiencies are diagnosed in young adults.

## Selective IgA Deficiency

IgA deficiency is one of the most common B-cell immunodeficiencies. Inheritance may be autosomal dominant or recessive; most cases are sporadic. Patients with selective IgA deficiency may be asymptomatic or present with recurrent sinopulmonary infections (otitis media, sinusitis, pneumonia) or gastrointestinal infections (giardiasis). Other common manifestations include inflammatory bowel disease; celiac disease; an increased frequency of autoimmune disorders, including rheumatoid arthritis, systemic lupus erythematosus, and chronic active hepatitis; and allergic disorders, including asthma, allergic rhinitis, and food allergies. Additionally, some patients may develop anti-IgA antibodies that may react with blood products containing IgA; anaphylactic transfusion reactions can occur. IgA deficiency is defined as a serum IgA level less than 7 mg/dL (0.07 g/L). A low level should be confirmed by repeat measurement. Levels of IgM and IgG are normal. IgA deficiency has no specific treatment; however, prophylactic antimicrobial agents may prevent recurrent sinus and pulmonary infections.

**KEY POINT**

- Patients with selective IgA deficiency may be asymptomatic; present with recurrent sinopulmonary infections, gastrointestinal infections, inflammatory bowel disease, or celiac disease; and have an increased frequency of autoimmune or allergic disorders.

## Common Variable Immunodeficiency

Common variable immunodeficiency involves B- and T-cell abnormalities and results in clinically significant immune dysregulation. The primary manifestation is hypogammaglobulinemia, and adults present with recurrent respiratory infections. The gastrointestinal tract is frequently involved and causes malabsorption or chronic diarrhea. Infection with *Giardia*, *Campylobacter*, or *Yersinia* species may occur, as may opportunistic infections. Concurrent autoimmune disorders occur in up to 25% of patients and include endocrinopathies; chronic active hepatitis; and neurologic, hematologic, or rheumatologic disorders. Pernicious anemia is also a potential complication. The risk for malignancy is increased, including gastrointestinal cancers and non-Hodgkin lymphoma. Patients also have a poor or absent response to protein and polysaccharide vaccines. Serum immunoglobulin levels are usually low, circulating B cells may be normal or low, and T-cell function varies. The diagnosis is made by confirming low levels of total IgG and IgA or IgM, as well as by a poor antibody response to vaccines. Early diagnosis and treatment with intravenous immune globulin improve survival.

**KEY POINTS**

- Common variable immunodeficiency primarily manifests with hypogammaglobulinemia, and patients present with recurrent respiratory infections and gastrointestinal tract involvement with malabsorption or chronic diarrhea.

- Common variable immunodeficiency is diagnosed by confirming low levels of total IgG and IgA or IgM, as well as by a poor antibody response to vaccines.

## Abnormalities in the Complement System

The complement system plays several important roles in host defense, including opsonization to improve phagocyte function, induction of the humoral immune response, clearance of immune complexes, and clearance of apoptotic cells. Complement deficiencies occur in approximately 5% of patients with primary immunodeficiency disorders. Complement deficiencies are classified as those affecting the early classic complement pathway, the alternative complement pathway, the mannose-binding proteins and proteases, and the late complement pathway (**Figure 17**). The most common of the early complement disorders is C2 deficiency; C6 deficiency is the most common of the late complement disorders. Patients lacking one of the early components usually present with a rheumatologic disorder, such as systemic lupus erythematosus, scleroderma, vasculitis, or dermatomyositis. Deficiencies of late complement components are sometimes associated with lupus-like illnesses or vasculitis. Those with late complement component deficiencies usually present with recurrent, invasive meningococcal or gonococcal infections. Patients with recurrent bloodstream infection with encapsulated bacteria or invasive meningococcal or gonococcal disease should be screened for complement deficiency by assaying for total hemolytic complement ($CH_{50}$) activity. If $CH_{50}$ is normal, alternate pathway function should be assessed with an alternative complement pathway ($AH_{50}$) assay. If results of either assay are abnormal, specific component concentrations should be determined. Patients with late complement deficiency should be immunized with a quadrivalent conjugate meningococcal vaccine. Pneumococcal vaccination is also indicated for patients with complement deficiencies (in particular, C1, C2, C3, and C4 deficiencies) (see MKSAP 17 General Internal Medicine).

> **KEY POINT**
> - Patients with recurrent bloodstream infection with encapsulated bacteria or invasive meningococcal or gonococcal disease should be screened for complement deficiency by assaying for total hemolytic complement ($CH_{50}$) activity.

# Bioterrorism

## Introduction

Bioterrorism is the intentional release of pathogens or toxins for the purpose of harming or killing civilians. Agents that could potentially be used in bioterrorist events have been prioritized into three groups (**Table 27**). Because they have the highest risk for use, group A agents are discussed here.

Epidemiologic characteristics that distinguish a bioterrorism attack from a naturally occurring infection include sudden onset; large number of cases; increased severity or uncommon clinical presentation; and unusual geographic, temporal, or demographic clustering of cases.

## Anthrax

Anthrax is caused by *Bacillus anthracis*, a gram-positive, aerobic organism. It is ubiquitous in soil and causes human

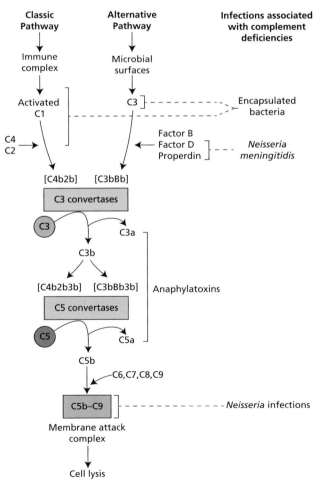

**FIGURE 17.** The complement reaction sequence and infections associated with deficiency states.

Redrawn with permission from Nairn R. Immunology. In: Brooks GF, Butel JS, Morse SA, eds. Jawetz, Melnick, and Adelberg's Medical Microbiology. 23rd ed. New York: Lange Medical Books/McGraw Hill; 2004.

| TABLE 27. | Potential Agents of Bioterrorism | |
|---|---|---|
| **Class A[a]** | **Class B[b]** | **Class C[c]** |
| Anthrax | Q fever | Emerging infectious diseases |
| Botulism | Brucellosis | |
| Plague | Glanders | Nipah virus |
| Smallpox | Melioidosis | Hantavirus |
| Tularemia | Viral encephalitis | |
| Viral hemorrhagic fever | Typhus fever | |
| | Ricin toxin | |
| | Staphylococcal enterotoxin B | |
| | Psittacosis | |
| | Foodborne illness | |
| | Waterborne illness | |

[a]Greatest potential, easy dissemination or person-to-person spread, high mortality, and profound public health implications.

[b]Less easily spread, fewer illnesses and deaths, fewer public health preparation measures.

[c]Future ability to engineer for mass dissemination and significant mortality.

infection by spore exposure (**Figure 18A** and **18B**). Spores may be acquired by cutaneous contact, resulting in a distinctive black eschar (**Figure 18C**); ingestion; or inhalation (most likely to be used for bioterrorism). Spores are easily dispersed by aerosolization and can be sent by mail. Even a single case of inhalational anthrax should raise the suspicion of bioterrorism.

Patients with inhalational anthrax present with low-grade fever, malaise, myalgia, and headache accompanied by cough, dyspnea, and chest pain. Chest radiograph showing mediastinal widening (**Figure 18D**) from hemorrhagic lymphadenitis is characteristic. Diagnosis is confirmed by culture or polymerase chain reaction (PCR) of blood, tissues, or fluid samples. Initial treatment is outlined in **Table 28**. Ciprofloxacin, levofloxacin, moxifloxacin, or doxycycline should be provided as soon as possible following any actual or suspected case of anthrax that raises concern for a bioterrorism attack. Raxibacumab, a monoclonal antibody that neutralizes *B. anthracis* toxin, is approved for the treatment and prevention of inhalational anthrax. Uncomplicated cutaneous anthrax is defined as the absence of systemic symptoms and involvement of the head or neck in the absence of extensive swelling. A non–FDA-licensed, cell-free anthrax vaccine is available for postexposure immunization. **H**

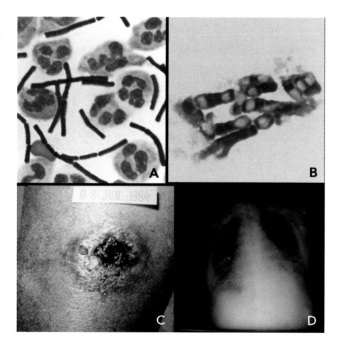

**FIGURE 18.** (*A*) "Box-car"-shaped, gram-positive *Bacillus anthracis* bacilli in the cerebrospinal fluid of the index case of inhalational anthrax resulting from bioterrorism in the United States. (*B*) Terminal and subterminal spores of *B. anthracis*. (*C*) Black eschar lesion of cutaneous anthrax. (*D*) Chest radiograph of a patient with anthrax showing a widened mediastinum due to hemorrhagic lymphadenopathy.

| TABLE 28. | Class A Bioterrorism Agents | | | |
|---|---|---|---|---|
| **Disease – Agent** | **Incubation Period** | **Clinical Features** | **Treatment** | **Prophylaxis** |
| Anthrax – *Bacillus anthracis* | 1-60 days | Inhalational: febrile respiratory distress<br><br>Cutaneous: necrotic eschar<br><br>Gastrointestinal: distention, peritonitis | Ciprofloxacin, levofloxacin, moxifloxacin, or doxycycline plus one or two additional agents[a] for 60 days | Ciprofloxacin, levofloxacin, moxifloxacin, or doxycycline |
| Smallpox virus – variola virus | 7-17 days | Fever followed by pustular cutaneous rash | Supportive care | Vaccine if exposure occurred in the previous 7 days |
| Plague – *Yersinia pestis* | 1-6 days | Fulminant pneumonia and sepsis | Streptomycin or gentamicin for 7 to 10 days<br><br>Alternatives: doxycycline or levofloxacin if aminoglycosides contraindicated | Doxycycline or levofloxacin for 7 days |
| Botulism – *Clostridium botulinum* | 2 hours to 8 days | Cranial nerve palsies and descending flaccid paralysis | Antitoxin and supportive care | Antibotulinum antitoxin (equine serum heptavalent botulism toxin) |
| Tularemia – *Francisella tularensis* | 3-5 days | Fever, respiratory distress, and sepsis | Streptomycin or gentamicin (severe disease) for 7 to 14 days<br><br>Doxycycline or ciprofloxacin (nonsevere disease) for 14 days | Doxycycline or ciprofloxacin |
| Viral hemorrhagic fevers – Ebola and Marburg viruses | Variable | Hemorrhage and multiorgan failure | Supportive care | None available |

[a]Penicillin, ampicillin, imipenem, meropenem, clindamycin, linezolid, rifampin, vancomycin, or clarithromycin.

## Smallpox (Variola)

Because smallpox was declared eradicated worldwide in 1979-1980, even a single case of suspected or proven disease justifies concern for bioterrorism. Infection is acquired by inhalation; deliberate aerosolization into a largely nonimmunized population could potentially result in a disastrous epidemic.

Patients with severe illness develop high fever, headache, vomiting, and backache. The rash first appears on the buccal and pharyngeal mucosa followed by cutaneous spread to the hands and face and then the arms, legs, and feet. The skin lesions evolve synchronously (same stage or maturation on any one area of the body) from macules to papules to vesicles to pustules and eventually become crusted (**Figure 19**). Patients remain contagious until all scabs and crusts are shed.

Treatment of smallpox is supportive. The nucleotide analogue cidofovir possesses good in vitro activity and may offer some therapeutic benefit. Postexposure vaccination with vaccinia, targeting close contacts of patients with smallpox who will be at greatest risk for contracting the disease ("ring vaccination"), offers some protection from the infection and is best if provided within 3 days after exposure. 🄷

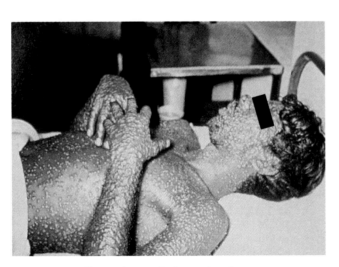

**FIGURE 19.** Diffuse synchronous skin lesions of smallpox.

## Plague 🄷

Infection with *Yersinia pestis* most often occurs by the bite of an infected flea but may also arise from inhalation of an intentional bioterrorism-related aerosol release of pathogen. Pneumonic plague most often arises through hematogenous spread from a bubo (an infected, swollen lymph node) but may be primary from direct inhalation. Patients present with sudden high fever, pleuritic chest discomfort, a productive cough, and hemoptysis. The chest radiograph is nonspecific. Sputum Gram stain (and possibly blood smear) may identify gram-negative bacilli demonstrating the classic bipolar staining or "safety pin" shape.

Pneumonic plague is universally and rapidly fatal unless prompt treatment is provided (see Table 28). Asymptomatic persons known to have been exposed to aerosolized *Y. pestis* or those known to have had close contact with an infected patient should be given postexposure prophylaxis (see Table 28). 🄷

## Botulism 🄷

*Clostridium botulinum* produces botulinum toxin, the most lethal biologic substance known. Inhalational botulism through the deliberate release of botulinum toxin or toxin ingestion following deliberate contamination of food would be most likely in a bioterrorism attack. The toxin blocks acetylcholine-mediated neurotransmission. Patients present with symmetric, descending flaccid paralysis with prominent bulbar signs (the "4 Ds": diplopia, dysarthria, dysphonia, and dysphagia), absence of fever, and normal mental status. Paralysis may progress to involve the respiratory muscles, necessitating ventilator-assisted support.

Confirmation of disease depends on identifying botulinum toxin from samples of blood, stool, and gastric contents, as well as from suspected foods. Treatment includes supportive care and early administration of antitoxin; antitoxin will not reverse existing paralysis. 🄷

- Symptoms of botulism usually occur within 24 to 72 hours of toxin exposure and consist of a classic triad of symmetric, descending flaccid paralysis with prominent bulbar signs, absence of fever, and normal mental status.

## Tularemia

*Francisella tularensis* is mainly a zoonotic disease; it is highly infectious and can cause significant illness through low inocula inhalation. Disease is heralded by the abrupt onset of fever, chills, myalgia, and anorexia.

Pneumonic tularemia is characterized by a nonproductive cough, dyspnea, and substernal or pleuritic chest pain. Severe respiratory failure may ensue. Chest radiographs reveal infiltrates, hilar lymphadenopathy, and pleural effusion.

Cultures of blood, sputum, pleural fluid, and tissue are frequently negative. PCR assays and direct fluorescent and immunohistochemical stains of clinical specimens assist in rapid diagnosis.

Treatment is outlined in Table 28. Mild or moderate infection can be treated with oral agents, which are also used for postexposure prophylaxis. Overall mortality is 1% with adequate treatment, but may be as high as 30% in untreated patients with pneumonic or typhoidal tularemia.

**KEY POINTS**

- *Francisella tularensis* disease onset is heralded by abrupt occurrence of fever, chills, myalgia, and anorexia followed by respiratory symptoms.
- Polymerase chain reaction assays and direct fluorescent and immunohistochemical stains applied directly to various clinical specimens have proven successful in making a rapid tularemia diagnosis.

## Viral Hemorrhagic Fever

Viral hemorrhagic fevers (VHFs) are caused by zoonotic RNA viruses (see Table 28). Characteristics such as high infectivity, virulence after low-dose exposure, capacity for causing significant morbidity and mortality, and limited prophylactic and therapeutic options render them likely candidates for use as biologic weapons.

Outside of a known epidemiologic exposure or travel to an endemic area, the occurrence or clinical suspicion of even one case of VHF should raise concern for bioterrorism, and simultaneous presentation of multiple patients should be expected.

A febrile prodrome, accompanied by myalgia and prostration occurs. Early signs of infection include conjunctival injection, petechial hemorrhages, easy bruising, flushing, and mild hypotension. As the disease advances, patients experience shock and generalized bleeding from the mucous membranes, skin, and gastrointestinal tract. Ultimately, multiorgan failure ensues.

Diagnostic confirmation requires RNA detection by reverse transcription PCR, the presence of viral protein antigens, development of IgM antibodies, or isolation of the virus. Treatment is primarily supportive.

**KEY POINT**

- A high febrile prodrome universally occurs with viral hemorrhagic fever, accompanied by varying degrees of myalgia and prostration, with early signs of infection including conjunctival injection, petechial hemorrhages, easy bruising, flushing, and mild hypotension.

# Travel Medicine
## Introduction

The risk for specific travel-associated infections varies by destination; specialized travel clinics provide individualized advice tailored to itinerary and planned activities. Recommended immunizations for travel are listed in **Table 29**. Trip-specific

| TABLE 29. Immunizations for Travel[a] |
|---|
| **Recommended According to Destination, Itinerary, and Purpose of Travel** |
| Hepatitis A[b]: 1 month before travel, booster at 6-12 months |
| Hepatitis B[b]: 0, 1 month, 6 months; accelerated schedule: 0, 1 week, 3 weeks, and 12 months (combination vaccine with hepatitis A available) |
| Typhoid[c]: Live-attenuated oral vaccine (Ty21a); 0, 2 days, 4 days, 6 days; capsular Vi polysaccharide intramuscular vaccine; 1 dose (preferred for immunocompromised persons) |
| Cholera: Killed, whole-cell-B subunit; 0, 1 week (not available in the United States) |
| Rabies: Inactivated; 0, 7 days, 21-28 days |
| Japanese encephalitis: Inactivated; 0, 28 days |
| Tick-borne encephalitis: Inactivated; 0, 1-3 months, 9-12 months (not available in the United States) |
| **Required for Certain Destinations** |
| Yellow fever: Live attenuated; 1 dose |
| Meningococcal: Quadrivalent conjugate (MenACWY), or polysaccharide (MPSV4); 1 dose; travel to Saudi Arabia during the Hajj |

[a]All patients being evaluated for travel should receive or be up to date with all scheduled immunizations, including influenza, pneumococcal, tetanus-diphtheria-pertussis, polio, varicella, and zoster vaccines. See MKSAP 17 General Internal Medicine for routine immunization recommendations.

[b]If not received as part of routine scheduled immunizations. If the vaccine series was completed as part of scheduled immunization, repeat immunization is not required.

[c]Oral vaccine should not be administered within 24 hours of the antimalarial drug mefloquine because of the potential to decrease the vaccine's immunogenicity; patients must not take any antibiotic for at least 72 hours before receiving the vaccine.

Data from Centers for Disease Control and Prevention. CDC Health Information for International Travel 2014. New York: Oxford University Press; 2014. Available online at http://wwwnc.cdc.gov/travel/page/yellowbook-home-2014. Accessed December 2014.

information is also available from the Centers for Disease Control and Prevention (CDC) Travel Health website (http://wwwnc.cdc.gov/travel/). A consultation should be scheduled at least 1 month before departure to assess the traveler's risk based on underlying medical conditions, travel destination, and planned activities and to provide appropriate immunizations.

The most significant and potentially severe travel-associated infections are listed in **Table 30**, with several key infections discussed in the following sections.

# Malaria

The *Anopheles* mosquito transmits malaria. Transmission is minimized by limiting outdoor exposure between dusk and dawn, using bed nets and insect repellents containing 30% to 50% N,N-diethyl-3-methylbenzamide (DEET), and adhering to chemoprophylaxis. Despite these measures, malaria remains a common cause of febrile illness, particularly in travelers returning from sub-Saharan Africa and large parts of Asia.

The incubation period is 12 to 35 days. Patients commonly present with fever (characterized by paroxysms occurring in 48- or 72-hour cycles), headache, myalgia, nausea, vomiting, abdominal pain, and diarrhea. Severe disease most often results from *Plasmodium falciparum* infection. Hyperparasitemia (5%-10% parasitized erythrocytes) results in sequestration in small blood vessels, causing infarcts, capillary leakage, and organ dysfunction. Complications include alterations in mentation, seizures, hepatic failure, disseminated

| TABLE 30. | Travel-Associated Infections |
|---|---|
| **Condition** | **Clinical Clues** |
| **Febrile illnesses** | |
| Malaria | Paroxysmal fever, intraerythrocytic parasites, thrombocytopenia |
| Dengue fever | "Saddleback" (biphasic) fever pattern, frontal headache, lumbosacral pain, extensor surface petechiae |
| Typhoid fever | Prolonged fever, diarrhea or constipation, "rose spot" rash (faint salmon-colored macules on the abdomen and trunk) |
| Rickettsial infection | Tick or flea exposure, maculopapular or petechial rash, eschar, lymphadenopathy |
| *Coxiella* infection (Q fever) | Animal contact, atypical pneumonia, elevated aminotransferases |
| Yellow fever | Abrupt fever and headache, relative bradycardia, jaundice |
| Viral hepatitis | Fatigue and anorexia, low-grade fever, hepatomegaly, dark urine, clay-colored stools |
| Mononucleosis syndrome (cytomegalovirus and Epstein-Barr virus) | Sore throat, fever, lymphadenopathy, splenomegaly, atypical lymphocytes |
| Brucellosis | Zoonotic exposure, undulant fever, arthralgia, hepatosplenomegaly |
| Leptospirosis | Conjunctival suffusion (conjunctival erythema without inflammatory exudates), calf and lumbar spine muscle tenderness, aseptic meningitis, jaundice, kidney failure |
| Chikungunya fever | Fever, rash, and small joint polyarthritis |
| Histoplasmosis | Nonproductive cough, chest pain, fever |
| Legionellosis | Pneumonia, diarrhea, fever, elevated aminotransferases, hyponatremia |
| Novel coronaviruses (severe acute respiratory syndrome [SARS], Middle East respiratory syndrome [MERS-CoV]) | Flu-like syndrome prodrome, diarrhea, dry cough with progressive dyspnea, lymphopenia, thrombocytopenia, elevated lactate dehydrogenase |
| Japanese encephalitis | High fever, altered consciousness, cranial nerve palsies |
| Hemorrhagic fever viruses (Ebola, Marburg, and Lassa) | Fever, malaise, myalgia, vomiting, diarrhea, coagulation disorders and bleeding |
| Rabies | Paresthesias or pain at wound site, fever, nausea and vomiting, hydrophobia, delirium, agitation |
| **Travelers' diarrhea** | |
| Bacterial agents: *Escherichia coli*, *Campylobacter* species, *Salmonella* species, *Vibrio* species, *Shigella* species | Abrupt onset, crampy diarrhea, blood in stools |
| Viral agents: rotavirus, norovirus | Closed setting (such as cruise ship or classroom) acquisition, vomiting, diarrhea, short duration |
| Protozoa: *Cryptosporidium* species, microsporidia, *Giardia* species, *Entamoeba histolytica*, and *Isospora* species | Gradual onset, progressive and prolonged diarrhea, foul-smelling and greasy stools, mucus or visible blood in stools |

**CONT.**

intravascular coagulation, brisk intravascular hemolysis, metabolic acidosis, kidney insufficiency and hemoglobinuria, and hypoglycemia. Patients may develop anemia and splenomegaly and frequently have elevated aminotransferases and thrombocytopenia. Various *Plasmodium* species infections are summarized in **Table 31**.

Diagnosis relies primarily on identifying parasitized erythrocytes on a peripheral blood smear. Morphologic features determine the malarial species. Rapid diagnostic tests capable of detecting malaria antigens are available. Tests differ in their ability to detect *P. falciparum* or other *Plasmodium* species and provide only qualitative information. Polymerase chain reaction (PCR) and other molecular tests for malaria detection are increasingly available for clinical use.

Accurate identification of *P. falciparum* and *Plasmodium knowlesi* is critical because of the risk for severe and potentially lethal infection. *P. falciparum* should be suspected if the patient travelled to Africa; symptoms begin soon after return from an endemic area, and the peripheral blood smear shows a high level of parasitemia with typical morphologic features (thin, delicate rings on the inner surface of erythrocytes, banana-shaped gametocytes). *P. knowlesi* is a more recently recognized human pathogen; infection may be severe because of high levels of parasitemia. Examination of the peripheral blood smear reveals all stages of the parasite; the findings may be difficult to distinguish from those for *Plasmodium malariae*, a milder form of malaria. The epidemiologic history is helpful because *P. knowlesi* is not encountered in Africa. **H**

Recommendations for chemoprophylaxis depend on the travel destination and are outlined in **Table 32**. Detailed information about malaria prophylaxis and treatment is provided in the CDC's Yellow Book (http://wwwnc.cdc.gov/travel/page/yellowbook-home).

---
**KEY POINTS**

- The most common symptoms of malaria are fever, headache, myalgia, nausea, vomiting, abdominal pain, and diarrhea.

*(Continued)*

---
**KEY POINTS** *(continued)*

- *Plasmodium falciparum* malaria should be suspected if the patient travelled to Africa and the peripheral blood smear shows a high level of parasitemia with typical morphologic features.

# Typhoid Fever

Typhoid fever is caused by *Salmonella enterica* serotype Typhi. Most cases occur from consuming water or food contaminated by human feces. Travelers to South and East Asia are at especially increased risk for infection. Nontyphoidal *Salmonella* infection is discussed elsewhere (see Infectious Gastrointestinal Syndromes).

The incubation period is 8 to 14 days. Patients present with gradual onset of fever, headache, arthralgia, pharyngitis, anorexia, and abdominal pain and tenderness. Diarrhea may occur early and resolve spontaneously but can become severe late in disease. However, numerous patients have constipation at diagnosis. Without treatment, temperature increases progressively and may remain elevated (up to 40 °C [104 °F]) daily for 4 to 8 weeks ("enteric fever"). Relative bradycardia and prostration may occur. In at least 20% of patients, discrete, pink, blanching lesions (rose spots) appear in crops on the chest and abdomen. Hepatosplenomegaly, leukopenia, anemia, thrombocytopenia, and liver chemistry abnormalities are common and pulmonary infiltrates may be present. Occasionally, secondary bacteremia leads to extraintestinal infection. Serious complications, including intestinal hemorrhage or perforation, may occur 2 to 3 weeks after infection develops. Invasion of the gallbladder by typhoid bacilli may result in a long-term carrier state. Patients with gallstones and chronic biliary disease are at greatest risk.

Diagnosis is made by isolating the organism from blood, stool, urine, or bone marrow. Serologic assays that detect specific *S. enterica* serotype Typhi antibodies have good sensitivity and specificity.

Preferred antibiotics include ceftriaxone, fluoroquinolones, and azithromycin; in consideration of increasing antibiotic resistance, in vitro susceptibility testing should always be

---

| TABLE 31. | Characteristics of *Plasmodium* Species | | | | |
|---|---|---|---|---|---|
| **Characteristics** | *P. vivax* | *P. ovale* | *P. malariae* | *P. falciparum* | *P. knowlesi* |
| Incubation period | 10-30 days | 10-20 days | 15-35 days | 8-25 days | Indeterminate |
| Geographic distribution | Tropical and temperate zones | West Africa and Southeast Asia | Tropical zones | Tropical and temperate zones | South and Southeast Asia |
| Parasitemia | Low | Low | Very low | High | Can be high |
| Risk for disease severity | Low risk | Low risk | Very low risk | High risk | High risk |
| Disease relapse risk | Yes | Yes | Yes | No | No |
| Chloroquine resistance | Yes | No | Rare | Yes | No |

**TABLE 32.** Antimalarial Chemoprophylaxis Regimens

| Drug | Dose | Time of Prophylaxis Initiation (before Travel) | Time of Prophylaxis Discontinuation (after Returning) |
|---|---|---|---|
| **For endemic areas with chloroquine-resistant *Plasmodium falciparum*** | | | |
| Atovaquone/proguanil[a] | 250 mg/100 mg once daily | 1-2 days | 7 days |
| Mefloquine | 250 mg once weekly | ≥2 weeks | 4 weeks |
| Doxycycline[a] | 100 mg once daily | 1-2 days | 4 weeks |
| **For endemic areas with chloroquine-sensitive *P. falciparum*** | | | |
| Chloroquine | 500 mg once weekly | 1-2 weeks | 4 weeks |
| Hydroxychloroquine | 400 mg once weekly | 1-2 weeks | 4 weeks |
| Atovaquone/proguanil | 250/100 mg once daily | 1-2 days | 7 days |
| Mefloquine | 250 mg once weekly | ≥2 weeks | 4 weeks |
| Doxycycline | 100 mg once daily | 1-2 days | 4 weeks |
| Primaquine[b] | 26.3 mg once daily | 1-2 days | 1 week |
| **For endemic areas with *Plasmodium vivax*** | | | |
| Primaquine[b] | 52.6 mg once daily | 1-2 days | 7 days |
| Chloroquine | 500 mg once weekly | 1-2 days | 4 weeks |
| Hydroxychloroquine | 400 mg once weekly | 1-2 weeks | 4 weeks |
| Atovaquone/proguanil | 250/100 mg once daily | 1-2 days | 7 days |
| Mefloquine | 250 mg once weekly | ≥2 weeks | 4 weeks |
| Doxycycline | 100 mg once daily | 1-2 days | 4 weeks |
| **Prophylaxis for relapse due to *Plasmodium vivax* or *Plasmodium ovale*** | | | |
| Primaquine[b] | 52.6 mg once daily | As soon as possible | 14 days |

[a]Should not be used in pregnant women.

[b]Contraindicated in persons with severe forms of glucose-6-phosphate dehydrogenase deficiency or methemoglobin reductase deficiency; should not be administered to pregnant women.

NOTE: Chloroquine is safe during pregnancy; however, pregnant women are advised against entering malarial areas because they experience more severe disease that often leads to maternal and perinatal adverse outcomes. If travel is essential to areas where chloroquine-resistant malaria is present, mefloquine may be safely prescribed.

Recommendations from Centers for Disease Control and Prevention. CDC Health Information for International Travel 2016. http://wwwnc.cdc.gov/travel/yellowbook/2016/infectious-diseases-related-to-travel/malaria. Updated July 10, 2015. Accessed July 17, 2015.

performed. Glucocorticoids may be added to treat severe toxicity, which can manifest as shock or encephalopathy. Vaccination is outlined in Table 29. Vaccination provides protection to 55% to 75% of recipients. **H**

**KEY POINTS**

- Typhoid fever has an incubation period of 8 to 14 days and presents with fever, headache, arthralgia, pharyngitis, anorexia, and abdominal pain and tenderness.
- Preferred antibiotics for typhoid fever include ceftriaxone, fluoroquinolones, and azithromycin.

## Travelers' Diarrhea

Diarrhea secondary to infection is estimated to occur in 40% to 60% of travelers to developing areas of the world. It is defined as three or more unformed stools per day with at least one other clinical sign (fever, cramps, nausea, vomiting, or blood in the stools); most episodes develop within 2 weeks of travel. It is usually self-limited; however, life-threatening volume depletion or severe colitis with systemic manifestations can occur. A few travelers develop chronic diarrhea or a postinfective irritable bowel syndrome. *Escherichia coli* is the most common causative agent. Other pathogens are outlined in Table 30. Persons who take gastric acid–reducing medications or have abnormal gastrointestinal motility or altered anatomy are at increased risk.

Travelers should be advised to avoid consuming tap water (through drinks and ice made with it or brushing teeth with it), undercooked meats and poultry, unpasteurized dairy products, and fruits that are not peeled just before eating. Wine, beer, and carbonated drinks are considered safe. Water can be purified by boiling for 3 minutes or by adding 2 drops of sodium hypochlorite (bleach) or 5 drops of tincture of iodine per 1.89 L of water. Antimicrobial prophylaxis for traveler's diarrhea is effective, but it is generally not recommended because of the potential for adverse effects. Prophylaxis should be considered in persons with coexisting inflammatory bowel disease, immunocompromised states (including advanced HIV), and comorbidities that would be adversely affected by significant dehydration. Antimicrobial agents appropriate for prophylaxis are listed in **Table 33**. Bismuth subsalicylate can be used to prevent diarrhea, but the doses required are inconvenient and can lead to salicylate toxicity.

Fluid replacement is the mainstay of treatment in patients who develop travelers' diarrhea, and most cases will resolve within 3 to 5 days with this therapy alone. Antimicrobials reduce the duration of diarrhea by 1 to 2 days but are recommended only in severe disease, generally defined as more than four unformed stools daily, fever, or blood or pus in the stool. Treatment may also be considered in patients with milder disease if symptoms significantly disrupt a vacation or business trip. Appropriate antimicrobial agents for use in treating traveler's diarrhea are listed in Table 33. Prior to travel, travelers can be given a prescription for antibiotics that can be self-administered according to specific guidelines given to the patient if severe diarrhea develops. Self-treatment with a fluoroquinolone, azithromycin (preferred in South and Southeast Asia), or rifaximin is usually sufficient in most cases. Antimotility drugs, such as loperamide and diphenoxylate, should be given only in conjunction with antimicrobial therapy but should not be used in cases of dysentery or bloody diarrhea because of increased risk for colitis and colonic perforation.

**TABLE 33. Oral Treatment and Prophylaxis of Travelers' Diarrhea**

| Agent | Regimen |
| --- | --- |
| **Treatment** | |
| Bismuth subsalicylate | 1 oz every 30 min for 8 doses |
| Norfloxacin | 400 mg twice daily for 3 days |
| Ciprofloxacin | 500 mg twice daily for 3 days |
| Ofloxacin | 200 mg twice daily for 3 days |
| Levofloxacin | 500 mg once daily for 3 days |
| Azithromycin | 1000 mg, single dose |
| Rifaximin | 200 mg three times daily for 3 days |
| **Prophylaxis** | |
| Bismuth subsalicylate | Two tablets chewed 4 times daily |
| Norfloxacin | 400 mg daily[a] |
| Ciprofloxacin | 500 mg daily[a] |
| Rifaximin | 200 mg once or twice daily[a] |

[a]Chemoprophylaxis is recommended for no more than 2 to 3 weeks (the duration studied in trials and a period short enough to minimize the risk for antimicrobial-associated adverse effects).

Adapted with permission from Hill DR, Ericsson CD, Pearson RD, et al; Infectious Diseases Society of America. The practice of travel medicine: guidelines by the Infectious Diseases Society of America. Clin Infect Dis. 2006 Dec 15;43(12):1499-539. [PMID: 17109284] Copyright 2006 Oxford University Press.

## Dengue Fever

Dengue fever, transmitted by the *Aedes aegypti* mosquito (a daytime feeder that prefers urban environments) is the most prevalent arthropod-borne viral infection in the world. Endemic areas are Southeast Asia, the South Pacific, South and Central America, and the Caribbean.

The incubation period is 4 to 7 days. Patients may be asymptomatic or present with acute febrile illness associated with frontal headache, retro-orbital pain, myalgia, and arthralgia, with or without minor spontaneous bleeding (purpura, melena, conjunctival injection). Gastrointestinal or respiratory symptoms may predominate. Severe lumbosacral pain is characteristic ("breakbone fever"). As the fever abates, a macular or scarlatiniform rash, which spares the palms and soles and evolves into areas of petechiae on extensor surfaces, may develop. Fever resolves after 5 to 7 days; however, a small percentage of patients experience a second febrile period ("saddleback" pattern). A prolonged period of severe fatigue may follow. In patients with severe infection, life-threatening hemorrhage (dengue hemorrhagic fever) or shock may develop, along with liver failure, encephalopathy, and myocardial damage. This syndrome appears to be related to previous dengue viral infection, often of a different serotype. Common laboratory abnormalities include leukopenia, thrombocytopenia, and elevated serum aminotransferase levels.

The diagnosis is based on clinical suspicion in a patient who traveled to an endemic area and presents with fever and other typical signs, symptoms, and laboratory abnormalities. Diagnosis is confirmed by serologic testing (IgM and IgG) or reverse transcriptase PCR. Therapy is supportive. A potential tetravalent dengue vaccine is undergoing trial.

## Hepatitis Virus Infection

Hepatitis A virus (HAV) is the most common cause of viral liver disease in the world. Infection often occurs though ingestion of contaminated food or water. Travel to Central and South America, Mexico, South Asia, and Africa poses the greatest risk for infection. Vaccination is recommended for persons traveling to developing countries and persons not already immune (see Table 29). Serum immune globulin is indicated for persons aged 12 months or younger and for those who decline vaccination or are allergic to its components. It has also been recommended for immunocompromised persons (who are less responsive to hepatitis A vaccine), patients with chronic liver disease, and those planning to depart within 2 weeks of their vaccination.

The risk for travel-associated acquisition of hepatitis B virus is low. Previously unvaccinated persons who have insufficient time before travel to receive the standard three-dose/6-month vaccination series can complete an accelerated vaccination schedule (0, 7, and 21 to 30 days); these persons require a booster dose at 12 months to ensure long-term protection. A combined hepatitis A/B vaccine is also available for this rapid three-dose schedule.

No vaccine prevents hepatitis C virus infection, and prophylactic immune globulin offers no protection. Avoidance of exposure to unscreened blood and nonsterile medical or injection practices is paramount in infection prevention. Tattooing and unprotected sexual practices may also pose an infection risk.

**KEY POINTS**

- Hepatitis A vaccine is available for travelers to endemic areas and should be administered 1 month before travel, with a second booster dose to be given 6 to 12 months later.

- An accelerated vaccination schedule for hepatitis B is available for persons who have insufficient time before planned travel to receive the standard 6-month dosing.

# Rickettsial Infection

Rickettsial infection is transmitted by small vectors (fleas, lice, mites, and ticks). Outbreaks have been associated with war and natural disasters and are promoted by suboptimal hygiene conditions and tick infestation; travel is now well recognized as a risk for infection. *Rickettsia typhi* causes endemic or murine typhus, is transmitted by fleas from a rat reservoir and is prevalent in tropical and subtropical areas. *Rickettsia prowazeki*, the cause of epidemic or louse-borne typhus, is transmitted by human body lice and has a worldwide distribution.

Clinical presentation includes fever, headache, and malaise, often accompanied by a maculopapular, vesicular, or petechial rash. Extensive vasculitic-appearing lesions may occur. Infection with *Rickettsia africae* (African tick typhus) is second only to malaria as the reason for fever in travelers to Africa, especially South Africa. Following the bite of an infected tick or mite, an eschar with regional lymphadenopathy develops at the site of inoculation with *R. africae*, *Rickettsia conorii*, and *Orientia tsutsugamushi*.

Diagnosis is confirmed by PCR, immunohistochemical analysis of tissue samples, or culture during the acute stage of illness before antibiotics are initiated. Empiric therapy is warranted, however, when clinical suspicion of disease is high because these diagnostic tools are not readily available. Serologic tests for convalescent antibodies against many of the common rickettsial pathogens can confirm the diagnosis. The treatment of choice for all rickettsial infections is doxycycline. H

**KEY POINT**

- Rickettsial infection presents with fever, headache, and malaise, often accompanied by a maculopapular, vesicular, or petechial rash.

# Brucellosis

Brucellosis occurs by ingestion of unpasteurized dairy products or undercooked meat, by direct contact with fluids from infected animals through skin wounds or mucous membranes, or by inhalation of contaminated aerosols. *Brucella* species are present in animal reservoirs worldwide.

The Mediterranean basin, Indian subcontinent, Arabian Peninsula, and parts of Central and South America, Mexico, Asia, and Africa are high-prevalence areas. After a variable incubation period, patients develop fever, myalgia, arthralgia, fatigue, headache, and night sweats. Depression is frequent. Focal infection may occur, most commonly osteoarticular involvement. Infection with *B. melitensis* and *B. suis* causes the most severe disease. Hepatosplenomegaly and lymphadenopathy may be apparent on physical examination. Disease relapse and chronic infection occur in few patients, most often from persistent foci of infection or inadequate antibiotic treatment.

Diagnosis relies on isolating the organism from cultures of blood, bone marrow, other body fluids, or tissue. The serum agglutination test is the most widely used serologic test available. An initial elevated titer of 1:160 or greater or demonstration of a fourfold increase from acute to convalescent titers is considered diagnostic. The treatment of choice is a combination of doxycycline, rifampin, and streptomycin (or gentamicin), often given for several weeks. H

**KEY POINT**

- Patients with brucellosis develop fever, myalgia, arthralgia, fatigue, headache, and night sweats, often with depression.

# Travel-Associated Fungal Diseases

The endemic fungi are generally limited to specific geographic areas (**Table 34**). Unlike most other travel-related infections, disease may not become clinically evident until months or even years after returning from travel. Histoplasmosis and coccidioidomycosis are the most frequently reported travel-related fungal infections (see Fungal Infections chapter for a full discussion of these diseases).

**TABLE 34. Common Travel-Associated Acquired Fungal Infections**

| Organism | Geographic Distribution |
|---|---|
| *Coccidioides* species | Southwest United States |
| | Mexico |
| | Central and South America |
| *Histoplasma* species | Mississippi and Ohio River Valleys |
| | Mexico |
| | Central America |
| *Penicillium marneffei* | Southeast Asia |
| | Southern China |

## Other Important Diseases

### Yellow Fever

Yellow fever is a flavivirus transmitted by the *Aedes* mosquito. Countries in tropical South America and sub-Saharan Africa are the geographic areas with the highest endemicity. After a 3- to 5-day incubation period, most patients present with fever, headache, myalgias, and backache. Serious multisystem disease (jaundice, hemorrhage, and shock) may develop. Immunization (see Table 29) is indicated for travelers to at-risk areas and to specific countries requiring proof of vaccination before entry.

### Rabies

Rabies is found worldwide, except in Antarctica. Although dogs are the major source of infection in developing countries, specific enzootic hosts may predominate in various geographic areas. Preexposure vaccination (see Table 29) is recommended for those traveling to any high-risk international destination with the intention of a prolonged stay. Short-term travelers who may be at risk include adventure travelers and cave explorers. When determined that the bite poses a risk for rabies, two doses of rabies vaccine should be given to persons who have previously completed a preexposure vaccine series. Unvaccinated persons require rabies immune globulin followed by rabies vaccination.

### Leptospirosis

The zoonosis leptospirosis is endemic worldwide. Infection occurs by direct exposure to urine or tissues of infected animals or indirectly through contaminated water or soil. Rodents and other small mammals are the most significant sources of human disease. Bacteria may be introduced through cuts and abrasions of the skin, mucous membranes or conjunctivae, or inhalation of aerosolized droplets. Acute systemic illness is manifested by high fever, headache, severe myalgias (especially in the lumbar region and calf muscles), conjunctival injection, abdominal pain, diarrhea, pharyngitis, and occasionally a pretibial rash. A second immune phase of illness is heralded by the production of antibodies and may include jaundice, kidney disease, pneumonitis, cardiac arrhythmia, hemorrhage, and aseptic meningitis.

Diagnosis relies on clinical suspicion and confirmatory serologic assays. Doxycycline is effective in treating mild disease, whereas intravenous penicillin or ceftriaxone is recommended for moderate to severe cases. Travelers at increased risk for infection may be given weekly chemoprophylaxis with doxycycline.

### Q Fever

*Coxiella burnetii* is the causative bacterial agent of Q fever, a zoonotic illness acquired through inhalation of aerosols contaminated by the infected placenta of cattle, sheep, and goats. Travel to Middle Eastern and African countries poses the greatest risk. Most infections manifest as a self-limited febrile illness, although some patients develop an atypical pneumonia with hepatitis. The diagnosis is often confirmed serologically, and doxycycline is the treatment of choice.

### Ebola

Ebola is a Filovirus associated with the viral hemorrhagic fever syndrome. Human outbreaks have sporadically occurred in regions of central Africa since 1976; however, the largest epidemic is ongoing in West African countries, which increases the risk for travel-associated disease. Infection can spread through direct contact with bodily fluids of symptomatic patients or improper infection control practices. Disease is often severe and manifested by abrupt fever, headache, prostration, coagulopathy, and multiorgan failure. Ill travelers at risk for Ebola infection must be rapidly identified and isolated when they present for care. Treatment consists of supportive measures. Potential antiviral medications are in trials. Artificial, passive immunity using antibodies from recovered patients has met with some success, and vaccine trials are ongoing.

# Infectious Gastrointestinal Syndromes

Diarrhea (the passage of three or more unformed stools per day) is a common reason for acute medical evaluation. Diarrhea can be subclassified as acute (symptoms <14 days), subacute (14-30 days), or chronic (>30 days), with the duration of symptoms guiding appropriate testing. Most bacterial and viral gastrointestinal infections cause an acute diarrheal syndrome. Chronic diarrhea is unlikely to be infectious, with the exception of parasitic syndromes. Most infectious diarrhea is self-limited and resolves without directed intervention. Otherwise healthy patients with mild illness who present with less than 72 hours of symptoms can often be treated supportively, with no additional diagnostic evaluation or antimicrobial treatment. More severe presentations, including fever, significant abdominal pain, or dysentery (visible blood or mucus in stool), suggest inflammatory diarrhea caused by an invasive pathogen. Antimotility agents, such as loperamide, are discouraged for the treatment of inflammatory diarrhea or *Clostridium difficile* colitis but may relieve symptoms for patients with noninfectious diarrhea.

Patients with acute diarrhea who are immunocompromised, require hospitalization, or have inflammatory diarrhea should have stool cultures performed. Routine stool cultures can identify the most common bacterial pathogens causing diarrhea (**Table 35**); however, when enterotoxigenic *Escherichia coli*

**TABLE 35.** Causative Agents, Clinical Presentation, and Treatment of Infectious Colitis

| Agent | Clinical Findings | Diagnosis | Antimicrobial Treatment[a] |
|---|---|---|---|
| **Bacterial** | | | |
| *Campylobacter* | Fevers, chills, diarrhea (watery or bloody), crampy abdominal pain | Standard stool culture | Azithromycin or erythromycin × 3-5 days |
| *Shigella* | Dysentery (fevers, abdominal cramps, tenesmus, bloody/mucusy stools) | Routine stool culture | Fluoroquinolone × 3 days; azithromycin × 3 days |
| *Salmonella* | Fever, chills, diarrhea (watery or bloody), cramps, myalgia; bacteremia in 10%-25% of cases | Routine stool culture; blood cultures (with moderate to severe illness) | Mild: none<br><br>Underlying disease or severe illness: fluoroquinolone plus parenteral third-generation cephalosporin |
| STEC including *Escherichia coli* O157:H7 | Bloody stools in >80% of cases; fever often absent or low grade; may be associated with HUS | *E. coli* O157:H7: stool culture with specialized media followed by serologic testing<br><br>Other STEC: stool culture with specialized media followed by Shiga toxin serologic testing or PCR | None |
| ETEC (travelers' diarrhea) | Nonbloody, watery stools; constitutional symptoms rare | None | Fluoroquinolone × 3 days, azithromycin × 1 dose, or rifaximin × 3 days |
| *Yersinia* | Fever, diarrhea, right lower quadrant pain (may mimic appendicitis) | Routine stool culture | Fluoroquinolone × 3 days; trimethoprim-sulfamethoxazole × 3 days |
| *Vibrio* | Bloody stools (>25% of cases), fever, vomiting (>50% of cases) | Stool culture with specialized media | Fluoroquinolone × 3 days; azithromycin × 3 days |
| *Clostridium difficile* | Diarrhea, fever, abdominal pain/cramping, colonic distention (including toxic megacolon in severe cases), leukocytosis, sepsis; gross blood uncommon | PCR or stool EIA for toxin | Mild: metronidazole<br><br>Severe: oral vancomycin |
| **Viral** | | | |
| Norovirus | Watery, noninflammatory diarrhea; vomiting in >50% of cases; short incubation period and high attack rate; fever rare | None (PCR for outbreak investigations) | None |
| **Parasitic** | | | |
| *Giardia* | Watery diarrhea, abdominal cramping, vomiting, steatorrhea, flatulence, weight loss | Stool O & P microscopy or stool antigen | Metronidazole × 5-10 days or tinidazole |
| *Cryptosporidium* | Watery diarrhea | Modified acid-fast stain, stool antigen | Supportive care |
| Amebiasis | Dysentery | Stool O & P microscopy, stool antigen | Tinidazole or metronidazole |
| *Cyclospora* | Watery diarrhea, bloating, flatulence, weight loss | Modified acid-fast stain | Trimethoprim-sulfamethoxazole |

EIA = enzyme immunoassay; ETEC = enterotoxigenic *Escherichia coli*; HUS = hemolytic uremic syndrome; O & P = ova and parasites; PCR = polymerase chain reaction; STEC = shiga toxin–producing *E. coli*.

[a]Empiric treatment with final choice of antimicrobial guided by in vitro susceptibility testing.

**CONT.**

(ETEC, including *E. coli* O157:H7) or *Vibrio* infection is suspected, the laboratory should be notified because these organisms require special media for growth. Even with testing restricted to this select population, a pathogen is identified in less than 5% of all stool cultures. Molecular tests using a multiplex panel to identify common bacterial, viral, and parasitic organisms on a single stool sample are increasingly available and may have improved sensitivity but are costly. Diagnostic testing for *Clostridium difficile* should be performed in this subgroup of patients, regardless of a history of recent antibiotic use. Blood cultures should be obtained in patients requiring hospitalization or when *Salmonella* gastroenteritis is suspected. **H**

**KEY POINTS**

- Most infectious diarrhea is self-limited and resolves without directed intervention; otherwise healthy patients with mild illness who present with less than 72 hours of symptoms can often be treated supportively, with no additional diagnostic evaluation or antimicrobial treatment.

- Diagnostic testing, including stool bacterial cultures, is appropriate for patients who are immunocompromised, sick enough to require hospitalization or those with inflammatory diarrhea.

## *Campylobacter* Infection

*Campylobacter* gastroenteritis is primarily a foodborne illness particularly associated with consumption of undercooked poultry products. Person-to-person transmission is rare. Symptoms are indistinguishable from other causes of invasive diarrhea (see Table 35). Immunocompromised patients are at increased risk for associated sepsis and extraintestinal infections. Routine stool culture is typically diagnostic, and blood cultures may be positive with extraintestinal disease.

Antibiotic treatment guided by in vitro susceptibility testing is recommended to hasten resolution of symptoms when *Campylobacter* is isolated in stools. Empiric therapy is controversial because antibiotics are contraindicated for other causes of dysentery, such as Shiga toxin–producing *E. coli* (STEC), but is indicated in patients who are immunocompromised or severely ill. Because of increasing resistance to fluoroquinolones, macrolides are the preferred empiric treatment if *Campylobacter* infection is suspected. Often, symptoms have spontaneously improved by the time culture results are obtained, so no therapy is needed.

Diarrhea may persist for a prolonged duration in the absence of ongoing bacterial infection, suggesting a postinfective irritable bowel syndrome. *Campylobacter* is one of several enteric pathogens associated with reactive arthritis in patients positive for HLA-B27 antigen. The most serious postinfective complication is Guillain-Barré syndrome, which is thought to be caused by production of an antibody directed against the bacteria that cross-reacts with host neuronal tissue, causing peripheral nerve demyelination. Although Guillain-Barré syndrome can be linked to previous *Campylobacter* infection in numerous patients, the risk for neurologic complications after this infection is less than 1%. **H**

**KEY POINT**

- Antibiotic treatment guided by in vitro susceptibility testing is recommended to hasten resolution of symptoms when *Campylobacter* is isolated in stools; if indicated, macrolides are the preferred empiric antibiotics for symptomatic patients suspected of having *Campylobacter* gastroenteritis.

## *Shigella* Infection

Shigellosis is caused by one of four species of *Shigella*, with disease severity varying depending on the infecting organism. The number of ingested bacteria necessary to cause infection is low (<100 organisms), and person-to-person transmission through fecal-oral spread is common. Outbreaks of shigellosis are most frequent in settings with close contact and poor hygiene or inability to use a toilet, such as day care centers or nursing homes. Other routes of infection include ingestion of contaminated food or water and sexual transmission among men who have sex with men. The clinical presentation is summarized in Table 35. Vomiting is occasionally present. Reactive arthritis may be seen in up to 3% of patients with *Shigella flexneri* infection, but not with other species. *Shigella dysenteriae* produces a Shiga toxin similar to that of STEC and is a rare cause of hemolytic uremic syndrome (HUS).

Stool cultures should be obtained in all patients with significant illness or dysentery at presentation. *Shigella* infection can be diagnosed by standard stool cultures or molecular assay; the latter may be more sensitive. Blood cultures should be obtained in patients with severe disease or sepsis syndromes. Antibiotics reduce the duration of gastrointestinal symptoms. Empiric therapy (see Table 35) should be considered for patients with a compatible epidemiologic history (such as day care workers) or severe symptoms. In most cases, infection is self-limited and resolves without treatment; however, because asymptomatic shedding may be prolonged after infection, antibiotics are recommended for all patients with positive stool cultures to reduce the risk for secondary transmission. **H**

**KEY POINT**

- Empiric therapy for *Shigella* infection should be considered for patients with a compatible epidemiologic history or severe symptoms and is recommended for all patients with positive stool cultures to reduce the risk for secondary transmission.

## *Salmonella* Infection

*Salmonella* causes typhoidal (serotypes Typhi or Paratyphi) or nontyphoidal (all other serotypes) infections. Nontyphoidal serotypes are the leading cause of foodborne illness in the

United States, with a broad array of implicated sources, including eggs, raw meat, dairy products, peanut butter, and fresh fruits and vegetables. Zoonotic infections associated with reptile exposure account for less than 5% of infections. Clinical manifestations of *Salmonella* gastroenteritis are summarized in Table 35. Occult blood is common, but grossly bloody stools are infrequent and suggest infection with *Shigella* or STEC.

Bacteremia occurs in 1% to 4% of immunocompetent patients with gastrointestinal salmonellosis and is significantly more common in older adults or immunocompromised patients. Bacteremia is associated with endothelial infection in 10% to 25% of patients, including aortitis, arteritis, or mycotic aneurysm. Vascular complications are associated with pre-existing atherosclerosis, placing older adults at especially high risk. *Salmonella* osteomyelitis is an unusual complication seen primarily in patients with sickle cell disease.

Treatment decisions must consider the severity of the infection and the risk for extraintestinal disease (**Table 36**). Antibiotic treatment of otherwise healthy patients with mild symptoms does not hasten recovery and may lead to prolonged asymptomatic shedding of bacteria. However, treatment of patients with severe disease, characterized by high fever, sepsis syndrome, or hemodynamic instability, is associated with shorter duration of symptoms and is presumed to decrease the risk for extraintestinal spread. Patients who have underlying health conditions or use medications that place them at increased risk for bacteremia or endovascular infection should also be treated to prevent these life-threatening complications (see Table 36).

Fluoroquinolones remain the most reliably effective class of antibiotics for empiric therapy, although increasing resistance has been reported. Other agents that often have activity include amoxicillin, trimethoprim-sulfamethoxazole, and azithromycin. Patients with severe illness requiring hospitalization should be treated with a fluoroquinolone and a third-generation cephalosporin, pending in vitro susceptibility testing. Endovascular infections typically require surgical removal of prosthetic material or infected valves and a 6-week course of antibiotic treatment.

**KEY POINTS**

- Antibiotic treatment of otherwise healthy patients with mild symptoms does not hasten recovery and may lead to prolonged asymptomatic shedding of *Salmonella* bacteria. **HVC**

- Treatment of patients with severe salmonellosis, characterized by high fever, sepsis syndrome, or hemodynamic instability, is associated with shorter duration of symptoms and is presumed to decrease the risk for extraintestinal spread.

## *Escherichia coli* Infection

*E. coli* is universally present in the healthy intestinal microbiota; however, particular pathotypes are associated with diarrheal illnesses. Two pathotypes, STEC and ETEC, are particularly significant. STEC (also called enterohemorrhagic *E. coli*) infection is a significant cause of dysentery; clinical findings are provided in Table 35. The prototypical STEC agent is *E. coli* O157:H7, which has been associated with numerous foodborne outbreaks of diarrhea and HUS. STEC causes inflammation through production of Shiga toxin but does not invade the colonic mucosa. *E. coli* O157:H7 requires specialized media for culture. Diagnostic testing depends on laboratory protocol. Some laboratories routinely plate all stool samples on media capable of detecting *E. coli* O157:H7; other laboratories restrict testing to

**TABLE 36.** Antibiotic Treatment Considerations for Salmonellosis

| Host | Clinical Presentation | Antibiotic Treatment[a] | Comments |
|------|----------------------|------------------------|----------|
| Healthy adults age ≤50 years | Mild to moderate gastrointestinal symptoms | None | No significant decrease in duration of symptoms, potential for prolonged shedding |
| | Severe gastrointestinal symptoms, sepsis syndrome | Fluoroquinolone plus parenteral third-generation cephalosporin | Treatment in severely ill patients associated with decreased duration of symptoms |
| Healthy adults age >50 years | Mild to severe gastroenteritis | Fluoroquinolone | Increased risk for bacteremia |
| Vascular grafts or prosthetic material (including prosthetic heart valves) | Mild to severe gastroenteritis | Fluoroquinolone | Increased risk for endovascular infection |
| Prosthetic joint | Mild to severe gastroenteritis | Fluoroquinolone | Increased risk for secondary infection with bacteremia |
| Immunocompromised hosts[b] | Mild to severe gastroenteritis | Fluoroquinolone | Increased risk for bacteremia or extraintestinal infection |
| Any | Bacteremia | Fluoroquinolone plus parenteral third-generation cephalosporin | Evaluation for endovascular infection if prosthetic material or sustained bacteremia |

[a]Empiric treatment, with final choice of antibiotic guided by in vitro susceptibility testing.

[b]Includes patients with HIV/AIDS, recent chemotherapy, use of immunosuppressing medications (such as glucocorticoids or tumor necrosis factor-α inhibitors), or hemoglobinopathies (such as sickle cell disease).

**CONT.**

only grossly bloody stools or to clinician request. Considering this variability, the laboratory should be notified when STEC is a concern to ensure appropriate testing is performed. When *E. coli* is isolated, confirmatory testing for the O157:H7 antigen is performed reflexively. Other strains of STEC, such as *E. coli* O104:H4, which caused a large outbreak in Europe, are increasingly recognized as causing dysentery, and additional testing for Shiga toxin production may be pursued in these cases. Molecular tests of stool using a multiplex panel capable of detecting numerous pathogens causing dysentery, including STEC organisms, are increasingly being used for rapid diagnosis. Administration of antibiotics and antimotility medications for STEC infection has been associated with increased risk for HUS. Therefore, decisions about treatment of dysentery with empiric antibiotics should be made with caution, weighing the probability of STEC versus other causes of invasive colitis.

ETEC is the most frequent cause of travelers' diarrhea but is also increasingly recognized as a cause of foodborne illness in developed countries. Laboratory testing for this organism is lacking outside of research settings, so determining the incidence of ETEC is difficult. ETEC causes disease through toxin production, resulting in a secretory diarrhea. Clinical manifestations are outlined in Table 35. Even without treatment, illness lasts less than 1 week. Preemptive treatment aimed at shortening the duration of symptoms is common when travelers to a developing region develop diarrhea. Recommended agents include fluoroquinolones, azithromycin, and rifaximin. **H**

**KEY POINT**

- Administration of antibiotics and antimotility medications for Shiga toxin–producing *Escherichia coli* infection has been associated with increased risk for hemolytic uremic syndrome.

## **H** *Yersinia* Infection

Enterocolitis due to *Yersinia* infection is uncommon. Most cases are associated with *Yersinia enterocolitica*, and infection usually occurs through ingestion of contaminated food products, especially undercooked pork. *Yersinia* infection causes acute inflammatory enteritis and is indistinguishable from other causes of inflammatory diarrhea. However, grossly bloody stools are uncommon. *Yersinia* is trophic for gastrointestinal lymphoid tissue. When mesenteric lymph nodes become infected, abdominal pain may localize to the right lower quadrant; this may mimic the presentation of appendicitis, so the diagnosis is often made at surgery. Postinfectious arthritis may occur in patients positive for HLA-B27. Stool culture is typically diagnostic; the organism may also be cultured from surgical specimens if appendectomy is performed. Treatment has not been clearly associated with improved clinical outcomes but does lead to more rapid eradication of bacteria from stool. Most strains are resistant to amoxicillin and macrolides but sensitive to fluoroquinolones and trimethoprim-sulfamethoxazole. **H**

**KEY POINT**

- *Yersinia* is trophic for gastrointestinal lymphoid tissue, and infection can mimic the presentation of appendicitis.

## *Vibrio* Infection **H**

Non-cholera-causing species of *Vibrio*, particularly *Vibrio parahaemolyticus* and *Vibrio vulnificus*, are significant causes of foodborne gastrointestinal infections. These bacteria live in salt water, and human infection most commonly occurs through ingestion of raw or undercooked seafood, particularly shellfish. *Vibrio* gastroenteritis is indistinguishable from other bacterial causes. Clinical findings are outlined in Table 35. Severe infections may be seen in patients with hepatic dysfunction and heavy alcohol use. In this population, bloodstream infection with resultant sepsis is common, with a fatality rate approaching 30%. Skin and soft tissue infections caused by *Vibrio* usually occur through cutaneous exposure to contaminated water and not through ingestion. *Vibrio* does not grow well on routine stool cultures; specialized media with high saline content are required. Most isolates are sensitive to fluoroquinolones and macrolides. **H**

**KEY POINT**

- Severe disease may occur in patients with *Vibrio* infection who have hepatic dysfunction and heavy alcohol use; bloodstream infection with resultant sepsis is common in this population, with a fatality rate approaching 30%.

## *Clostridium difficile* Infection **H**

*Clostridium difficile* infection (CDI) is the most common cause of health care–associated colitis. The incidence of this potentially devastating infection has more than doubled in the last decade. CDI is increasingly recognized as a significant cause of diarrhea outside of the hospital. National surveillance data identified half of all cases of CDI as community onset, and greater than 5% had no known previous health care or antibiotic exposure. Asymptomatic carriage of *C. difficile* is identified in more than 20% of patients hospitalized without diarrhea. These patients are an important source of secondary transmission in health care settings through fecal-oral spread of bacteria or spores. Antibiotic use is the strongest risk factor for CDI. It is most highly associated with antimicrobial agents that have activity against anaerobic colonic flora but are not effective against *C. difficile* (such as clindamycin). Antibiotic-associated diarrhea in these cases is thought to occur by suppression of the intestinal microbiota, with resultant overgrowth of *C. difficile* organisms and production of toxin (toxins A and B). Strains of *C. difficile* causing particularly fulminant infection have been identified, and disease in these cases is related to elevated production of toxins A and B and production of a novel binary toxin. These hypervirulent strains have been associated with severe or even fatal disease and may occur in patients without any known antibiotic use or health care exposure.

The clinical presentation of CDI is broad (findings shown in Table 35). CDI frequently causes a pronounced leukemoid reaction and is identified in 25% of hospitalized patients with leukocyte counts of 30,000/μL (30 × 10⁹/L) or more. Determination of CDI severity has prognostic and treatment ramifications. Features associated with severe infections are listed in **Table 37**.

Diagnosis relies on laboratory identification of *C. difficile* in stool samples; however, the presence of this organism does not necessarily imply disease because asymptomatic colonization may occur. Therefore, many laboratories perform testing only on unformed or liquid stool specimens. Enzyme immunoassays (EIAs) to detect toxin are specific, but sensitivity using a single stool sample is 75% to 85%. EIA results may be false negative when toxin production is low or if a strain does not produce the particular toxin the test is optimized to detect. Polymerase chain reaction (PCR) assays to detect the genes responsible for production of toxins A and B are increasingly used for diagnosis and allow improved sensitivity compared with EIAs. Considering the high sensitivity of PCR testing, repeat testing within 1 week of a negative result is unlikely to provide additional information; a negative result essentially rules out this infection. In patients with negative PCR results, an alternative cause should be considered. Stool cultures and cell culture cytotoxicity assays are not useful for clinical management. Visualization of colonic pseudomembranes may suggest CDI, but endoscopy is not recommended for purely diagnostic purposes.

**TABLE 37.** Clinical Features Associated with Severity of *Clostridium difficile* Infection

| Variable | Mild to Moderate CDI | Severe CDI |
|---|---|---|
| Leukocytes (cells/μL [cells × 10⁹/L])ᵃ | ≤15,000 (15 × 10⁹/L) | >15,000 (15 × 10⁹/L) |
| Serum creatinineᵃ | <1.5 times the baseline level | ≥1.5 times the baseline level |
| Age (y)ᵃ | ≤60 | >60 |
| Temperature (°C [°F]) | ≤38.3 (100.9) | >38.3 (100.9) |
| Serum albumin (g/dL [g/L]) | ≥2.5 (25) | <2.5 (25) |
| Endoscopic visualization of pseudomembranes | Absent | Present |
| Admission to ICU | No | Yes |
| Ileus or megacolon | No | Yes |

CDI = *Clostridium difficile* infection.

ᵃFactors noted as indicating severity of disease in Society for Healthcare Epidemiology of America/Infectious Diseases Society of America guidelines.

All patients with confirmed CDI require antimicrobial treatment, but optimal management depends on whether the episode represents the initial presentation or a recurrence and the severity of the illness (**Figure 20**). Oral metronidazole and vancomycin are equally effective in the treatment of

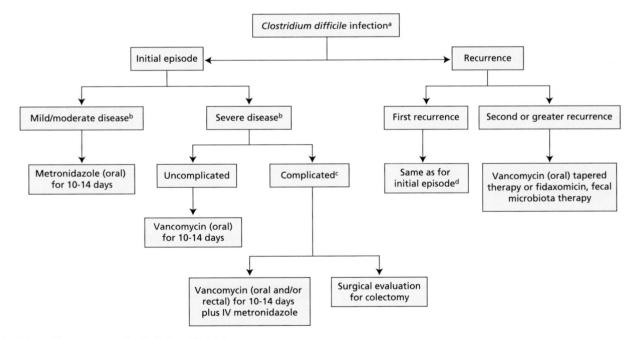

**FIGURE 20.** Treatment options for *Clostridium difficile* infection.

IV = intravenous.

ᵃDefined as diarrhea with a confirmatory laboratory test.

ᵇSevere disease is defined as any of the following: (1) leukocyte count >15,000/μL (15 × 10⁹L); (2) serum creatinine level ≥1.5 times baseline level; (3) age >60 years.

ᶜAssociated with ileus, megacolon, or hypotension.

ᵈBased on disease severity at the time of recurrence (e.g., a mild-to-moderate first recurrence would be appropriately treated with the same regimen as for an initial mild-to-moderate case).

CONT.

mild-to-moderate CDI, with the former preferred because of its lower cost.

Relapse is seen in approximately 20% of patients regardless of antibiotic given. At initial relapse, a repeat course of the same medication may be used, assuming disease severity remains the same. In patients with a second relapse, treatment options include oral vancomycin given as a prolonged taper over more than 6 weeks or fidaxomicin, a nonabsorbable macrolide. Fidaxomicin has been associated with lower rates of subsequent relapses compared with oral vancomycin when used to treat the initial episode, but it is significantly more expensive. A terminal course of 2 weeks of rifaximin after pronged vancomycin pulsed taper (antibiotic given at the end of the course every other or every third day) has been beneficial in some case series.

Severe CDI is associated with significant medical costs, morbidity, and mortality. Oral vancomycin is superior to metronidazole in this subgroup and should be the initial treatment of choice. Ileus is frequently present, limiting colonic transit of orally dosed medications; therefore, a vancomycin enema through a rectal tube should be considered to maximize colonic luminal concentrations. Parenteral vancomycin does not penetrate intraluminally; however, intravenous metronidazole achieves detectable fecal levels and can be used in combination with oral or rectal vancomycin in critically ill patients. Fidaxomicin has not been well studied in severe CDI but may be indicated as salvage therapy in patients not responding to standard therapy. Surgical consultation for emergent colectomy is indicated in patients with toxic megacolon, colonic perforation, or severe sepsis.

Fecal microbiota transplant (FMT) has been advocated as a treatment approach for patients with multiple relapses of CDI. The rationale is that exogenous feces will restore the normal colonic microbiota. Numerous studies have documented improved outcomes in patients treated with FMT. Issues related to choice of donor, potential transmission of infectious agents in donor stool, method of administration, and logistics have limited the widespread implementation of FMT. Because of these challenges, increasing interest has focused on probiotic regimens to repopulate the bowel flora in patients with CDI. Probiotics have been effective in reducing the risk for CDI among patients prescribed antibiotics. The data on use of probiotics for treatment of CDI are less compelling; initial studies have not found a benefit in probiotics for treatment of CDI, but subsequent studies suggest some role for adjuvant probiotics in treatment of mild-to-moderate relapsing disease. Concern exists that use of probiotics in immunocompromised patients may be associated with development of extraintestinal infections.

*C. difficile* spores are stable for prolonged periods in the environment, which allows secondary spread of infection. This is a particular concern in health care settings. Alcohol-based hand gels are inferior to soap and water for eradication of spores, and hand washing is indicated for all health care workers interacting with infected patients. Hospitalized patients with CDI should be placed in contact isolation at least until diarrhea resolves. Documenting clearance of *C. difficile* through testing serial stool samples after an initial positive test result has no role in management.

**KEY POINTS**

- Enzyme immunoassays for *Clostridium difficile* infection have good specificity, but sensitivity using a single stool sample is only 75% to 85%; polymerase chain reaction assays to detect the genes responsible for production of toxins A and B are increasingly used for diagnosis with better sensitivity.

- Oral metronidazole and vancomycin are equally effective in treating mild-to-moderate *Clostridium difficile* infection, with the former preferred because of its lower cost; oral vancomycin is recommended for severe disease. **HVC**

- Fecal microbiota transplant is an effective treatment approach for patients with multiple relapses of *Clostridium difficile* infection and is effective in reducing the risk for this infection among patients prescribed antibiotics.

- Documenting clearance of *C. difficile* through testing serial stool samples after an initial positive test result has no role in management. **HVC**

# Viral Gastroenteritis

Most cases of gastroenteritis are caused by viral pathogens. In immunocompetent patients, viral gastroenteritis is typically a mild, self-limited illness, and neither laboratory diagnosis nor directed treatment is indicated. The most significant viral cause of diarrhea in adults is norovirus, which has been associated with large outbreaks of gastrointestinal disease. Most cases are believed to be spread through fecal-oral transmission following ingestion of contaminated foods or water. Transmission via contact with contaminated surfaces is common. Clinical manifestations are outlined in Table 35. Diarrhea typically lasts less than 72 hours, which may distinguish viral from bacterial causes of gastroenteritis. Laboratory confirmation is indicated only for epidemiologic investigation of outbreaks. People with suspected infections should not handle food, and their clothing and bedding should be thoroughly washed.

**KEY POINT**

- Norovirus-caused viral gastroenteritis is most likely spread through ingestion of contaminated food or water.

# Parasitic Infections

Parasitic gastrointestinal infections are most common in developing countries but can occur throughout the world.

Protozoan infections cause subacute or chronic diarrhea. The yield of stool parasitic tests varies according to local prevalence, host immune status, history of travel, and duration of symptoms. In developed countries, stool microscopy has positive results in less than 10% of cases. Testing for parasites is not recommended for diarrhea lasting less than 7 days or for patients who develop diarrhea more than 3 days into a hospital stay.

### *Giardia* Infection

*Giardia* is widespread in zoonotic reservoirs, and infections occur worldwide through ingestion of contaminated food and water. Excretion of cysts by beavers and other animals leads to contamination of natural water supplies, and persons who drink untreated fresh water are at particular risk for giardiasis. Infection is asymptomatic in up to two thirds of cases, but cysts may be shed for many months, with the potential for secondary spread. Clinical manifestations are outlined in Table 35. In many cases, symptoms resolve spontaneously without treatment, but a subset of patients will develop chronic symptoms with significant weight loss owing to malabsorption and anorexia. Hypogammaglobulinemia and IgA deficiency are risk factors for prolonged infection.

Because *Giardia* cysts are intermittently shed, stool microscopy is less sensitive than stool antigen testing. Treatment with metronidazole is curative in more than 85% of patients. Another nitroimidazole, tinidazole, is curative in approximately 90% of patients and offers the advantage of single-dose therapy. Occasionally, nitroimidazole resistance causes treatment failures with these agents; in this case, nitazoxanide may be effective. Infection in pregnant women is particularly problematic because nitroimidazoles are contraindicated during the first trimester. Paromomycin is an alternative. Even after eradication of the protozoa, diarrhea may persist because of infection-induced lactose intolerance, and diet modification in the months after treatment will minimize postinfective symptoms.

**KEY POINTS**

HVC
- Testing for parasites is not recommended for diarrhea lasting less than 7 days or for patients who develop diarrhea more than 3 days into a hospital stay.

- Treatment of giardiasis with metronidazole is curative in more than 85% of patients.

### *Cryptosporidium* Infection

Cryptosporidia infections are ubiquitous in the environment. Infection can occur in humans by close contact with infected animals, as can happen in petting zoos or through consumption of contaminated water or food. Immunocompromised patients, especially those with HIV/AIDS, are particularly susceptible to infection. Large community outbreaks following contamination of municipal water supplies have been reported. Infections in immunocompetent persons are usually asymptomatic or associated with a self-limited diarrheal illness. Among patients with AIDS, diarrhea may be prolonged and the large volume of stools may lead to dehydration and pronounced weight loss. Oocysts are not well visualized with conventional microscopy for ova and parasites but may be seen with modified acid-fast staining. Because oocytes may be shed intermittently, stool antigen testing is more sensitive than microscopy. Most immunocompetent patients do not require treatment, but nitazoxanide should be considered in symptomatic patients. Those with HIV often clear chronic infection with initiation of antiretroviral therapy.

**KEY POINT**

- Immunocompromised patients, especially those with HIV/AIDS, are particularly susceptible to *Cryptosporidium* infection; in patients with AIDS, diarrhea may be prolonged, and the large volume of stools may lead to dehydration and pronounced weight loss.

### Amebiasis

*Entamoeba histolytica* causes amoebic dysentery. Other species of *Entamoeba* may colonize the gastrointestinal tract but are not pathogenic and, when identified, do not mandate treatment. In developed countries, amebiasis is usually seen in immigrants or travelers returning from extended stays in endemic areas. Infections may be seen in institutional settings, where poor hygiene may predispose to spread of oocytes. Although most infected patients are asymptomatic, a subset develops dysentery with prolonged shedding in stool with visible blood or mucus. Stool microscopy for ova and parasites may detect the protozoa and is most sensitive if sequential samples are submitted, but stool antigen testing is more sensitive. Serum antibodies may also be useful in suggesting the diagnosis but cannot distinguish recent from remote infection. Tinidazole or metronidazole is effective as initial treatment, followed by a second agent, such as paromomycin, for eradication of intraluminal cysts.

**KEY POINT**

- Stool antigen testing is more sensitive than ova and parasite examination for the diagnosis of amebiasis.

### *Cyclospora* Infection

*Cyclospora* species are widespread in the environment. Infections in the United States are most commonly associated with ingestion of contaminated fruits and vegetables imported internationally. Sporadic cases and outbreaks of cyclosporiasis have been identified. Symptoms are outlined in Table 35. Persons with HIV infection may have more severe illness associated with wasting. Modified acid-fast stains are required to visualize oocytes. Trimethoprim-sulfamethoxazole is the treatment of choice for symptomatic patients, with ciprofloxacin an alternative for patients intolerant to sulfa antimicrobials.

**KEY POINT**

- Trimethoprim-sulfamethoxazole is the treatment of choice for *Cyclospora* infection in patients with symptoms; ciprofloxacin is an alternative for anyone intolerant of sulfa antimicrobial agents.

# Infections in Transplant Recipients

## Introduction

Rates of transplantation of solid organs or hematopoietic stem cells continue to rise in the United States, as do survival rates after transplantation. With increasing long-term survival, many of these patients are being integrated back into community medical settings, with regular medical care being transferred back to primary care providers. Consequently, all physicians are increasingly likely to be involved in the care of patients who have undergone transplantation, and an awareness of posttransplant complications, including infections, is increasingly important.

## Antirejection Drugs in Transplant Recipients

Antirejection drugs are required after solid organ transplantation (SOT) or hematopoietic stem cell transplantation (HSCT). In general, the intensity of therapeutic immunosuppression is highest in the first few months after transplantation (induction therapy) to ensure initial graft survival and is then gradually decreased (maintenance therapy), although it may need to be increased later to manage episodes of rejection or graft-versus-host disease (GVHD). Additionally, some induction regimens include treatment with lymphocyte-depleting agents in association with lower doses of conventional immunosuppressants to further decrease the initial immune response to the transplant.

Because antirejection drugs work through suppression of different aspects of the immune system, various agents carry different risks for specific infections (**Table 38**). Glucocorticoids (such as prednisone) interfere with the immune response broadly, increasing the risk for infection from a wide range of organisms, including bacteria, viruses, and fungi. Lymphocyte-depleting agents also act broadly and are associated with increased risk for infection with cytomegalovirus (CMV), polyoma BK virus, *Pneumocystis* species, and other fungi. However, agents providing more focused T-cell suppression tend to have a narrower risk for infection. For example, mycophenolate regimens with lower glucocorticoid doses have a lower risk for *Pneumocystis* infection, whereas sirolimus is associated with lower rates of CMV disease but an increase in viral and bacterial respiratory infections.

**TABLE 38.** Immunosuppressive Agents Used in Transplantation

| Class | Agents |
|---|---|
| Glucocorticoids | Prednisone, others |
| Cytotoxic agents (DNA synthesis inhibitors, antimetabolites) | Mycophenolate mofetil |
| | Mycophenolate sodium |
| | Azathioprine |
| | Methotrexate |
| | Cyclophosphamide |
| Calcineurin pathway inhibitors | Cyclosporine |
| | Tacrolimus |
| mTOR inhibitors | Sirolimus (rapamycin) |
| | Everolimus |
| Lymphocyte-depleting antibodies | |
| Polyclonal | Antithymocyte globulins |
| Monoclonal | Muromonab (anti-CD3) |
| | Basiliximab (anti–IL-2 receptor) |
| | Daclizumab (anti–IL-2 receptor) |
| | Rituximab (anti-CD20) |
| | Alemtuzumab (anti-CD52) |

IL-2 = interleukin-2; mTOR = mammalian target of rapamycin.

Epstein-Barr virus (EBV)–associated posttransplant lymphoproliferative disease (PTLD) is also a potential complication with variable risk depending on specific immunosuppressive drug therapy. PTLD risk is higher in patients with a history of preexisting EBV infection treated with lymphocyte-depleting agents and in those receiving sirolimus and tacrolimus than in those receiving mycophenolate and cyclosporine.

Many immunosuppressive agents have significant drug interactions, which can be pharmacokinetic (affecting drug levels and metabolism) or pharmacodynamic (additive toxicity). Pharmacokinetic interactions are usually mediated through inhibition of, competition for, or induction of the cytochrome P-450 system (especially the 3A isoenzymes) or the membrane transporter P-glycoprotein. Additionally, individual genetic polymorphisms affect enzyme activity and can result in different rates of drug metabolism among patients. Pharmacokinetic interactions are very common and involve a long list of drugs; thus, possible interactions should be checked before any new drug is prescribed to a transplant recipient. Additive toxicity may result in nephrotoxicity or cytopenias and may also affect the risk for infection.

**KEY POINT**

- Pharmacokinetic interactions are very common and involve a long list of drugs, so possible interactions must be checked before any new drug is prescribed to a transplant recipient.

# Posttransplantation Infections

Infections after transplantation may present in atypical fashion and are more likely to disseminate. They may manifest with subtle signs and symptoms owing to altered anatomy associated with the transplant or to immunosuppression, so a high level of suspicion must be maintained. Additionally, noninfectious complications, such as graft rejection, GVHD, and drug toxicity, may present similarly to and be confused with infection.

## Timeline and Type of Transplant

The risk for specific infections varies somewhat predictably with the type of transplant, the immunosuppressive regimen used, time after transplant, recipient and donor characteristics (such as seropositivity for certain microbes), and posttransplant complications, including GVHD or rejection. Before transplantation, donor and recipient should be evaluated for active infection and screened for CMV, EBV, hepatitis B and C viruses, HIV, and tuberculosis.

Risk for infection in patients with SOT can be divided into three time periods (**Table 39**). In the first month after transplantation, patients are at risk for surgical site and other nosocomial

**TABLE 39.** Timeline of Common Infections After Solid Organ Transplantation

| Early Period (<1 Month after Transplantation) | Middle Period (1-6 Months after Transplantation) | Late Period (>6 Months after Transplantation)[a] |
|---|---|---|
| Staphylococcus aureus infection (including methicillin-resistant) | Cytomegalovirus infection | Epstein-Barr virus (including PTLD) infection |
| Nosocomial Gram-negative bacterial infection | Epstein-Barr virus (including PTLD) infection | Varicella-zoster virus infection |
| Clostridium difficile colitis | Herpes simplex virus infection | Community-acquired pneumonia |
| Candida infection | Varicella-zoster virus infection | Urinary tract infections |
| Aspergillus infection | Polyoma BK virus infection | Polyoma BK virus infection |
| Surgical site infections | Pneumocystis jirovecii infection | Cytomegalovirus infection |
| Nosocomial pneumonia | Toxoplasma gondii infection | Listeria infection |
| Catheter-related bacteremia | Listeria infection | Nocardia infection |
| Urinary tract infections | Legionella infection | |
| | Nocardia infection | |
| | Tuberculosis reactivation | |
| | Fungal infections | |
| | Hepatitis B and C | |

PTLD = posttransplant lymphoproliferative disorder.

[a]For opportunistic infections in the late period, risk depends on level of immunosuppression.

infections, which may include resistant bacteria or *Candida* species. Specific sites at highest risk for infection are usually related to the transplanted organ, for example urinary tract infection after kidney transplantation. With the intensive use of antimicrobials, *Clostridium difficile* colitis is an increasing problem in this group.

Between 1 and 6 months after SOT, the highest risk is for infection resulting from suppressed cell-mediated immunity. This is the most likely time for CMV reactivation and disease and other viruses (see Table 39). Opportunistic pathogens, such as *Pneumocystis* species, other fungi, and certain bacteria, also are relatively common in this time period.

Six months after SOT, opportunistic infections become less common unless episodes of rejection occur or need for high-level immunosuppression continues. In these instances (or with chronic allograft dysfunction), certain infections may present late (see Table 39). Patients may also present with more severe episodes of typical community-acquired infections.

Risk for infection after HSCT also follows a timeline (**Figure 21**). The most significant additional risk, compared with risk for infection after SOT, results from the significant period of neutropenia that occurs in the preengraftment phase after transplantation, with increased risk for bacterial (especially gram-negative and streptococcal) and invasive fungal disease.

**KEY POINT**

- The risk for specific infections varies somewhat predictably with the type of transplant, immunosuppressive regimen used, time after transplantation, recipient and donor characteristics (such as seropositivity for certain microbes), and posttransplant complications, including graft-versus-host disease or rejection.

## Specific Posttransplantation Infections
### Viral Infections

Although numerous viral infections can complicate transplantation, CMV is the most significant. The risk for reactivation is related to serologic status of the donor and recipient and is most likely in seronegative recipients from a seropositive donor; it is unlikely when donor and recipient are both negative. CMV disease after transplantation may manifest as a nonspecific febrile illness; may cause leukopenia and thrombocytopenia; or may cause specific organ disease, most often pneumonitis, colitis, esophagitis, or hepatitis. CMV is an immunomodulatory virus (active infection also results in nonspecific changes in immune system function), and CMV reactivation is associated with organ rejection, secondary infection and PTLD, and an increased risk for graft loss and death.

Other important viruses include EBV, human herpes virus (HHV) 6, and HHV-8, also known as Kaposi sarcoma herpes virus. The most significant consequence of EBV infection is PTLD resulting from B-lymphocyte proliferation. PTLD should be considered in any patient presenting with fever and

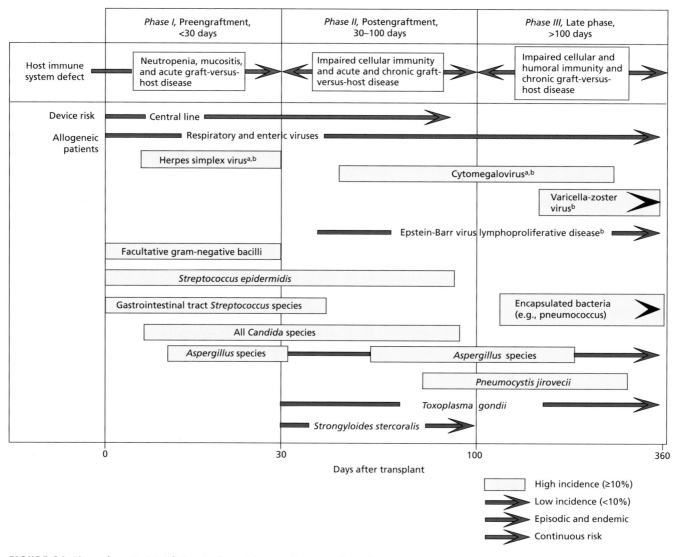

**FIGURE 21.** Phases of opportunistic infections in allogeneic hematopoietic stem cell transplant recipients.

[a]Without standard prophylaxis.

[b]Primarily among persons who are seropositive before transplantation.

Reprinted with permission from CDC, Infectious Diseases Society of America, and the American Society of Blood and Marrow Transplantation. Guidelines for preventing opportunistic infections among hematopoietic stem cell transplant recipients. Recommendations of CDC, the Infectious Diseases Society of America, and the American Society of Blood and Marrow Transplantation. Cytotherapy. 2001;3(1):41-54. [PMID: 12028843]

lymphadenopathy or an extranodal mass; treatment includes reduction of immunosuppression and rituximab or other chemotherapy. HHV-6 reactivation is common after SOT and HSCT, although its correlation to specific disease is not always clear. Syndromes associated with HHV-6 include fever, myelosuppression, hepatitis, encephalitis, and pneumonitis. Recently, hepatitis E virus, previously thought to only cause acute hepatitis, has been shown to cause chronic hepatitis after SOT and may be associated with hepatic fibrosis and glomerulonephritis.

## Bacterial Infections

Bacterial infections are common early after transplantation because of nosocomial and surgical infections after SOT and because of neutropenia after HSCT. Sites of infection are most often related to the specific organ after SOT. The most common causative agents for nosocomial infections are antibiotic-resistant staphylococci and gram-negative organisms. Pathogens may be present in the recipient before transplantation, including *Pseudomonas* and *Burkholderia* species in patients with cystic fibrosis receiving lung transplantation. *C. difficile* colitis is common considering the frequent and intense antibiotic use in these patients, especially in the second week after SOT, and in patients with GVHD after HSCT.

Even in the late period after HSCT, patients remain at risk for encapsulated organisms, such as *Streptococcus pneumoniae*. These and other community-acquired infections may be more severe than in patients without transplant. *Legionella*

**CONT.**

species cause a more extensive and rapidly progressive multi-lobar pneumonia in transplant recipients. *Listeria* species usually cause meningoencephalitis. *Nocardia* infection most commonly presents with lung nodules but may be disseminated at presentation, often to the brain. Tuberculosis usually occurs as a reactivation of latent infection after transplantation; all patients undergoing transplantation should be screened for latent tuberculosis and, if positive, treated for this before transplantation if feasible. In transplant recipients with tuberculosis, two thirds of cases occur in the first year, and 30% to 50% are extrapulmonary or disseminated at presentation. Treatment of tuberculosis after transplantation is complicated by increased risk for hepatotoxicity and drug interactions.

### Fungal Infections

Fungal infections are common after transplantation, especially in the neutropenic phase after HSCT, or with GVHD. Early-phase fungal disease is most often due to invasive *Candida* infection or *Aspergillus* infection. Invasive aspergillosis is also more common after lung transplantation. Pulmonary aspergillosis may present with fever, dry cough, or chest pain, and may disseminate to the brain, causing headache, focal deficits, or mental status changes. With prophylaxis against these fungi, other molds are becoming increasingly common, such as *Mucor* species, which can present in a fashion similar to that of aspergillosis.

Meningitis due to *Cryptococcus neoformans* is most common in the later period after SOT and presents with subacute or chronic onset of fever, headache, and mental status changes. Infection with geographic fungi–*Histoplasma* in the Midwest and *Coccidioides* in the Southwest–may also occur late after SOT in their endemic areas in the United States, presenting with fever and pulmonary infection, although both may disseminate. *Blastomycosis* infection is not significantly increased in incidence or mortality in transplant recipients.

*Pneumocystis jirovecii* pneumonia can be significantly reduced by use of prophylaxis but may occur in the middle or late periods after transplant. In transplant recipients, *Pneumocystis* pneumonia is a more acute and rapidly progressive illness than is typical in those with AIDS.

### Protozoa and Helminths

*Toxoplasma gondii* is a protozoan that can cause reactivation disease in the middle or late period after transplantation, most often with multiple brain abscesses with fever, headache, focal deficits and seizures, and multiple ring-enhancing lesions on brain imaging. Immunosuppression after transplantation can lead to a hyperinfection syndrome with *Strongyloides* species, which is associated with pneumonia, gram-negative bacteremia, and a high mortality rate. Trypanosomiasis and leishmaniasis can be seen in transplant recipients who are from endemic areas outside the United States.

**KEY POINTS**

- Cytomegalovirus infection after transplantation may manifest as a nonspecific febrile illness or may cause leukopenia and thrombocytopenia, pneumonitis, colitis, esophagitis, or hepatitis.
- The most significant consequence of Epstein-Barr virus infection is posttransplant lymphoproliferative disease resulting from B-lymphocyte proliferation.
- Bacterial infections are common early after transplantation because of nosocomial and surgical infections (after solid organ transplantation) and because of neutropenia (after hematopoietic stem cell transplantation).
- Early-phase fungal disease is most often due to invasive *Candida* infection or *Aspergillus* infection, *Cryptococcus neoformans* meningitis is most common in the later period, and *Pneumocystis* pneumonia may occur in the middle or late periods after transplant.

## Prevention of Infections in Transplant Recipients

Prevention of infection after transplantation relies primarily on prophylactic antimicrobial agents and immunizations. Prophylaxis after SOT and HSCT can reduce incidence of bacterial and candidal infections in the early period. During neutropenia, prophylaxis usually includes an antifungal with mold activity, such as voriconazole, which is often continued for 3 months or longer if GVHD is present. Trimethoprim-sulfamethoxazole is the preferred agent for *Pneumocystis* prophylaxis and also has activity against some bacteria, including *Listeria* and *Nocardia* species, and *Toxoplasma* species. It is often continued for 12 months and sometimes longer.

Reducing the burden of CMV disease after transplantation remains important, usually through true prophylaxis (valganciclovir for those at risk on the basis of serologic results) or preemptive therapy (monitoring for reactivation by nucleic acid amplification testing and initiating therapy when results are positive). Both strategies are effective; prophylaxis is usually used for seronegative recipients of an organ from a seropositive donor (highest risk). If donor and recipient are both seronegative, CMV preventive therapy need not be given.

Immunizations are important for transplant recipients (**Table 40**). These are preferably given before patients undergo SOT. Because they receive myeloablative therapy, patients undergoing HSCT need revaccination with complete series after immune system reconstitution. Recommendations concerning pneumococcal vaccination have been revised, and immunocompromised patients should receive the 13-valent pneumococcal conjugate vaccine first followed by the 23-valent pneumococcal polysaccharide vaccine (see MKSAP 17 General Internal Medicine for complete recommendations). Live vaccines are typically contraindicated for patients receiving immunosuppression after transplantation.

**TABLE 40.** Immunization Recommendations for Adult Recipients of Transplants[a]

| Immunization | Recommendations for Solid Organ Transplantation | Recommendations for Hematopoietic Stem Cell Transplantation[b] |
|---|---|---|
| Pneumococcal | Before transplantation: PCV13 followed 8 weeks later by PPSV23 | 3-6 months after transplantation: 3-4 doses of PCV13 |
| | 5 years after transplantation: 1 dose PPSV23 | 12 months after transplantation: 1 dose of PPSV23 |
| Influenza (inactivated only) | Annually | Annually |
| Tdap | Before transplantation: complete series, including Tdap booster | 6 months after transplantation: 3 doses Tdap |
| MMR | Contraindicated after transplantation | 24 months after transplantation: 1-2 doses, only if no GVHD or immune suppression |
| Inactivated polio | Before transplantation: complete series | 6-12 months after transplantation: 3 doses |
| *Haemophilus influenzae* type B | No recommendation | 6-12 months after transplantation: 3 doses |
| Meningococcal | Per recommendations for nontransplant patients | Per recommendations for nontransplant patients |
| Hepatitis B | Before transplantation: complete series if not already immune | 6-12 months after transplantation: 3 doses if indications for nontransplant patients are met |
| Hepatitis A | Before transplantation: complete series if not already immune | Per recommendations for nontransplant patients |
| Varicella-zoster | >4 weeks before transplantation: varicella if not immune | >4 weeks before transplantation: varicella if not immune |
| | >4 weeks before transplantation: zoster if same indications as nontransplant patients are met | 24 months after transplantation: 2 doses varicella if seronegative and only if no GVHD or immunosuppression |
| | Both contraindicated after transplantation | |
| Human papillomavirus | Before transplantation: per recommendations for nontransplant patients | Per recommendations for nontransplant patients |

GVHD = graft-versus-host disease; MMR = measles, mumps, and rubella; PCV13 = 13-valent pneumococcal conjugate vaccine; PPSV23 = 23-valent pneumococcal polysaccharide vaccine; Tdap = tetanus, diphtheria, and pertussis.

[a]See MKSAP 17 General Internal Medicine for more information on vaccination recommendations and schedules.

[b]For multiple-dose immunizations, the time period between doses is generally 1-2 months.

**KEY POINTS**

- Infection prevention after transplantation relies primarily on prophylactic antimicrobial agents and immunizations, although live vaccines are typically contraindicated for patients receiving immunosuppression.
- Patients undergoing hematopoietic stem cell transplantation require revaccination with complete series after immune system reconstitution, but live vaccines are contraindicated.

# Health Care-Associated Infections

## Epidemiology

Health care–associated infections are acquired while receiving care in a health care setting (hospital, dialysis center, ambulatory surgery center, long-term care facility). Hospital-acquired infections (HAIs) are a subset of health care–associated infections. An HAI is an infection that was neither present nor incubating upon admission to the hospital, usually defined as developing 48 hours after admission, depending on the implicated organism and the type of infection. HAIs are associated with the use of indwelling medical devices, surgery, invasive procedures, injections, transmission of organisms/infections between patients and health care personnel (HCP), and inappropriate use of antimicrobial agents. Bloodstream infections, pneumonia, surgical site infections, and urinary tract infections account for most HAIs. The Centers for Disease Control and Prevention estimates that 1 in 20 hospitalized patients will develop an HAI resulting in 1.7 million infections and 98,000 deaths per year. It is estimated that the direct costs of HAIs range from $35.7 billion to $45 billion annually, and, therefore, reduction of HAIs is a top health care priority. Approximately 65% to 70% of catheter-associated bloodstream infections and urinary tract infections and 55% of cases of ventilator-associated pneumonia and surgical site infections may be preventable. Hospitals have been challenged to eliminate preventable HAIs by aiming for 100% adherence to evidence-based practices and strategies shown to prevent these infections.

HVC

> **KEY POINT**
>
> - Approximately 65% to 70% of catheter-associated bloodstream infections and urinary tract infections and 55% of ventilator-associated pneumonia cases and surgical site infections may be preventable.

## Prevention

Hand hygiene remains the cornerstone for preventing infection. According to the World Health Organization, hand hygiene should be performed before clean/aseptic procedures and after bodily fluid exposure, touching a patient, and touching patient surroundings. Hand washing with soap and water should be performed for at least 15 seconds, being careful to cover all surfaces of the hands up to the wrists, between the fingers, and finger tips. Alcohol-based hand rubs are acceptable alternatives to soap and water, except after contact with patients who have *Clostridium difficile* infection or their environment. Standard precautions (wearing gloves, gowns, masks, eye protection) should be practiced in the care of every patient to protect HCP from exposure to bloodborne pathogens. All body fluids except sweat are potentially infectious, and HCP should use these barriers to protect themselves from anticipated exposure depending on the activity being performed. Transmission-based precautions (airborne, contact, droplet) are used in addition to standard precautions to prevent transmission of epidemiologically significant organisms (**Table 41**).

Appropriate and judicious device use, safe injection practices, following aseptic technique for invasive procedures and surgery, and maintaining a clean environment are important components of reducing HAIs. Many HAI prevention initiatives over the last decade have been successful, several of which have relied on bundling processes of care to improve outcomes. "Bundles" are usually three to five evidence-based processes of care that, when performed together, consistently have a greater effect on decreasing HAIs than individual components

performed inconsistently. A multifaceted and multidisciplinary approach is required to prevent HAIs.

> **KEY POINT**
>
> - Hand hygiene remains the cornerstone for preventing infection and should be performed, at minimum, before and after every patient contact.

## Catheter-Associated Urinary Tract Infections

### General Information

Catheter-associated urinary tract infections (CAUTIs) account for the largest proportion of HAIs (40%). Urinary catheters are used in 15% to 25% of hospitalized patients and are associated with most hospital-acquired urinary tract infections (UTIs). Urinary catheters are often placed for inappropriate indications, and physicians are frequently unaware that their patients have a urinary catheter, leading to prolonged and unnecessary use. It is well established that the duration of catheterization is directly related to the risk for a UTI. With a catheter in place, the daily risk for a UTI ranges from 3% to 7%. CAUTI is the leading cause of secondary hospital-acquired bacteremia, and 17% of hospital-acquired bacteremias are from a urinary source (2.3% mortality). The pathogens most often associated with CAUTI are *Escherichia coli*, *Pseudomonas aeruginosa*, *Klebsiella pneumoniae/oxytoca*, *Candida albicans*, and *Enterococcus faecalis*. As with other HAIs, risk factors can be divided into modifiable and nonmodifiable categories (**Table 42**). Catheters should be used for appropriate indications only, which include urinary retention and bladder outlet obstruction, measurement of urinary output in critically ill patients, perioperative use for selected surgical procedures, assistance with healing of perineal or sacral wounds in patients with incontinence, use in patients requiring prolonged immobilization, and contribution to comfort at the end of life.

| TABLE 41. | Transmission-Based Precautions[a] | | |
|---|---|---|---|
| **Precaution Type** | **Indications** | **Precaution** | **Examples** |
| Airborne | Organisms transmitted from respiratory tract by small droplet nuclei (≤5 microns) that travel long distances on air currents | Airborne infection isolation room (negative-pressure room); HCP wear fit-tested N95 respirator | Chickenpox (plus contact precautions), tuberculosis, measles |
| Contact | Organisms transmitted by direct or indirect contact | Single room; gloves and gown for HCP entering room | Multidrug-resistant organisms (such as MRSA, VRE, ESBL-producing gram-negative organisms), *Clostridium difficile*, rotavirus |
| Droplet | Organisms transmitted from respiratory tract by large droplet nuclei (>5 microns) that travel less than 3 feet on air currents | Single room; HCP wear face/surgical mask when within 3 feet of patient | Influenza, *Bordetella pertussis*, *Neisseria meningitidis* for first 24 hours of therapy, mumps |

ESBL = extended-spectrum β-lactamase; HCP = health care personnel; MRSA = methicillin-resistant *Staphylococcus aureus*; VRE = vancomycin-resistant enterococci.

[a]Some organisms/infections require a combination of transmission-based precautions (adenovirus: contact and droplet; disseminated varicella zoster virus: airborne and contact).

| TABLE 42. Risk Factors for Catheter-Associated Urinary Tract Infection |
| --- |
| **Nonmodifiable** |
| Female sex |
| Age >50 years |
| Diabetes mellitus |
| Severe underlying illness |
| Nonsurgical illness |
| Serum creatinine level >2.0 mg/dL (176.8 µmol/L) |
| **Modifiable** |
| Duration of catheterization |
| Nonadherence to aseptic technique (e.g., opening a closed system) |
| Less experienced catheter inserter |

**KEY POINT**

HVC
- Urinary catheters are often placed for inappropriate indications in health care settings, and use is frequently prolonged and unnecessary, which increases the risk for urinary tract infection.

 ## Diagnosis

Pyuria and bacteriuria are common in hospitalized patients with indwelling urinary catheters, even in those without infection; therefore, routine urinalysis and culture should not be performed in patients without symptoms or signs of infection. Patients considered to have a CAUTI are those with an indwelling urethral or suprapubic catheter, those in whom a catheter was removed in the 48 hours before symptom onset, or those undergoing intermittent catheterization who have signs and symptoms compatible with UTI (see Urinary Tract Infections), no other identifiable source, and bacteriuria ($10^3$ or more colony-forming units/mL of one or more bacterial species in a urine specimen). Patients with spinal cord injury may have increased spasticity or autonomic dysreflexia as symptoms related to a CAUTI. Bacteriuria in patients without signs or symptoms of UTI is called catheter-associated asymptomatic bacteriuria; most patients do not develop signs or symptoms of infection and generally do not require treatment, and the catheter may remain in place if still indicated. **H**

**KEY POINT**

HVC
- Routine urinalysis and culture should not be performed for patients with indwelling urinary catheters without symptoms or signs of urinary tract infection.

## Treatment

A urine specimen for culture should be obtained before antimicrobial treatment begins to guide definitive therapy based on culture results. Part of the treatment for CAUTI includes removing or replacing the urinary catheter, especially if it has been in place for 2 weeks or longer. The presence of biofilm on the catheter makes it difficult to eradicate bacteriuria or funguria and may lead to antimicrobial resistance if organisms cannot be eradicated. When culture data are available, therapy should be adjusted to the narrowest coverage spectrum possible. Treatment should be given for 7 days if symptoms resolve promptly and longer (10-14 days) for patients with delayed response (fever, unresolved symptoms after several days of therapy). CAUTIs caused by *Candida* species should be treated for 14 days; however, patients with candiduria alone do not require treatment. **H**

**KEY POINT**

- When culture data are available, therapy for catheter-associated urinary tract infections should be adjusted to the narrowest coverage spectrum possible. HVC

## Prevention

Avoiding urinary catheter use, when possible, is the mainstay of CAUTI prevention. Condom catheters for men and intermittent catheterization are alternative strategies associated with a decreased risk for infection. An estimated 17% to 69% of CAUTIs may be preventable by following recommended infection prevention measures (**Table 43**). Antimicrobial or antiseptic coated catheters may be considered if the CAUTI rate is not decreasing after implementing, and complying with, core prevention strategies, including aseptic insertion and maintenance. The effect of these catheters in reducing CAUTIs and which patient populations may be most likely to benefit require further study. CAUTI prevention strategies are summarized by the acronym ABCDE: Adhere to general infection control principles, perform Bladder ultrasonography to potentially avoid catheterization, use Condom catheters or intermittent catheterization when appropriate, Do not use an indwelling catheter if criteria for use are not met, and remove catheters Early when they are no longer indicated using computerized reminders or nurse-driven removal protocols. **H**

**KEY POINT**

- Avoiding urinary catheter use and considering alternatives are important components of catheter-associated urinary tract infection prevention. HVC

# Surgical Site Infections

## General Information

An estimated 80 million surgical procedures are performed in the United States each year, 32 million of which are in ambulatory settings. The overall risk for a surgical site infection (SSI) after surgery is 1.9%. SSIs account for 23% of HAIs and add 7 to 10 days to hospital stays. The excess cost per patient is estimated to be from $10,443 to $25,546 and can be up to $90,000 when an antimicrobial-resistant organism or prosthetic joint implant is involved. The overall mortality rate associated with SSIs is 3%, with 75% of deaths directly attributable to the SSI.

**TABLE 43.** Prevention of Catheter-Associated Urinary Tract Infection

| Period | Preventive Measures |
|---|---|
| Before catheterization | Avoid catheterization whenever possible |
| | Insert catheter only for appropriate indications |
| | Consider alternatives, such as condom catheters and intermittent catheterization |
| At time of catheter insertion | Ensure that only properly trained persons insert and maintain catheters |
| | Adhere to hand hygiene practices and standard (or appropriate isolation) precautions according to CDC HICPAC/WHO guidelines |
| | Use proper aseptic techniques and sterile equipment when inserting the catheter (acute care setting) |
| After catheter insertion | Promote early catheter removal whenever possible |
| | Secure the catheter |
| | Use aseptic technique when handling the catheter, including for sample collection from the designated port (not collecting bag) |
| | Maintain a closed drainage system |
| | Avoid unnecessary system disconnections |
| | Maintain unobstructed urine flow |
| | Keep the collecting bag below the level of the bladder |
| | Empty the collecting bag regularly, using a separate collecting container for each patient |

CDC = Centers for Disease Control and Prevention; HICPAC = Healthcare Infection Control Practices Advisory Committee; WHO = World Health Organization.

Patient and procedure risk factors affect the overall SSI risk (Table 44), and surgical wound classification correlates with the infection rate. SSIs typically occur in the first 30 days after surgery and up to 90 days after surgery with implants or prosthetic joints. The major sources of organisms causing SSIs are from the patient's skin and possibly the alimentary tract or female genital tract depending on the type of surgery. The organism most often isolated is *Staphylococcus aureus* (30.4%), followed by coagulase-negative staphylococci (11.7%), *E. coli* (9.4%), *E. faecalis* (5.9%) and *P. aeruginosa* (5.5%).

**KEY POINT**

- *Staphylococcus aureus* is the organism most often responsible for surgical site infection.

## Diagnosis

The clinical signs and symptoms vary by the site and type of SSI and the implicated organism. Inflammatory changes at the surgical site (signs and symptoms of pain/tenderness, warmth, swelling, erythema) and the presence of

**TABLE 44.** Risk Factors for Surgical Site Infection

| Endogenous | Exogenous (usually modifiable) |
|---|---|
| Diabetes mellitus | Prolonged preoperative stay |
| Advanced age | Preoperative hair removal by shaving |
| Obesity | Inadequate surgical scrub/antiseptic skin preparation |
| Smoking | Length of operation |
| Malnutrition, recent weight loss | Surgical technique |
| Cancer | Prophylactic antimicrobials and timing |
| Immunosuppression (glucocorticoid use, chemotherapy, radiation therapy) | Hypothermia |
| Remote site of infection | Hypoxia |
| Wound class[a] | Hyperglycemia |
| | Blood transfusion |

[a]Surgical wound classification is based on risk for infection: Clean: does not enter a hollow organ (gastrointestinal [GI], genitourinary [GU], respiratory tract), no inflammation at surgical site, site closed at end of surgery (infection rate <2%); Clean contaminated: hollow organ(s) (GI, GU, respiratory tract) entered, area appropriately prepared before surgery, no unusual events leading to additional risk for contamination, minimal spillage, no infected bile or urine (infection rate <10%); Contaminated: significant break in sterile technique (minor break during clean procedure), entry into infected hollow organ, gross spillage from GI tract, infected urine or bile encountered, inflammation (nonpurulent) at surgical site, penetrating trauma (<4 hours old) (infection rate 20%); Dirty/infected: surgical site grossly contaminated, preexisting infection (purulent inflammation, perforation of an unprepared hollow viscus, chronic open wound to be grafted/covered, penetrating trauma (>4 hours old) (infection rate 30%-40%).

**H**
CONT.

purulent drainage suggest a superficial incisional infection. Deep incisional SSIs may have more extensive tenderness, including outside the area of erythema, and more systemic signs of infection, such as fever and leukocytosis. A deep incisional SSI also should be considered with wound dehiscence or if the surgeon deliberately opens the incision, unless the wound/drainage culture is negative. Organ/deep space SSIs generally present with more systemic signs of infection and local symptoms related to a deep abscess or infected fluid collection. When organ/deep space SSIs are suspected, CT imaging is helpful to localize the infection and determine the best approach to for drain the fluid/abscess. When an SSI is suspected, wound drainage fluid, purulent fluid, or infected tissue should be obtained and sent for culture. Deep tissue or wound cultures are preferable to superficial wound swab cultures, which are more likely to reflect skin or wound colonization and not necessarily yield the causative pathogen (sensitivity, <30%). **H**

### KEY POINT

- When a surgical site infection is suspected, wound drainage material, purulent fluid, or infected tissue should be obtained and sent for culture.

### **H** Treatment

The choice of antimicrobial agent should be guided by culture results; the duration of treatment varies by the anatomic site of infection and the depth of the infection. Patients with signs of sepsis may require empiric therapy pending culture results, with antibiotics chosen to cover the most likely pathogens based on surgical type and site. Therapy should be revised after culture results are available. Superficial incisional infections can usually be managed with antimicrobial agents without tissue debridement. Treatment of deep incisional and organ/deep space SSIs generally requires a combination of surgical debridement to remove necrotic tissue or drain abscesses or infected fluid and specific antimicrobial therapy. Surgical debridement or drainage of infected fluid and abscess material may need to be repeated for the infection to be controlled and resolved, even with appropriate antimicrobial therapy. When an SSI involves an implant, removing the implant should be considered. However, depending on the patient and the site, organism, and severity of infection, a trial of antimicrobial therapy may be appropriate before implant removal. **H**

### KEY POINT

- Treatment of deep incisional and organ or deep space surgical site infections generally requires a combination of specific antimicrobial therapy and surgical debridement to remove necrotic tissue or drain abscesses or infected fluid.

### Prevention

Preventing SSIs can be divided into preoperative, intraoperative, and postoperative measures. Although many host risk factors for SSIs are not modifiable, several are and should be optimized before surgery. Hyperglycemia should be controlled, doses of immunosuppressive agents should be lowered as much as possible or stopped completely if feasible, patients who are obese should be encouraged to lose weight, and patients who smoke should cease tobacco use. Patients should shower with soap or an antiseptic agent the night before surgery. Hair around the planned incision site should be clipped, not shaved, if it must be removed. Skin preparation at the planned incision site should be performed at the time of surgery using an alcohol-based antiseptic; studies support the efficacy of alcohol combined with either chlorhexidine or povidone iodine–based antiseptics. If antimicrobial prophylaxis is indicated, the correct agent should be given at the correct dose at the correct time (for example, in the 60 minutes before incision or 2 hours before incision for vancomycin or fluoroquinolones, respectively) and discontinued within 24 hours after surgery. Continuing antimicrobial agents postoperatively has not shown benefit, even in cases of intraoperative spillage of gastrointestinal contents. During surgery, patient normothermia and adequate volume replacement help maximize tissue oxygen delivery. Perioperative blood glucose levels should be maintained at less than 200 mg/dL (11.1 mmol/L). A primarily closed incision should remain covered with a sterile dressing for 24 to 48 hours. **H**

### KEY POINT

- Continuing prophylactic antimicrobial agents postoperatively has not shown benefit in preventing surgical site infections.

**HVC**

# Central Line-Associated Bloodstream Infections  **H**

Central line–associated bloodstream infections (CLABSIs) originate from a central venous catheter (including peripherally inserted central catheters) without another recognizable source of infection and cause bacteremia. Approximately 250,000 CLABSIs occur in the United States every year, with 80,000 occurring in the intensive care unit (ICU). CLABSIs increase length of hospital stay up to 24 days and have an attributable mortality rate of 35%. Approximately 55% of patients in the ICU and 24% of those in other units have a central line. Antimicrobial resistance is a problem for most CLABSI-associated pathogens. CLABSI risk factors are shown in **Table 45**.

### Diagnosis

A CLABSI should be suspected in patients with a central line who do not have an obvious source of bacteremia due to an infection at another site. At least two sets of blood cultures

**TABLE 45.** Risk Factors for Central Line-Associated Bloodstream Infections

**Nonmodifiable (Intrinsic) Risk Factors**

Age (highest risk in neonates)

Male sex

Underlying diseases or conditions (for example, hematologic and immunologic deficiencies)

Neutropenia

**Modifiable (Extrinsic) Risk Factors**

Prolonged hospitalization before catheterization

Prolonged catheterization

Multiple CVCs

Multilumen CVC

Heavy microbial colonization at insertion site and catheter hub

Femoral vein (followed by internal jugular vein) catheterization

Lack of maximal sterile barriers for insertion and breaks in aseptic technique

Emergent insertion

Total parenteral nutrition

Poor catheter care and maintenance

CVC = central venous catheter.

*Enterococcus faecium*, *C. albicans*, *Enterobacter* species, *E. coli*, and *P. aeruginosa*. Blood cultures from central lines have a higher rate of false positivity; they may falsely identify a CLABSI by surveillance data definitions that are different from clinical definitions. However, negative cultures from central lines have a high negative predictive value for infection. **H**

**KEY POINT**

- A central line–associated bloodstream infection should be suspected in patients with a central line who do not have an obvious source of bacteremia due to an infection at another site.

**Treatment**

The infected central line should be removed, especially when *S. aureus*, *P. aeruginosa*, or a *Candida* species is involved. Most cases of uncomplicated CLABSI are treated for 7 to 14 days (**Table 46**); *S. aureus* CLABSI may require treatment for 4 to 6 weeks after catheter removal. Shorter therapy durations (14 days) may be considered in select patients with *S. aureus* CLABSI whose catheters have been removed and do not have diabetes mellitus, are not immunosuppressed, have no implanted prosthetic devices, have no evidence of endocarditis by echocardiography (preferably transesophageal), and have no evidence of infected thrombophlebitis ; whose fever and bacteremia resolve within 72 hours of starting appropriate therapy; and whose physical examination and/or diagnostic tests do not suggest the presence of metastatic infection. Blood cultures should become negative after removal of the central line and appropriate antimicrobial therapy is given in all cases of CLABSI. When bacteremia persists, evaluation for

**H**
CONT.

should be obtained (at least one peripherally) from different sites after appropriate skin disinfection and before starting antimicrobial therapy. Primary CLABSI pathogens include coagulase-negative staphylococci, *S. aureus* (including methicillin-resistant *S. aureus* [MRSA]), *E. faecalis*, other *Candida* species, *K. pneumoniae* and *Klebsiella oxytoca*,

**TABLE 46.** Management of Central Venous Catheter-Related Bloodstream Infection Based on Pathogen[a]

| Organism | Treatment |
|---|---|
| **Uncomplicated**[b] | |
| Coagulase-negative staphylococci | Remove catheter, antimicrobial therapy 5-7 days |
| | If catheter is not removed, systemic antimicrobials and antimicrobial lock treatment[c] 10-14 days |
| *Staphylococcus aureus* (no active malignancy or immunosuppression) | Remove catheter, antimicrobials ≥14 days |
| *Enterococcus* species | Remove catheter, antimicrobials 7-14 days |
| Gram-negative bacilli | Remove catheter, antimicrobials 7-14 days |
| *Candida* species | Remove catheter, antifungal agent 14 days after first negative blood culture |
| **Complicated** | |
| Suppurative thrombophlebitis, endocarditis, osteomyelitis, other site of metastatic or deep-seated infection | Remove catheter, antimicrobials 4-6 weeks (6-8 weeks for osteomyelitis) |

[a]Short-term catheters.

[b]Bloodstream infection and fever resolves in 72 hours, no intravascular hardware, no endocarditis or suppurative thrombophlebitis.

[c]For detailed information on this procedure, refer to Mermel LA, Allon M, Bouza E, et al. Clinical practice guidelines for the diagnosis and management of intravascular catheter-related infection: 2009 update by the Infectious Diseases Society of America [errata in Clin Infect Dis. 2010 Apr 1;50(7):1079; Clin Infect Dis. 2010 Feb 1;50(3):457]. Clin Infect Dis. 2009 Jul 1;49(1):1-45. [PMID: 19489710]

CONT.

a deeper source of infection, including endocarditis, should be performed. **H**

**KEY POINT**

- The first step in treating a central line–associated bloodstream infection is to remove the infected central line, followed by appropriate antimicrobial therapy.

**H** **Prevention**

Preventing CLABSIs begins with inserting and accessing central lines only when absolutely necessary and removing them as soon as possible. Hospitalized patients with central lines should be assessed daily to determine whether the line can be removed. Basic catheter insertion techniques should be followed, including hand hygiene, chlorhexidine skin antisepsis following recommended application methods and contact time for maximal effect, maximal barrier precautions, and optimal catheter site selection (with a subclavian site preferred and femoral sites avoided). Insertion techniques, checklists, and staff education significantly reduce CLABSIs. Although most prevention efforts and research have focused on CLABSIs occurring in ICUs, similar prevention strategies and precautions should be applied for all central lines. **H**

**KEY POINT**

HVC
- Hospitalized patients with central lines should be assessed daily to determine whether the line can be removed.

## **H** *Staphylococcus aureus* Bacteremia

*S. aureus* is a leading cause of hospital-acquired bacteremia. Source control, with removal or drainage of the focus of infection (such as an infected central venous access catheter, a foreign body, or an abscess), is important for treatment success. Bacteremia that persists longer than 72 hours after the start of appropriate antimicrobial therapy suggests a complicated *S. aureus* infection and requires additional evaluation and a longer course of therapy. Endocarditis and vertebral osteomyelitis are two important complications of *S. aureus* bacteremia. Patients with complicated bacteremia should undergo evaluation for endocarditis with echocardiography, preferably transesophageal. Additionally, when bacteremia is related to an infected central line, 71% of patients have thrombosis of the affected vein and require a longer course of antimicrobial therapy to clear the infection. Complicated *S. aureus* bacteremia should be treated for 4 to 6 weeks with an appropriate antimicrobial agent. Blood cultures should be repeated every 2 to 4 days until they are negative in order to document clearance of bacteremia. Bacteremia caused by methicillin-sensitive *S. aureus* (MSSA) should be treated with a penicillinase-resistant semisynthetic penicillin (nafcillin) or a first-generation cephalosporin (cefazolin) given at maximal doses. Vancomycin leads to higher rates of relapse and microbiologic failure in the treatment of MSSA bacteremia because it has slow bactericidal activity compared with β-lactam antibiotics.

For complicated bacteremia with MRSA, vancomycin and daptomycin are the preferred antimicrobial agents for treatment. Vancomycin trough concentrations of 15 to 20 µg/mL are recommended. For isolates with a vancomycin minimum inhibitory concentration (MIC) of 2 µg/mL or less, the patient's clinical response determines whether to continue vancomycin or change to an alternate agent, independent of the MIC. An alternative to vancomycin should be considered if no clinical or microbiologic (such as persistent bacteremia) response occurs despite adequate source control. Bacteremia may persist owing to the slow bactericidal activity of vancomycin, inadequate dosing, or poor tissue penetration. Vancomycin should not be used when the isolate has an MIC greater than 2 µg/mL; daptomycin is an acceptable alternative if the isolate is susceptible, although resistance has developed in patients taking daptomycin. Some experts recommend trying high-dose daptomycin (8-10 mg/kg per day) if bacteremia persists despite adequate source control. The median time to clearance of MRSA bacteremia is 7 to 9 days.

Management of persistent MSSA and MRSA bacteremia includes a search for, and removal of, all foci of infection, including surgical debridement of infected wounds and abscess drainage. It is important to remember that foci of infection not present on initial evaluation may develop with persistent bacteremia. Combination antimicrobial agents (for example, β-lactams and aminoglycosides, vancomycin and rifampin) to enhance bacterial killing do not improve outcomes and should not be given. Daptomycin should not be used in patients with concomitant *S. aureus* pneumonia because it is inactivated by surfactant. **H**

**KEY POINTS**

- Bacteremia caused by methicillin-sensitive *Staphylococcus aureus* should be treated with a penicillinase-resistant semisynthetic penicillin (nafcillin) or a first-generation cephalosporin (cefazolin); for complicated bacteremia caused by methicillin-resistant *S. aureus*, vancomycin and daptomycin are the preferred antimicrobial agents for treatment.

- The median time to clearance of methicillin-resistant *Staphylococcus aureus* bacteremia is 7 to 9 days.

## Hospital-Acquired Pneumonia and **H** Ventilator-Associated Pneumonia
### General Information

Hospital-acquired pneumonia (HAP) is defined as pneumonia occurring more than 48 hours after admission that was not incubating at admission. Ventilator-associated pneumonia (VAP) is defined as pneumonia developing 48 hours after endotracheal intubation. HAP accounts for 15% of HAIs (the second most common HAI) and has an estimated attributable

**H**
**CONT.**
mortality rate of 27% to 50%. It increases hospital length of stay by 7 to 9 days at an additional cost of $40,000. Risk factors for developing HAP are listed in **Table 47**. The most significant risk factor is intubation and mechanical ventilation. In patients receiving mechanical ventilation, the incidence of HAP increases 6-fold to 21-fold. VAP is the most common HAI in critically ill patients and occurs in 5% to 15% of patients using ventilators. Bacteria are the most commonly isolated pathogens. Viral and fungal pathogens also play a role, primarily in immunocompromised patients. Early onset (<5 days after admission/intubation) generally results from antimicrobial-sensitive organisms (*Streptococcus pneumoniae, Haemophilus influenzae, S. aureus,* and antibiotic-susceptible gram-negative bacteria); late onset (≥5 days after admission/intubation) is more likely with multidrug-resistant organisms (MDROs), including *P. aeruginosa, K. pneumoniae, Acinetobacter* species, *Stenotrophomonas maltophilia, Burkholderia cepacia,* and MRSA. **H**

**KEY POINT**

- The most significant risk factor for hospital-acquired pneumonia is intubation and mechanical ventilation.

**H** ## Diagnosis

Diagnosing HAP and VAP can be difficult because no reliable tests exist to make a definitive diagnosis. Instead, diagnosis is based on clinical, radiologic, and microbiologic findings. Clinical findings include temperature greater than 38.0 °C (100.4 °F), leukocytosis or leukopenia, purulent sputum, and a decrease in arterial oxygen saturation. A new or progressing lung infiltrate on chest radiograph is also required; if clinical findings are present without radiographic findings, tracheobronchitis should be considered. A specimen from the lower respiratory tract should be obtained before starting antimicrobial therapy; however, inability to obtain a specimen should not delay therapy in critically ill patients. Alternatively, quantitative cultures of specimens obtained by bronchoalveolar lavage can be used to diagnose VAP (and confirm the microbiology of the infection). Bronchoalveolar lavage is similar to

**TABLE 47.** Risk Factors for Hospital-Acquired Pneumonia and Ventilator-Associated Pneumonia

| Modifiable Risk Factors | Nonmodifiable Risk Factors |
|---|---|
| Depressed level of consciousness | Age >70 years |
| Enteral nutrition | Immunosuppression |
| Malnutrition | Thoracic or abdominal surgery |
| Mechanical ventilation | Underlying chronic lung disease |
| Oropharyngeal colonization | |
| Reintubation | |
| Stress ulcer prophylaxis | |
| Supine position | |

diagnosis by clinical findings in terms of antimicrobial use and outcomes. **H**

**KEY POINT**

- Clinical findings of ventilator-associated pneumonia include temperature greater than 38.0 °C (100.4 °F), leukocytosis or leukopenia, purulent sputum, and a decrease in arterial oxygen saturation.

### Treatment

**H**

Therapy should be started promptly when HAP is suspected. Empiric treatment guidelines depend on whether HAP is early or late onset. Combination antimicrobial therapy may be considered for empiric therapy to provide a broader spectrum of coverage when MDROs are possible pending microbiologic testing results. No evidence indicates that HAP or VAP caused by *Pseudomonas* species requires combination therapy or that a synergistic combination improves outcomes. If a patient had a witnessed aspiration event or recent surgery, antimicrobial coverage for oral anaerobes may be considered. Cephalosporins should be avoided as monotherapy in situations in which extended-spectrum β-lactamase (ESBL)–producing gram-negative organisms (such as *K. pneumoniae*) are prevalent; a carbapenem may be a more appropriate empiric antimicrobial choice in such settings. All patients should be re-evaluated for clinical improvement and review of microbiologic results at 48 to 72 hours and considered for de-escalation (changing to narrow-spectrum or oral therapy) or discontinuation of antimicrobial therapy when the diagnosis is in doubt. De-escalation of antimicrobial therapy is considered when culture results are available and the patient has stabilized (clinical improvement usually takes 48-72 hours) to prevent the emergence of antimicrobial resistance. The duration of therapy for HAP and VAP is generally 7 to 8 days except in cases caused by *P. aeruginosa* or *Acinetobacter* species, for which treatment should continue for 14 days. Patients who do not improve within 72 hours of appropriate antimicrobial therapy initiation should be evaluated for infectious complications, an alternate diagnosis, or another site of infection to explain the clinical picture. (For example, a patient with moderate to large pleural effusions should be evaluated for infection with a diagnostic thoracentesis.) **H**

**KEY POINTS**

- No evidence indicates that hospital-acquired pneumonia or ventilator-associated pneumonia caused by *Pseudomonas* species requires combination therapy or that a synergistic combination improves outcomes. **HVC**

- Patients suspected of having hospital-acquired or ventilator-associated pneumonia who do not improve within 72 hours of appropriate antimicrobial therapy initiation should be evaluated for infectious complications, an alternate diagnosis, or another site of infection to explain the clinical picture.

## Prevention

Avoiding intubation, if possible, and using noninvasive positive-pressure ventilation as an alternative, when feasible, can decrease the risk for HAP. Sedation should be minimized and interrupted once daily if not clinically contraindicated in patients who are mechanically ventilated, and patients should be assessed for readiness for extubation using spontaneous breathing trials. This practice has been shown to decrease the duration of intubation by 1 to 2 days. The head of the bed should be elevated 30 to 45 degrees; a supine position, particularly in patients receiving enteral nutrition, increases the risk for VAP. Daily oral care with chlorhexidine may benefit some patients. Additional components of commonly used ventilator guidelines include subglottic suctioning, peptic ulcer disease and deep venous thrombosis prophylaxis, and avoiding gastric overdistention. One study showed that using a multifaceted intervention and ventilator guidelines decreased VAP rates by 71%.

### KEY POINT

HVC
- Avoiding intubation (if possible) and using noninvasive positive-pressure ventilation as an alternative (when feasible) can significantly decrease the risk for hospital-acquired pneumonia.

## Hospital-Acquired Infections Caused by Antimicrobial-Resistant Organisms

Up to 75% of HAIs are associated with organisms resistant to first-line antimicrobial agents. Infections with MDROs are associated with increased morbidity, mortality, and cost (up to $20 billion per year). Antimicrobial resistance has been noted in nearly all bacterial pathogens. However, antimicrobial resistance has dramatically increased among gram-negative organisms in the last 10 years. ESBL-producing Enterobacteriaceae, carbapenem-resistant Enterobacteriaceae (production of *K. pneumoniae* carbapenemase enzyme is most common in the United States), and pan-resistant strains of *P. aeruginosa* and *Acinetobacter* species are particularly concerning. Among gram-positive organisms, more than two thirds of *E. faecium* isolates in the United States are vancomycin resistant. Vancomycin-intermediate *S. aureus* is a global concern. Vancomycin-resistant *S. aureus* remains rare. Infections caused by these organisms are particularly difficult and challenging to treat and are associated with mortality rates estimated to be up to four times higher than mortality seen with infections caused by non–antimicrobial-resistant strains. Resistance to antimicrobial agents is not limited to the hospital setting. It occurs in other health care settings and to a lesser extent in the community (such as community-associated MRSA). Limiting transmission of these organisms in any health care setting must be a priority and is best accomplished by full compliance with hand hygiene protocols and contact precautions, cleaning and disinfecting the environment and patient care equipment before it

is used for another patient, and judicious use of antimicrobial agents. Although *C. difficile* is not technically an MDRO, it is often listed with MDROs as a problematic pathogen in health care settings.

### KEY POINT

- Limiting transmission of antimicrobial-resistant    HVC
organisms in health care settings is best accomplished by full compliance with hand hygiene protocols and contact precautions, cleaning and disinfecting the environment and patient care equipment before it is used for another patient, and judicious use of antimicrobial agents.

# HIV/AIDS

## Epidemiology and Prevention

More than 33 million persons worldwide are estimated to be infected with the retrovirus HIV-1, including more than 1 million persons in the United States. More than 50,000 persons are newly infected each year in the United States. HIV-2 is another retrovirus infecting humans, but almost all HIV-2 infections to date have been acquired in Africa; infection with HIV-2 remains uncommon in the United States. Although infection with HIV-2 can cause a positive result on screening serologic tests, the HIV-1/HIV-2 antibody differentiation immunoassay now recommended for HIV testing will differentiate HIV-2 from HIV-1 infection (see following section on Screening and Diagnosis). Because the remainder of this chapter deals specifically with HIV-1, the term *HIV* is used throughout.

HIV is spread by sexual contact (estimated to be responsible for >80% of all infections), by contact with infected blood (transfusions, shared needles, occupational exposures), or perinatally. Transmission can be reduced by use of condoms and clean needle exchange programs. Transmission is also reduced (although not to zero) with attainment of undetectable viral load levels in the blood of infected patients. Treatment of a pregnant woman significantly reduces perinatal transmission. Prophylaxis with antiretroviral agents can reduce HIV infection in the postexposure and preexposure settings.

### KEY POINT

- HIV is spread by sexual contact or by contact with infected blood, such as transfusions, shared needles, occupational exposures, or perinatal transmission.

## Pathophysiology and Natural History

HIV can infect numerous cell types, most significantly CD4 T-helper lymphocytes. HIV integrates into the host cell genome, and long-lived cells can serve as a reservoir of virus, which contributes to the challenge of developing a cure for HIV infection. Replication of HIV contributes to early death of T cells, depletion of CD4 cells, and immunocompromise, resulting in increased risk for opportunistic infections and development of AIDS.

### Acute HIV Infection

Most persons who develop HIV infection experience an acute symptomatic illness, referred to as acute retroviral syndrome, within a few weeks of acquiring the infection. Severity varies, but presentation is most often consistent with an infectious mononucleosis syndrome. Signs and symptoms and their frequency are listed in **Table 48**. Differential diagnosis includes acute infection with Epstein-Barr virus, cytomegalovirus, influenza, and a hepatitis virus and syphilis. Patients with acute infection may not yet be producing antibodies against HIV antigen (the "window period"), which results in negative results on traditional HIV serologic testing. Therefore, diagnosis of acute HIV infection during this time period relies on detecting the virus by RNA polymerase chain reaction or p24 antigen testing. Because levels of virus are usually very high in patients with acute infection, treatment is recommended to reduce the rate of transmission and possibly to reduce the progression of disease. **H**

> **KEY POINT**
> - Diagnosis of acute HIV infection relies on detecting the virus by RNA polymerase chain reaction or p24 antigen testing.

### Chronic HIV Infection and AIDS

Whether patients with acute HIV infection are treated or not, signs and symptoms of infection resolve and the disease enters a chronic stage. Although patients may be asymptomatic for years, active viral replication and destruction of CD4 T-helper lymphocytes continue. Signs and symptoms of chronic HIV infection include the following:

- Lymphadenopathy
- Fever, night sweats
- Fatigue
- Weight loss
- Chronic diarrhea
- Seborrheic dermatitis, psoriasis, tinea, onychomycosis
- Oral aphthous ulcers, oral hairy leukoplakia, gingivitis/periodontitis
- Peripheral neuropathy
- Leukopenia, anemia, thrombocytopenia
- Nephropathy

AIDS is diagnosed when certain indicator opportunistic infections or malignancies develop or when the CD4 cell count falls below 200/μL. Even before reaching this cell count level, however, patients may develop recurrent or refractory infections, such as vaginal candidiasis, oral or genital herpes simplex virus infection, pneumococcal pneumonia, and herpes zoster. **H**

> **KEY POINT**
> - In patients with chronic HIV infection, AIDS is diagnosed when certain indicator opportunistic infections or malignancies develop or when the CD4 cell count falls below 200/μL.

## Screening and Diagnosis

The recommended algorithm for diagnosing HIV infection has changed significantly with the recent implementation of the fourth-generation HIV test. This test combines an immunoassay for HIV antibody with a test for HIV p24 antigen (**Figure 22**). This improves the ability of the test to detect early HIV infection because p24 antigen becomes detectable a week before antibody in acute infection. Detection of antigen may help diagnose patients as early as 2 weeks after infection. Western blot testing is no longer recommended. Combined antibody/antigen testing with the approved assay has a specificity of 99.6% but must be confirmed with additional testing.

A positive result on HIV-1/2 antigen/antibody combination assay is followed by testing of the sample with the HIV-1/HIV-2 antibody differentiation immunoassay. Detection of HIV-1 or HIV-2 antibody confirms the diagnosis. Samples negative on the antibody differentiation immunoassay are tested with an HIV-1 nucleic acid amplification test (NAAT); if the NAAT result is positive with a negative antibody, then acute HIV infection is diagnosed. Specimens positive on the initial antigen/antibody combination immunoassay but negative on the antibody differentiation immunoassay and NAAT represent false-positive results. Although false-positive findings are rare, in a population with low pretest probability (such as in

**TABLE 48.** Signs and Symptoms of Acute HIV Infection (Acute Retroviral Syndrome)

| Sign/Symptom | Frequency (%) |
| --- | --- |
| Fever | 96 |
| Lymphadenopathy | 74 |
| Pharyngitis | 70 |
| Rash | 70 |
| Myalgia/arthralgia | 54 |
| Diarrhea | 32 |
| Headache | 32 |
| Nausea/vomiting | 27 |
| Hepatosplenomegaly | 14 |
| Weight loss | 13 |
| Thrush | 12 |
| Neurologic symptoms | 12 |

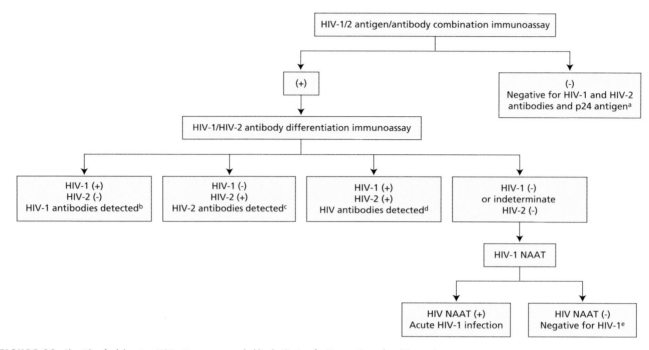

**FIGURE 22.** Algorithm for laboratory HIV testing recommended by the Centers for Disease Control and Prevention.

NAAT = nucleic acid amplification test. (+) indicates reactive test result; (−) indicates nonreactive test result.

[a]No evidence of HIV infection.

[b]HIV-1 infection.

[c]HIV-2 infection.

[d]HIV infection (undifferentiated).

[e]HIV-1/2 antigen/antibody combination immunoassay result was false-positive.

Centers for Disease Control and Prevention, Association of Public Health Laboratories. Laboratory testing for the diagnosis of HIV infection: updated recommendations. http://stacks.cdc.gov/view/cdc/23447. Published June 27, 2014. Accessed July 9, 2015.

**CONT.** screening), false-positive results on the initial antigen/antibody combination assay may be seen with higher frequency than true-positive results; waiting for the confirmatory testing results is crucial to avoid misdiagnosis.

Rapid HIV tests, which give results from salivary samples in about 20 minutes, are also available for clinic and home use. These are enzyme immunoassay antibody tests and, if results are positive, must be confirmed by using the HIV testing algorithm described previously.

**Table 49** lists indications for HIV testing. In addition to diagnostic testing when HIV infection is suspected, screening for HIV infection is recommended for all persons aged 13 to 65 years by the Centers for Disease Control and Prevention, American College of Physicians, Infectious Diseases Society of America, and U.S. Preventive Services Task Force. HIV testing should be "opt-out" (the person is informed of the proposed test and testing proceeds unless the person declines). Those at higher risk for HIV infection (injection drug users and their sexual partners, persons who exchange sex for money or drugs, sexual partners of HIV-infected persons, and those with more than one sexual partner since their most recent HIV test) should have repeat testing at least annually (some experts recommend every 3-6 months) to detect incidental infection as early as possible.

Universal testing is especially important for pregnant women so that treatment can be initiated to reduce perinatal transmission.

**KEY POINTS**

- Fourth-generation HIV testing combines an HIV antibody enzyme immunoassay with a test for HIV p24 antigen; a positive test result is followed by HIV-1/HIV-2 antibody differentiation immunoassay.

- Screening for HIV infection is endorsed for all persons aged 13 to 65 years.

## Initiation of Care

### Initial Evaluation and Laboratory Testing

Initial evaluation of a patient with newly diagnosed HIV infection includes a complete history, including social and sexual history, and physical examination, with particular attention to symptoms and signs of infections or other complications. Counseling is also essential regarding the transmission and prevention of HIV infection and the natural history and prognosis of treated infection. Initial laboratory evaluation includes testing for infections that may be transmitted concurrently with HIV or may complicate HIV infection, as well as routine

## TABLE 49. Indications for HIV Testing

Symptoms/signs of acute HIV infection (acute retroviral syndrome)

Symptoms/signs of chronic HIV infection

Opportunistic infection

Severe, recurrent, or persistent infection that does not qualify as opportunistic

Presence of tuberculosis, HBV infection, HCV infection, other sexually transmitted infections, hemophilia

History of at-risk behavior (multiple sex partners, men having sex with men, injection drug use) or sexual partner of someone who engages in at-risk behavior

Persons aged 13-65 years, unless in population areas with low (<0.1%) prevalence

Known or suspected HIV exposure

Victim of sexual assault

Patient request

All pregnant women

Child born to mother infected with HIV

Occupational exposure to blood/body fluids (both source patient and exposed worker)

Blood/semen/organ donor

HBV = hepatitis B virus; HCV = hepatitis C virus.

testing to evaluate organ function and metabolic status before beginning antiretroviral therapy (**Table 50**). Quantitative HIV RNA (viral load) testing and measurement of T-cell subsets (CD4 cell count) are important baseline studies to help guide decisions regarding initiation of therapy and to assess response after therapy is begun. Repeat testing (HIV viral load, CD4 cell count, complete blood count, and tests of kidney function and

## TABLE 50. Laboratory Testing as Part of the Evaluation of HIV Infection

Repeat HIV antibody testing if no documentation

Viral resistance testing at baseline and for treatment failure

Quantitative HIV RNA assay (viral load)

T-cell subsets (CD4 cell count)

Complete blood count with differential

Chemistries, including kidney function studies and fasting plasma glucose

Liver chemistry studies/liver enzymes

Fasting serum lipid profile

Urinalysis

Tuberculin skin test or interferon-$\gamma$ release assay

Serologic testing for hepatitis A, B, and C virus infection

Serologic testing for syphilis; testing for other sexually transmitted infections

Serologic testing for toxoplasmosis

Pap test

liver chemistries) should be performed before any modification in current therapy, 2 to 8 weeks after starting or changing therapy, and every 3 to 6 months in patients who remain stable with their current therapy. In patients with persistent undetectable viral loads and a CD4 cell count that has normalized and whose therapy is stable, further monitoring of T-cell subsets is no longer recommended. ⊞

### KEY POINTS

- Quantitative HIV RNA (viral load) testing and measurement of CD4 cell count are important baseline studies to help guide decisions regarding initiation of therapy and to assess therapy response.

- In patients with persistent undetectable viral loads and a CD4 cell count that has normalized and whose therapy is stable, further monitoring of T-cell subsets is no longer recommended.

## Immunizations and Prophylaxis for Opportunistic Infections

Patients with HIV infection, regardless of CD4 cell counts, are at increased risk for invasive infection with *Streptococcus pneumoniae* and should be vaccinated with the 13-valent pneumococcal conjugate vaccine and the 23-valent pneumococcal polysaccharide vaccine (see MKSAP 17 General Internal Medicine). All patients should receive three doses of hepatitis B virus (HBV) vaccine unless testing confirms that they already have HBV infection or are immune to HBV. Indications for influenza, tetanus-diphtheria-pertussis, hepatitis A virus, human papillomavirus, and meningococcal vaccines are the same as for the general population. Although patients with HIV infection generally should not receive live vaccines, the measles-mumps-rubella and varicella vaccines are considered safe for those with CD4 cell counts greater than 200/µL.

Recommendations for primary prophylaxis against opportunistic infections are outlined in **Table 51**. Before latent tuberculosis treatment is begun, active tuberculosis infection must be ruled out in patients with a positive tuberculin skin test result or a positive result on interferon-$\gamma$ release assay; single-agent therapy used to treat latent infection would be ineffective and would also select for resistance, making active infection more difficult to treat. For the same reasons, active *Mycobacterium avium* complex infection must be ruled out in patients with a CD4 cell count less than 50/µL before prophylaxis for this infection begins.

### KEY POINTS

- Patients with HIV infection, including those with higher CD4 cell counts, are at increased risk for invasive infection with *Streptococcus pneumoniae* and should be vaccinated with the 13-valent pneumococcal conjugate vaccine and the 23-valent pneumococcal polysaccharide vaccine.

*(Continued)*

**TABLE 51.** Prophylaxis against Opportunistic Infections in HIV/AIDS[a]

| Opportunistic Infection | Indication | Preferred Drug |
|---|---|---|
| *Pneumocystis jirovecii* | CD4 cell count <200/µL | TMP-SMX, double-strength tablet once daily or three times weekly |
| Toxoplasmosis | CD4 cell count <100/µL and positive serologic results | TMP-SMX, double-strength tablet once daily |
| *Mycobacterium avium* complex | CD4 cell count <50/µL | Azithromycin, 1200 mg/week |
| Tuberculosis | TST >5 mm or positive IGRA results | INH, 300 mg/d for 9 months |

IGRA = interferon-γ release assay; INH = isoniazid; TMP-SMX = trimethoprim-sulfamethoxazole; TST = tuberculin skin test.

[a]Also recommended are the 23-valent pneumococcal polysaccharide vaccine and 13-valent pneumococcal conjugate vaccine, influenza vaccine annually, hepatitis B vaccine in susceptible persons, and hepatitis A vaccine for persons at high risk.

**KEY POINTS** *(continued)*

- Before treatment for latent tuberculosis or prophylaxis against *Mycobacterium avium* complex (MAC) infection begins, active tuberculosis infection must be ruled out in patients with a positive tuberculin skin test result or a positive result on interferon-γ release assay; active MAC infection must be ruled out in patients with a CD4 cell count less than 50/µL.

# Complications of HIV Infection in the Antiretroviral Therapy Era

## Metabolic Disorders

Management of metabolic disorders, including hyperlipidemia and diabetes mellitus, is of increasing importance in treating patients with HIV infection. This is partly for the same reasons that metabolic disorders are increasing in the general population and partly related to HIV infection and treatment. HIV infection is associated with decreases in serum total cholesterol, HDL cholesterol, and LDL cholesterol levels and increases in serum triglyceride levels. Treatment of HIV infection leads to increases in total cholesterol and LDL cholesterol levels. Additionally, certain antiretroviral agents, including some protease inhibitors, directly contribute to further increases in cholesterol and triglyceride levels. Although some antiretroviral agents, notably certain protease inhibitors, may contribute directly to insulin resistance, HIV treatment often leads to regaining of weight lost before the start of therapy; thus, it contributes to impaired fasting plasma glucose levels or development of diabetes. Results of lipid panels and fasting plasma glucose or hemoglobin $A_{1c}$ measurements should therefore be monitored periodically as part of treatment.

Older antiretroviral agents are also associated with lipodystrophy, which refers to changes in fat distribution causing lipoatrophy in the face and extremities and fat accumulation centrally. Lipodystrophy is associated with adverse cosmetic and metabolic effects. Nucleoside analogues are also associated with mitochondrial toxicity, which can lead to lactic acidosis and may be fatal if not recognized. Avoidance of the nucleoside analogues stavudine and zidovudine has decreased the occurrence of lipodystrophy and mitochondrial toxicity.

Osteopenia and osteoporosis are increased in patients with HIV infection; however, the role of specific antiretroviral agents, such as tenofovir, in these conditions is unclear. Bone densitometry assessment should be considered in specific patients with HIV infection (postmenopausal women, men older than 50 years, and all patients with other risk factors for osteopenia or osteoporosis).

Kidney dysfunction is increasingly being diagnosed in patients with HIV infection. Although HIV can cause associated nephropathy and chronic kidney disease, other factors contributing to kidney dysfunction include diabetes and certain antiretroviral agents, most notably tenofovir. Because proteinuria is usually the first manifestation of tenofovir nephrotoxicity, patients receiving tenofovir require urinalysis every 6 to 12 months. Additionally, certain agents used in antiretroviral regimens, notably cobicistat and dolutegravir, inhibit tubular secretion of creatinine. This can cause measured serum creatinine to increase without any true change in glomerular filtration rate and should not be mistaken for actual kidney dysfunction. Dialysis or kidney transplantation is an option for selected patients with HIV infection and end-stage kidney disease.

All patients with HIV infection should be evaluated for active hepatitis B and C because coinfection is associated with increased risk for progression and worse prognosis. Hepatitis C should be tested for annually. HIV infection and hepatitis B can both be treated with tenofovir, emtricitabine, and lamivudine, and including two of these agents in the medication regimen is crucial for managing coinfection. Treatment of hepatitis C (previously difficult because of overlapping toxicities of regimens for the two viruses) has become less problematic as a result of the new hepatitis C agents (sofosbuvir, simeprevir, ledipasvir, ombitasvir, paritaprevir, dasabuvir) (see MKSAP 17 Gastroenterology and Hepatology), although drug interactions between agents in both regimens will still require monitoring.

**KEY POINTS**

- HIV infection and its management are associated with increased incidence of hyperlipidemia, glucose intolerance, and diabetes mellitus.
- All patients with HIV infection should be evaluated for active hepatitis B and C because coinfection is associated with increased risk for progression and worse prognosis.

## Cardiovascular Disease

As patients with HIV infection age and develop metabolic risks, such as hyperlipidemia and diabetes, the incidence of cardiovascular disease increases. HIV infection is also associated with an increased risk for cardiovascular disease, which is thought to be caused by chronically high levels of inflammatory markers. Interrupting HIV therapy is associated with an increase in cardiovascular events and death, as well as more infectious complications. Therefore, even if HIV treatment regimens contribute to unfavorable metabolic effects, the net effect of antiretroviral therapy on risk for cardiovascular disease is very favorable because of benefits thought to be related to decreased inflammation. In patients with HIV infection, attention to the usual modifiable risk factors for cardiovascular disease is as important as, or more important than, in the general population.

> **KEY POINT**
>
> - Interrupting HIV therapy is associated with an increase in cardiovascular events and death, as well as more infectious complications.

## Immune Reconstitution Inflammatory Syndrome

Immune reconstitution inflammatory syndrome (IRIS) may develop in the first few months after initiation of antiretroviral therapy, most often in patients whose baseline CD4 cell count was low. IRIS is due to a vigorous inflammatory response, made possible by reconstitution of the immune system, to an infection that was already present, either known and receiving treatment or undiagnosed and asymptomatic. Patients may paradoxically appear to be presenting with a new infection or worsening of a previously diagnosed infection after undergoing successful treatment with antiretroviral agents. IRIS is associated with various infections but is most likely to be caused by infection with mycobacteria or fungi (such as cryptococcal meningitis). Therapy usually includes continued antiretroviral agents along with treatment of the specific infection. Adjuvant glucocorticoid therapy is sometimes needed to modulate the overactive inflammatory response.

> **KEY POINT**
>
> - Immune reconstitution inflammatory syndrome may develop in the first few months after initiation of antiretroviral therapy and is due to a vigorous inflammatory response, made possible by reconstitution of the immune system, to an infection that was already present, either known and being treated or undiagnosed and asymptomatic.

## Opportunistic Infections

In patients with untreated HIV infection, decreasing CD4 cell counts predispose them to infections that do not usually occur in persons with an intact immune system. These opportunistic infections usually develop when the CD4 cell count is less than 200/µL and become even more likely when the count is lower. However, mucocutaneous *Candida* infection can develop with CD4 cell counts greater than 200/µL. Oral candidiasis (thrush) most often can be treated with topical agents such as clotrimazole troches. Dysphagia or other swallowing symptoms indicate esophageal involvement, and treatment of esophageal candidiasis requires a systemic agent such as fluconazole.

*Cryptococcus* infection may be isolated to the lung but usually has disseminated before diagnosis and manifests as subacute or chronic meningitis. Cryptococcal meningitis is diagnosed by cerebrospinal fluid culture or by antigen testing of cerebrospinal fluid or serum. Treatment includes antifungal agents and control of increased intracranial pressure by serial lumbar punctures or shunting.

*Pneumocystis jirovecii* pneumonia is a common complication in patients with HIV infection who have not received prophylaxis. Patients present with subacute onset of fever, dyspnea, and dry cough, and chest radiographs most commonly show diffuse interstitial or alveolar infiltrates (**Figure 23**). Although the microorganisms may be found in induced sputum, diagnosis usually requires stains of bronchoalveolar lavage fluid. High-dose trimethoprim-sulfamethoxazole is the treatment of choice. During treatment, an immune response to dying microorganisms may actually worsen disease in the first few days. Adjunctive glucocorticoids are beneficial and should be used in patients with an arterial partial pressure of oxygen (breathing ambient air) of less than 70 mm Hg (9.31 kPa) or an alveolar-arterial gradient of greater than 35 mm Hg (4.66 kPa).

*Toxoplasma gondii* can cause encephalitis in patients with CD4 cell counts less than 100/µL. Diagnosis is typically

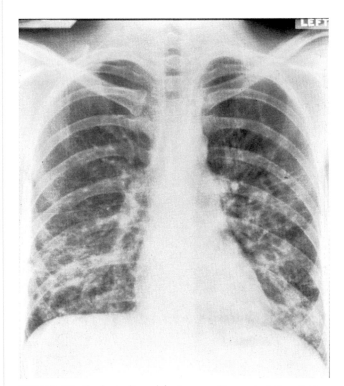

**FIGURE 23.** The chest radiograph for *Pneumocystis* pneumonia in a patient with AIDS typically shows diffuse bilateral interstitial or alveolar infiltrates. Diagnosis can be confirmed by identification of stains of the organism in sputum or bronchoalveolar lavage fluid.

based on signs and symptoms and imaging findings. Patients present with headache, fever, focal neurologic deficits, and possibly seizures. Multiple ring-enhancing lesions are seen on imaging studies (**Figure 24**). MRI is preferred to CT because of higher sensitivity. Toxoplasmosis in patients with AIDS is almost always a reactivation disease; therefore, results of serologic testing for anti-*Toxoplasma* IgG antibodies are usually positive. After presumptive treatment (with pyrimethamine plus either sulfadiazine or clindamycin), patients should be assessed for response within 1 or 2 weeks of starting therapy.

Tuberculosis and MAC infection are the most common mycobacterial infections in patients with AIDS. Tuberculosis may present at any CD4 cell count, is more likely to be extrapulmonary at presentation, and may not have the classic chest radiographic findings. Treatment of tuberculosis and HIV coinfection must take into account drug interactions between the rifamycins and many antiretroviral agents. MAC infection in patients with AIDS is usually disseminated at presentation and develops at CD4 cell counts less than 50/µL. Clinical features include fever, sweats, weight loss, lymphadenopathy, hepatosplenomegaly, and cytopenias. Treatment involves a multidrug regimen with clarithromycin or azithromycin as the cornerstone of therapy.

Cytomegalovirus (CMV) infection in patients with AIDS usually presents with specific end-organ dysfunction rather than a nonspecific systemic illness. The most common manifestations are retinitis, esophagitis or colitis, and polyradiculitis or encephalitis. The diagnosis may be made clinically or by demonstrating CMV by histopathologic studies or NAAT. Initial treatment of CMV infection is oral valganciclovir or intravenous ganciclovir.

Molluscum contagiosum is a poxvirus infection that most commonly causes multiple small papules on the face and trunk; it usually responds to immune reconstitution after treatment of the HIV infection. *Bartonella* infection causes bacillary angiomatosis and is characterized by skin lesions that resemble Kaposi sarcoma (KS). KS is caused by a herpes family virus (human herpesvirus 8) and presents with lesions that may vary in color from red to purple to brown and may be macules, papules, plaques, or nodules. KS is most often found on the skin but may also occur on mucous membranes of the respiratory and gastrointestinal tracts. **H**

**KEY POINTS**

- In patients with untreated HIV infection, opportunistic infections usually develop when the CD4 cell count is less than 200/µL.

- Diagnosis of *Pneumocystis jirovecii* pneumonia usually requires stains of bronchoalveolar lavage fluid.

- The most common manifestations of cytomegalovirus infection are retinitis, esophagitis or colitis, and polyradiculitis or encephalitis.

- In patients with AIDS, Kaposi sarcoma presents with lesions that may vary in color from red to purple to brown and may be macules, papules, plaques, or nodules.

## Management of HIV Infection
### When to Initiate Treatment

Recommendations regarding when to start treatment for HIV infection have changed over the years as new data and new regimens become available. Current recommendations from the U.S. Department of Health and Human Services are updated regularly and are available at the National Institutes of Health AIDSInfo Web site (www.aidsinfo.nih.gov). Newer regimens are better tolerated and easier to adhere to (with many single-pill options available). With the additional benefits of fewer complications and reduced transmission, the threshold for starting treatment is now earlier in the disease process and at higher CD4 cell counts. Guidelines recommend treatment for all patients with HIV who are ready to start treatment; the strength of the recommendation varies by CD4 cell count and is based on randomized controlled trials for patients with cell counts less than 350/µL, on cohort studies for those with cell counts between 350 and 500/µL, and on expert opinion for those with cell counts greater than 500/µL. Randomized controlled trials in patients with normal cell counts are in progress.

**KEY POINTS**

- Newer antiretroviral regimens are better tolerated and easier to adhere to, so the threshold for starting treatment is now earlier in the disease process and at higher CD4 cell counts.

- Antiretroviral treatment is recommended for all persons with HIV who are ready to start treatment.

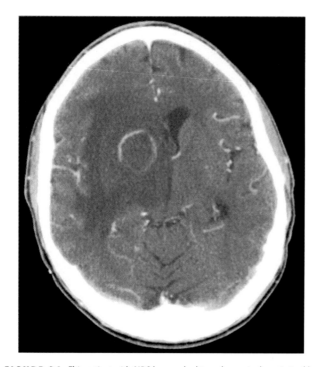

**FIGURE 24.** This patient with AIDS has cerebral toxoplasmosis characterized by a ring-enhancing brain lesion associated with edema and mass effect.

## Antiretroviral Regimens

The most important principle in treating HIV infection is that treatment must fully suppress viral replication to prevent the development of viral drug resistance. Generally, this involves treatment with three drugs from two different classes (**Table 52**). The effectiveness of therapy is determined by monitoring viral load levels, which should fall quickly and progressively within the first few weeks of treatment and reach undetectable levels within a few months. Viral loads should remain undetectable while the patient is receiving antiretroviral therapy, and any persistent detectable levels of virus should be considered as treatment failure. Such treatment requires a level of adherence that may be difficult to maintain for some patients, and adherence must be addressed before therapy begins and at every follow-up visit. The availability of single-pill, once-daily combination regimens has greatly simplified adherence.

Dosing frequency has also been reduced with the use of the pharmacologic "booster" drugs ritonavir and cobicistat. These drugs are not used as antiretroviral agents. Instead, they inhibit the metabolism of other drugs and improve therapeutic drug levels while requiring less frequent dosing. Cobicistat is coformulated with elvitegravir, an integrase inhibitor, and with the protease inhibitors darunavir and atazanavir. Ritonavir is given with most protease inhibitors. Many antiretroviral agents, and pharmacologic boosters especially, affect levels of many other drugs that are metabolized by the same pathways. Drug interactions are increasingly a concern, given the aging population with HIV infection and the increasing frequency in this population of other medical conditions that require treatment. Possible interactions must always be checked before any new drug is started (http://aidsinfo.nih.gov/guidelines/html/1/adult-and-adolescent-arv-guidelines/32/drug-interactions).

| **TABLE 52.** Antiretroviral Agents Used in the United States to Treat HIV Infection | | |
|---|---|---|
| **Class** | **Agent**[a] | **Adverse Effects** |
| Nucleoside RTIs | Abacavir | Hypersensitivity (test for and rule out HLA B5701 before prescribing) |
| | Didanosine | Nausea, neuropathy, pancreatitis, lactic acidosis |
| | Emtricitabine | Minimal toxicity, HBV activity |
| | Lamivudine | Minimal toxicity, HBV activity |
| | Stavudine | Neuropathy, lipodystrophy, lactic acidosis, dyslipidemia |
| | Tenofovir | Nausea, kidney disease and Fanconi syndrome, decreased bone density, HBV activity |
| | Zidovudine | Nausea, headache, anemia, leukopenia, lactic acidosis, lipodystrophy, myopathy |
| Nonnucleoside RTIs | Efavirenz | Neuropsychiatric symptoms (dizziness, somnolence, sleep disturbance, vivid dreams, mood changes), rash, dyslipidemia |
| | Etravirine | Nausea, rash |
| | Nevirapine | Hypersensitivity, rash, hepatitis |
| | Rilpivirine | Rash, headache, insomnia; requires food and gastric acid (no concomitant PPI use) for absorption |
| Protease inhibitors | Atazanavir | Nausea, hyperbilirubinemia, nephrolithiasis, rash; requires food and gastric acid (no concomitant PPI use) for absorption |
| | Darunavir | Nausea, diarrhea, rash |
| | Fosamprenavir | Nausea, diarrhea, rash |
| | Lopinavir | Nausea, diarrhea, hyperlipidemia, insulin resistance |
| | Saquinavir | Nausea, diarrhea, hyperlipidemia, QT prolongation |
| | Tipranavir | Nausea, diarrhea, hyperlipidemia, rash, hepatitis, intracranial hemorrhage |
| CCR5 antagonist | Maraviroc | Hypersensitivity, hepatitis |
| Integrase inhibitors | Dolutegravir | Elevated creatinine (decrease in tubular secretion, not GFR), insomnia, headache (otherwise well tolerated) |
| | Elvitegravir | Nausea, diarrhea (otherwise well tolerated) |
| | Raltegravir | Rash, myopathy (otherwise well tolerated) |
| Pharmacokinetic boosters | Cobicistat | Elevated creatinine (decrease in tubular secretion, not GFR), not recommended if CrCl <70 mL/min |
| | Ritonavir | Nausea, diarrhea, hyperlipidemia, insulin resistance, lipodystrophy |

CrCl = creatinine clearance; GFR = glomerular filtration rate; HBV = hepatitis B virus; PPI = proton-pump inhibitor; RTIs = reverse transcriptase inhibitors.

[a]Many agents are also available as components of combination medications.

Recommendations for initial HIV treatment include use of tenofovir and emtricitabine or abacavir and lamivudine as the dual nucleoside reverse transcriptase inhibitor "backbone." Options for a third agent to complete the regimen include the ritonavir-boosted protease inhibitor darunavir or the integrase inhibitors raltegravir, dolutegravir, or cobicistat-boosted elvitegravir. These regimens are effective and are associated with low toxicity. The choice between them is often based on patient preference and small differences in potential adverse effects.

**KEY POINTS**

- The most important principle in treating HIV infection is that the antiretroviral regimen must fully suppress viral replication to prevent the development of viral drug resistance.

- With effective antiretroviral therapy, viral load levels decrease quickly and progressively within the first few weeks of treatment, reach undetectable levels within a few months, and remain undetectable while therapy continues.

- Cobicistat and ritonavir are pharmacologic "booster" drugs that inhibit the metabolism of other drugs and improve therapeutic drug levels while requiring less frequent dosing.

- Recommendations for initial HIV treatment include three drugs from two different classes, usually two nucleoside reverse transcriptase inhibitors as a "backbone" plus a third agent, most commonly a protease inhibitor or an integrase inhibitor.

### Resistance Testing

Testing for HIV drug resistance can be genotypic (looking for specific mutations associated with resistance to specific drugs) or phenotypic (assessing whether HIV can replicate in the presence of achievable levels of specific drugs). Genotypic testing is cheaper and faster, but phenotypic test results may be easier to interpret, especially for drugs such as protease inhibitors that have complicated patterns of resistance involving multiple mutations. Resistance testing should always be done before an initial drug regimen is chosen and when treatment failure occurs, as indicated by failure to suppress viral load or an increase in viral load that was previously suppressed. Resistance testing should be done while the patient is still receiving the ineffective regimen because testing after therapy is discontinued may allow wild-type virus to outgrow the resistant virus population so that resistance will not be detected. A viral load level greater than 500 copies/mL is usually necessary to successfully perform resistance testing.

**KEY POINTS**

- Resistance testing should always be done when antiretroviral therapy is initiated and when treatment failures occur.

- Resistance testing should be done while the patient is still receiving the ineffective regimen.

## Management of Pregnant Patients with HIV Infection

All pregnant women should be tested for HIV infection; all those with HIV should be treated with antiretrovirals. Treatment for HIV infection during pregnancy will reduce the risk for perinatal transmission to the newborn from about 25% to less than 2%. About one third of transmissions occur in utero and about two thirds at delivery. Because the virus is also transmissible in breast milk, breast-feeding should be avoided in women with HIV infection, even those with undetectable viral load, if an alternative is available. Treatment of the mother after delivery is the same as in a nonpregnant patient with HIV infection.

**KEY POINTS**

- All pregnant women should be tested for HIV infection.

- All pregnant women with HIV infection should receive antiretroviral therapy to reduce perinatal transmission.

## Postexposure Prophylaxis and Preexposure Prophylaxis

Postexposure prophylaxis for HIV infection after an occupational exposure has been used since the 1990s. Antiretroviral agents must be started as soon as possible after exposure to maximize likelihood of successful prevention; treatment is continued for 4 weeks. Exposed workers should be counseled on transmission, symptoms of acute infection, and toxicity of the medications being prescribed. Testing for HIV should be done immediately and at follow-up in 6 weeks, 12 weeks, and 6 months. Prophylaxis should always include at least three drugs. Drug selection may depend on the history of viral resistance in the source patient, but the recommended regimen is tenofovir, emtricitabine, and raltegravir.

Prophylaxis against significant nonoccupational exposures is also recommended by the Centers for Disease Control and Prevention. **Table 53** outlines the risk for HIV transmission

| TABLE 53. | Risk for Transmission of HIV per Single Exposure |
|---|---|
| **Exposure** | **Risk (%)** |
| Occupational—needlestick | 0.3 |
| Occupational—mucous membrane | 0.09 |
| Needle-sharing injection drug use | 0.7 |
| Receptive anal intercourse | 0.5 |
| Receptive vaginal intercourse | 0.1 |
| Insertive anal intercourse | 0.07 |
| Insertive vaginal intercourse | 0.05 |
| Oral sex | 0.01 |

**CONT.**

associated with each type of single exposure. Prophylaxis is recommended for persons presenting with an exposure within the previous 72 hours. Counseling, recommended antiretroviral regimen, and testing are the same as for occupational exposure. **H**

Data also support the use of preexposure prophylaxis (PrEP) in certain populations with ongoing high risk for infection, such as sexual partners of infected persons. Studies have shown benefit in heterosexual partners of infected persons, men who have sex with men, and injection drug users, and consideration of PrEP is recommended for persons in such groups who can adhere to the daily regimen. Efficacy has varied depending on adherence to the regimen; rates of reduction in new infection ranged from 42% to 75% and as high as 92% in patients whose adherence was documented by monitoring blood levels of the drugs. The FDA-approved regimen for PrEP is combination tenofovir-emtricitabine taken once daily. Patients should be counseled regarding possible drug toxicity, the need for strict adherence to the regimen, and the need for continued barrier precautions during sex because the effectiveness of this regimen is less than 100%. They should also be tested for HIV infection, hepatitis B, and other sexually transmitted infections before initiating preventive therapy. Women also require a pregnancy test before starting any regimen. While receiving prophylaxis, patients should be monitored for HIV infection and kidney function (and pregnancy in women) every 2 to 3 months.

**KEY POINTS**

- Postexposure prophylaxis for HIV infection after an occupational exposure or a significant nonoccupational exposure must be started as soon as possible; prophylaxis should always include three drugs taken for 4 weeks.

- The FDA-approved regimen for preexposure prophylaxis is combination tenofovir-emtricitabine taken once daily.

# Viral Infections

## Influenza Viruses

### Overview

The influenza virus group consists of three enveloped RNA members of the family Orthomyxoviridae: influenza A, B, and C. Influenza A viruses are further classified into hemagglutinin (H) and neuraminidase (N) subtypes based on activity of their surface envelope glycoproteins. Influenza A viruses infect humans and other animal (for example, avian and swine) hosts. Influenza B viruses infect only humans. Influenza C viruses are rarely recognized in humans.

H and N surface envelope glycoproteins (antigenic variation) change frequently. Minor changes (antigenic drift) are partly responsible for seasonal outbreaks or epidemics that occur almost yearly. Major changes (antigenic shift) are alterations in the virus caused by reassortment of genes between human and animal influenza A strains. Emergence of a new influenza virus for which humans have no previous protective immunity may result in severe worldwide pandemics.

Influenza A outbreaks generally occur in winter, with attack rates of 10% to 20%. Seasonal influenza disproportionately affects persons 65 years of age or older. Very old persons, very young children, persons with chronic medical conditions, and pregnant women often develop severe disease, which accounts for most hospitalizations and deaths attributable to this infection. In pandemics, disease extends beyond the usual season with higher attack rates and increased mortality in all age groups, especially otherwise healthy young adults. The highly pathogenic H5N1 avian influenza virus predominantly affects children and young adults recently exposed to infected birds and poultry in Europe and Asia. Person-to-person human transmission appears to be limited. The novel H7N9 influenza virus in China is also believed to result from exposure to infected poultry or contaminated environments. To date, no evidence of sustained person-to-person spread has been found. **H**

**KEY POINT**

- Seasonal influenza disproportionately affects persons 65 years or older; more severe infection often develops in very old persons, very young children, persons with chronic medical conditions, and pregnant women.

### Clinical Features and Evaluation

Influenza virus is transmitted by sneezing and coughing. After an incubation period of 1 to 4 days, patients develop fever, headache, myalgia, pharyngeal irritation, and respiratory symptoms (dry cough and nasal discharge). Mild or asymptomatic infections occur, particularly with influenza B. Viral shedding begins 24 to 48 hours before symptom onset and may continue for 5 to 10 days. Patients with uncomplicated infection improve within 2 to 5 days. The most common complications are primary influenza pneumonia and secondary bacterial pneumonia, which are mainly responsible for increased morbidity and mortality in patients aged 65 years and older (see Community-Acquired Pneumonia).

During a confirmed local influenza outbreak, infection can be reliably diagnosed on the basis of clinical criteria alone. When confirmation is needed, rapid antigen tests of respiratory samples from nasopharyngeal swabs detect both influenza A and B. Positive test results are highly specific. However, sensitivity ranges from 40% to 80%. Detection of viral nucleic acid by polymerase chain reaction (PCR) is rapid, has high sensitivity and specificity, and can determine the type and subtype of influenza virus. Serologic assays are useful only for diagnosing infection retrospectively. Whether to test is based on how the result will influence management; testing is generally reserved for patients at high risk for complications, including adults older than 65 years, immunocompromised patients, pregnant and postpartum women, and health care workers. **H**

- The most common complications of influenza are primary influenza pneumonia and secondary bacterial pneumonia.
- During a confirmed local influenza outbreak, infection can be reliably diagnosed on the basis of clinical criteria alone; confirmatory testing is generally reserved for patients at high risk for complications.

## Management

Annual influenza vaccination is the most effective intervention for preventing influenza and is recommended for all persons 6 months of age or older. See MKSAP 17 General Internal Medicine for more information.

Prophylactic or therapeutic antiviral agents should be avoided in persons at low risk for or with equivocal clinical findings of influenza infection. Antiviral therapy begun within 48 hours of symptom onset reduces symptom duration, decreases hospitalization rates, and reduces the incidence and severity of complications; however, adults younger than 65 years without high-risk conditions are unlikely to benefit from antiviral therapy begun later. When treatment is required, the neuraminidase inhibitors oseltamivir and zanamivir are active against influenza A and B. Oseltamivir or zanamivir is recommended for patients with confirmed or highly suspected influenza infection who have an increased risk for complications. Peramivir, an intravenous neuraminidase inhibitor, was approved for use in adults in 2014. All hospitalized patients should receive a neuraminidase inhibitor promptly, even if 48 hours or more has elapsed since disease onset. Treatment duration is generally 5 days but may be longer in immunocompromised or severely ill patients.

Oseltamivir is also approved for pre- and postexposure chemoprophylaxis but is not a substitute for vaccination. Preexposure chemoprophylaxis is taken daily for the duration of potential exposure and, for unvaccinated persons at increased risk for disease complications, up to 10 days after the last known exposure to a person with active influenza. Household transmission is greatly decreased with good hand hygiene and facemasks. Respiratory droplet precautions are required for hospitalized patients.

HVC
- Annual influenza vaccination is the most effective intervention for preventing influenza and is recommended for all persons 6 months of age or older.
- Oseltamivir or zanamivir is recommended for patients with confirmed or highly suspected influenza infection who have an increased risk for complications.

## Novel Coronaviruses

RNA-containing coronaviruses cause upper and lower respiratory tract infections and, to a lesser extent, gastrointestinal disease manifested as diarrhea. In 2002, a novel coronavirus, severe acute respiratory syndrome–coronavirus (SARS-CoV), was reported in China and has now spread worldwide. SARS-CoV causes acute pneumonia with a high mortality rate. Treatment is supportive.

A second novel coronavirus, Middle East respiratory syndrome–coronavirus (MERS-CoV), was first isolated in autumn of 2012. Most reported cases have been linked to six Arabian Peninsula countries, with very limited spread outside these regions. Older persons with comorbid conditions have a mortality rate approaching 50%, whereas younger, healthy persons tend to have asymptomatic or mild disease. Human-to-human spread occurs.

- Novel RNA-containing coronaviruses cause severe acute respiratory syndrome–coronavirus infection and Middle East respiratory syndrome–coronavirus infection.

# Human Herpesvirus Infections
## Overview

The eight herpesviruses capable of infecting humans establish lifelong latency following acute infection and are capable of reactivation and oncogenesis under certain conditions. These DNA viruses are subdivided into groups according to their site of latency and their infectious manifestations. The human herpesviruses (HHVs) and their associated manifestations are summarized in Table 54.

HHV infections are acquired by direct contact with a clinically active infected person or through asymptomatic shedding of the virus. For many HHVs, infected saliva is a common source of spread. Sexual contact, intrauterine infection or exposure at the time of delivery, blood transfusion, and transmission with organ transplantation are modes of acquisition depending on HHV type. Airborne transmission occurs only with varicella-zoster virus (VZV). Humoral immunity is required to protect against primary infection; however, after infection is established, it does not control its spread. The cell-mediated immune system is responsible for controlling the spread, severity, and reactivation of HHV infections. Infection prevention relies mainly on screening, safe sexual practices, and infection control measures. Vaccines exist only for VZV. Effective antiviral medications are available for treatment and reducing reactivation of some of the HHVs. Immune globulin preparations for VZV and cytomegalovirus are indicated under certain circumstances in immunocompromised patients.

## Herpes Simplex Viruses

Although they are closely related and cause similar diseases, herpes simplex viruses 1 and 2 (HSV-1 and HSV-2) are genetically and serologically distinct. HSV-1 infection occurs earlier in life, with nearly 90% of adults worldwide having detectable antibodies by age 40 years. HSV-2 is less prevalent, ranging

**TABLE 54.** Human Herpesviruses and Associated Manifestations

| Type | Synonym | Subfamily | Manifestations | Latency Site |
|---|---|---|---|---|
| HHV-1 | Herpes simplex virus 1 | α | Primary infection: oral and/or genital herpes (predominantly orofacial: gingivostomatitis, pharyngitis, herpes labialis)<br><br>Reactivation: Bell palsy, viral encephalitis; other sites, including skin and eye (recurrent herpes labialis) | Nerve ganglion |
| HHV-2 | Herpes simplex virus 2 | α | Primary infection: oral and/or genital herpes (predominantly genital); meningitis, sacral radiculopathy, and transverse myelitis | Nerve ganglion |
| HHV-3 | Varicella-zoster virus | α | Varicella (chickenpox), herpes zoster (shingles) | Nerve ganglion |
| HHV-4 | Epstein-Barr virus | γ | Infectious mononucleosis, nasopharyngeal carcinoma; in immunocompromised patients: Burkitt lymphoma, central nervous system lymphoma (in patients with AIDS), posttransplant lymphoproliferative disease, hairy leukoplakia | B cell |
| HHV-5 | CMV | β | CMV mononucleosis; in immuno-compromised patients: CMV retinitis, leukopenia and thrombocytopenia, pneumonitis, colitis, esophagitis, or hepatitis | Monocyte, lymphocyte, endothelial cell, epithelial cell |
| HHV-6 (6A and 6B) | Roseolovirus, herpes lymphotropic virus | β | Mononucleosis-like syndrome, sixth disease (in children); may affect various organ systems in transplant patients | T cell |
| HHV-7 | Roseolovirus | β | Usually asymptomatic; may be associated with pityriasis rosea; sixth disease (in children) | T cell |
| HHV-8 | Kaposi sarcoma-associated virus | γ | Kaposi sarcoma, PEL, multicentric Castleman disease | B cell, endothelial cell |

CMV = cytomegalovirus; HHV = human herpesvirus; PEL = primary effusion lymphoma.

from 20% to 60% depending on number of sexual partners, sex, and geographic location.

Numerous infection syndromes are caused by HSV, depending on the virus type, host age, immune status, and anatomic site involved. HSV-1 most frequently manifests as gingivostomatitis and pharyngitis (**Figure 25**).

HSV-2 is a common cause of genital ulcer disease worldwide (see Sexually Transmitted Infections). Primary genital infection during pregnancy may be transmitted to the fetus and lead to spontaneous abortion. Although recurrent infection occurs more often during pregnancy, neonatal outcome is usually unaffected in seropositive women.

HSV-1 and HSV-2 may cause other cutaneous manifestations, including infection of the finger (herpetic whitlow) or skin (herpes gladiatorum) (see MKSAP 17 Dermatology). Involvement of the eye, with keratitis and acute retinal necrosis, occurs infrequently. Proctitis may occur secondary to anal intercourse. HSV infection (primarily HSV-1) is the most common cause of nonepidemic viral encephalitis. Aseptic (sometimes recurrent) meningitis, sacral radiculopathy, and transverse myelitis may also occur after HSV-2 genital infection. Infection of visceral organs, including the esophagus, lung, and liver, may result from viremia or direct extension from nearby mucosal surfaces. The common association of erythema multiforme and HSV infection is a consequence of the host's immune response to the virus.

## Management

The nucleoside analogues acyclovir, valacyclovir, and famciclovir are effective for treating episodic HSV-1 and HSV-2 infections and suppressing recurrent infections. Topical antiviral agents have limited usefulness for treating mucocutaneous disease; however, they are recommended for treatment of

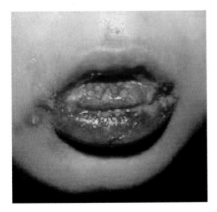

**FIGURE 25.** Herpes simplex virus 1 gingivostomatitis.

CONT.

HSV eye infections. Intravenous acyclovir is required to treat HSV encephalitis. No studies of efficacy of systemic antiviral therapy for HSV aseptic meningitis exist. **H**

**KEY POINTS**

- Primary infection with herpes simplex virus 1 most frequently manifests as gingivostomatitis and pharyngitis.
- Infection with herpes simplex virus 2 is a common cause of genital ulcer disease worldwide.
- Acyclovir, valacyclovir, and famciclovir are effective for treating episodic herpes simplex virus infections and suppressing recurrent infections.

## Varicella-Zoster Virus

### Overview

Varicella-zoster virus (HHV-3) causes a primary infection (varicella, or chickenpox) and a reactivation disorder (herpes zoster, or shingles). VZV establishes lifelong latency after the initial infection. Widespread pediatric varicella immunization has led to a 90% reduction in this once predominantly childhood disease. Varicella in adults and immunocompromised persons of any age is associated with greater morbidity and occasional mortality. Contact and airborne precautions should be used for hospitalized patients with varicella.

Herpes zoster occurs most often in persons older than 60 years. Up to 4% of persons who have had one episode of herpes zoster will experience a second episode; recurrence rates are increased in immunocompromised patients. Herpes zoster cannot be transmitted by contact with a person who has active herpes zoster lesions. However, persons lacking VZV immunity may develop varicella from close contact with viral particles in herpes zoster lesions. Hospitalized patients with herpes zoster must be placed in contact isolation; airborne isolation is required for patients who are immunocompromised.

### Clinical Features and Diagnosis

Varicella develops after an incubation period of 10 to 21 days following exposure. Fever, malaise, and rash (often pruritic) subsequently develop. Classically, the exanthem begins on the face and trunk and spreads centrifugally to the extremities. Oropharyngeal mucosa may also be involved. Characteristic lesions consist of macules, papules, vesicles, and scabs in different stages of development at the same time (**Figure 26A**).

Most infections resolve within 1 to 2 weeks. Complications, most often in adults, include pneumonitis, acute cerebellar ataxia, encephalitis, hepatitis, and secondary bacterial skin infections. Nonimmune pregnant women are especially prone to varicella pneumonitis during the second and third trimesters, and perinatal infection may occur if infection presents approximately 5 days before and up to 2 days after delivery. **H**

Herpes zoster presents with pain or paresthesias in a specific dermatome; the characteristic rash develops several days later (**Figure 26B**). In order of frequency, the thoracic, trigeminal, lumbar, and cervical cutaneous dermatomes are most

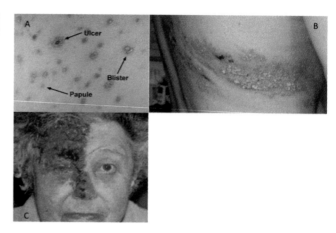

**FIGURE 26.** (*A*) Varicella (chickenpox) exanthem showing characteristic macules, papules, vesicles, and scabs in different stages of development at the same time. (*B*) Dermatomal herpes zoster showing vesicles and pustules on an erythematous base. (*C*) Trigeminal herpes zoster with nasociliary nerve involvement.

often involved. Lesions are similar to varicella, and the rash does not cross the midline. Scattered lesions may occur outside the affected dermatome, more commonly in immunocompromised patients.

Pain due to acute neuritis and postherpetic neuralgia is the most debilitating complication. Postherpetic neuralgia refers to pain that continues for more than 1 month after resolution of the rash. More than 50% of cases occur in persons older than 60 years. Herpes zoster ophthalmicus is a potentially serious sight-threatening condition that may develop when the first branch of the trigeminal nerve is involved (**Figure 26C**). Involvement of the geniculate ganglion may cause Ramsay Hunt syndrome (pain and vesicles in the external ear canal, ipsilateral peripheral facial palsy, and altered or absent taste). Other extracutaneous complications include central nervous system involvement (meningoencephalitis or encephalitis, transverse myelitis, Guillain-Barré syndrome, and stroke), visceral disease (pneumonitis and hepatitis), and secondary bacterial skin infections.

Diagnosis of varicella is clinical and is based on characteristic skin lesions. The lesions may sometimes be confused with disseminated HSV or enteroviral infections; direct fluorescent antibody tests or PCR of samples from active vesicular lesions may be useful in differentiating the infection. Serologic assays detecting IgG antibodies to VZV confirm both previous infection and immunity.

### Management

Acyclovir, valacyclovir, and famciclovir, if started within 72 hours of onset of VZV rash, accelerate the resolution of lesions, decrease new lesion formation and viral shedding, and lessen the severity of acute zoster pain. Valacyclovir and famciclovir also decrease the duration of postherpetic neuralgia. Intravenous acyclovir is indicated for hospitalized, immunocompromised patients and for patients with severe neurologic complications. The addition of glucocorticoids to antiviral therapy is controversial.

Primary prevention of VZV infection involves avoidance of close contact with actively infected persons, routine childhood vaccination, and vaccination for adults who lack a history or serologic evidence of previous VZV infection. Vaccination within 3 to 5 days of exposure is also recommended for postexposure prophylaxis in susceptible immunocompetent persons. Varicella-zoster immune globulin, given within 4 to 10 days of exposure, is recommended for postexposure prophylaxis of immunocompromised adults and pregnant women without evidence of VZV immunity. A zoster vaccine is available and recommended for immunocompetent persons aged 60 years and older that reduces the incidence and severity of herpes zoster and postherpetic neuralgia. The vaccine may also be given to persons with a previous episode of herpes zoster. ▐

**KEY POINTS**

- Acyclovir, valacyclovir, and famciclovir, if started within 72 hours of onset of varicella-zoster virus rash, accelerate the resolution of lesions, decrease new lesion formation and viral shedding, and lessen the severity of acute zoster pain.
- A zoster vaccine is available for immunocompetent persons aged 60 years and older that reduces the incidence and severity of herpes zoster and postherpetic neuralgia.

## Epstein-Barr Virus

Epstein-Barr virus (EBV) (HHV-5) infects oropharyngeal B-cell lymphocytes; latency is established locally and in lymphatic tissue throughout the body. Primary infection mainly occurs when asymptomatic persons shedding EBV in saliva have intimate contact with previously uninfected persons. Most often, infection is asymptomatic and transpires in children and adolescents; antibodies to EBV are present in 95% of adults worldwide. EBV is the most common cause of infectious mononucleosis, characterized by an exudative pharyngitis, fever, and lymphadenopathy (mostly cervical). Splenomegaly is present in approximately 50% of patients. Other, less frequent findings include jaundice, hepatomegaly, and an erythema multiforme–like rash. In most cases, disease spontaneously resolve within 2 to 3 weeks; however, subsequent asthenia may persist for variable periods. EBV is associated with the development of certain malignancies in immunosuppressed and immunocompetent hosts (see Table 54).

Diagnosis can be confirmed by the presence of EBV heterophile (Monospot) antibodies or by the detection of EBV-specific antibodies, particularly IgM, to the EBV viral capsid antigen. With mononucleosis, a lymphocytosis typically exists, classically consisting of atypical lymphocytes. Thrombocytopenia, elevated hepatocellular enzymes, lactate dehydrogenase, and bilirubin are other commonly found laboratory abnormalities.

Acyclovir and other antiviral agents have not proven beneficial in the treatment of infectious mononucleosis or EBV malignancies. Glucocorticoids should be reserved for complications of EBV, such as a compromised airway or autoimmune hemolytic anemia but in general are not recommended for the treatment of mononucleosis.

**KEY POINTS**

- Epstein-Barr virus is the most common cause of infectious mononucleosis, characterized by exudative pharyngitis, fever, and lymphadenopathy.
- Glucocorticoids should be reserved for complications of Epstein-Barr virus but in general are not recommended for the treatment of mononucleosis.

## Human Cytomegalovirus

Most cases of cytomegalovirus (CMV) infection (HHV-5) are asymptomatic, and the virus remains latent afterward. Serologic evidence of CMV is present in 60% to 100% of adults worldwide. CMV may spread by close contact through saliva, blood transfusion, organ transplantation, and breastfeeding. Disease acquisition can also occur through congenital or sexual transmission. Symptomatic primary infection usually manifests as a mononucleosis-like syndrome. Compared with patients who have EBV mononucleosis, patients are usually older and have pharyngitis less often. Fever alone may predominate, making CMV a consideration in persons with fever of unknown origin. The lung, liver, heart, and hematologic and central nervous systems may be involved during primary infection. Latent CMV frequently reactivates in immunocompromised patients. Manifestations of secondary infection include fever, retinitis, pneumonitis, hepatitis, esophagitis, gastritis, colitis, and meningoencephalitis.

Diagnosis relies on isolation of the virus from body fluids, such as urine; detection of CMV pp65 antigen in leukocytes; cytopathic demonstration of "owl's eye" intracellular inclusions; PCR; and serologic assays. Antiviral treatment is typically indicated in cases of disease reactivation in immunocompromised patients and occasionally in immunocompetent hosts with severe disease. Ganciclovir and valganciclovir are first-line agents and are also used as prophylaxis or preemptive therapy in certain transplant patients. Foscarnet and cidofovir are second-line agents. ▐

**KEY POINTS**

- Most cases of cytomegalovirus infection are asymptomatic; symptomatic primary infection usually manifests as a mononucleosis-like syndrome.
- Ganciclovir is typically indicated in cases of cytomegalovirus reactivation in immunocompromised patients.

# New Topics in Anti-infective Therapy

## Introduction

There is a critical shortage of new antimicrobial agents active against multidrug-resistant organisms, often referred to as the ESKAPE pathogens: *Enterococcus faecium,*

**CONT.** *Staphylococcus aureus*, *Klebsiella pneumoniae*, *Acinetobacter* species, *Pseudomonas aeruginosa*, and *Enterobacter* species. Few new agents address the growing problem of gram-negative antimicrobial resistance. Therefore, older antimicrobial agents with in vitro activity against resistant organisms are being used to address these therapeutic challenges.

## Newer Antibacterial Drugs

### Lipopeptides and Glycolipopeptides

Daptomycin is active in vitro against gram-positive organisms, such as *S. aureus* (including methicillin-resistant *S. aureus* [MRSA]), streptococci, and enterococci (including vancomycin-resistant *E. faecium* [VRE] but not vancomycin-resistant *Enterococcus faecalis*). It is an alternative for *S. aureus* bacteremia organisms with vancomycin minimum inhibitory concentrations of 2 µg/mL or more. Resistance to daptomycin occurs but is rare.

Telavancin is active in vitro against aerobic gram-positive organisms, such as *S. aureus* (including MRSA), streptococci, and vancomycin-susceptible *E. faecalis*. New or worsening kidney dysfunction may occur during telavancin therapy, so kidney function should be monitored and the dose adjusted as needed.

Dalbavancin and oritavancin are new agents (approved in 2014) that have pharmacokinetics allowing administration once per week. Both are approved only for the treatment of skin and soft-tissue infections.

Refer to **Table 55** for expanded information on each of the newer antibacterial drugs discussed throughout this section. **H**

**KEY POINTS**

- Daptomycin is approved for gram-positive complicated skin and soft tissue infections, *Staphylococcus aureus* bacteremia, and right-sided endocarditis.

- Telavancin is approved for complicated skin and soft tissue infections caused by aerobic gram-positive organisms (including methicillin-resistant *S. aureus*) and *S. aureus* hospital-acquired pneumonia.

- Dalbavancin and oritavancin are newly approved medications for the treatment of acute bacterial skin and skin structure infections and can be administered once per week.

### **H** Oxazolidinones

Oxazolidinone antibiotics exert a bacteriostatic effect. Linezolid has excellent bioavailability and is active in vitro against gram-positive aerobic organisms (including MRSA and VRE). Linezolid should not be used in patients taking monoamine oxidase inhibitors. Tedizolid is a new oxazolidinone that is more potent than linezolid against gram-positive organisms and has activity against linezolid-resistant *S. aureus*. It presents a lower risk for thrombocytopenia, lower potential for monoamine oxidase interaction, and shorter duration of treatment for skin and soft tissue structure infection (6 days versus 10 days) compared with linezolid. **H**

**KEY POINT**

- Tedizolid is a new oxazolidinone that is more potent against gram-positive organisms than linezolid, and has activity against linezolid-resistant *Staphylococcus aureus* and a lower risk for thrombocytopenia.

### β-Lactam Antibiotics **H**

Ceftaroline is an advanced-generation bactericidal cephalosporin with activity against MRSA (unique for β-lactam antibiotics), multidrug-resistant *Streptococcus pneumoniae*, and *S. aureus* (vancomycin-intermediate, linezolid-resistant, daptomycin-nonsusceptible strains). It has gram-negative activity similar to that of ceftriaxone and is not active against *P. aeruginosa* or extended-spectrum β-lactamase-producing or carbapenemase-producing Enterobacteriaceae species. Ceftolozane-tazobactam, a combination novel cephalosporin and well-established β-lactamase inhibitor, is approved to treat complicated urinary tract infection (including pyelonephritis) and complicated intra-abdominal infections (in combination with metronidazole). This new agent is active against multidrug-resistant strains of *Pseudomonas* and extended-spectrum β-lactamase producing *Escherichia coli*. **H**

**KEY POINTS**

- Ceftaroline is active against methicillin-resistant *Staphylococcus aureus*; multidrug-resistant *Streptococcus pneumoniae*; and vancomycin-intermediate, linezolid-resistant, daptomycin-nonsusceptible strains of *S. aureus* and has gram-negative activity similar to that of ceftriaxone.

- Ceftolozane-tazobactam is active against multidrug-resistant strains of *Pseudomonas* and extended-spectrum β-lactamase–producing *Escherichia coli*.

### Glycylcyclines **H**

Tigecycline is active in vitro against aerobic gram-positive organisms (including MRSA, VRE, and penicillin-resistant *S. pneumoniae*); many gram-negative organisms, including *Enterobacter cloacae*, carbapenem-resistant Enterobacteriaceae, and *Acinetobacter baumannii* (but not *P. aeruginosa* or *Proteus mirabilis*); anaerobes, including *Bacteroides fragilis*; and some atypical organisms (*Mycoplasma*). **H**

**KEY POINT**

- Tigecycline is a broad-spectrum antibiotic that should be used only when alternative treatments are not available. **HVC**

## Newer Uses for Older Antimicrobial Agents **H**

### Trimethoprim-Sulfamethoxazole

Trimethoprim-sulfamethoxazole (TMP-SMX) is used to treat *Pneumocystis jirovecii*, *Stenotrophomonas maltophilia*,

**TABLE 55.   Newer Antimicrobial Agents**

| Agent (class) | Adverse Events | Issues/Limitations | FDA Indications | Relative Cost |
|---|---|---|---|---|
| Ceftaroline (cephalosporin) | Similar to other cephalosporins | Limited clinical experience for MRSA outside of skin infections | Community-acquired pneumonia (not caused by MRSA, clinical trial data lacking), ABSSSI caused by susceptible organisms (including MRSA) | $$ |
| Ceftolozane-tazobactam (combination cephalosporin-β-lactamase inhibitor) | Similar to other cephalosporins | Approved at the end of 2014, so limited clinical experience | Complicated UTI (including pyelonephritis) and complicated intra-abdominal infections (in combination with metronidazole) | $$$ |
| Dalbavancin and oritavancin (glycolipopeptide) | Nausea, headache, diarrhea | Red man syndrome, elevated liver enzymes, cost | ABSSSIs caused by susceptible strains of gram-positive microorganisms (*Staphylococcus aureus* including MRSA, *Streptococcus pyogenes*, *Streptococcus agalactiae*, *Streptococcus anginosus* group) | $$$$ |
| Daptomycin (lipopeptide) | Creatinine kinase elevation | Inactivated by lung surfactant, not effective for pneumonia | Gram-positive complicated skin and soft tissue infections, *S. aureus* (including MRSA) bacteremia, and right-sided endocarditis | $$ |
| Linezolid (oxazolidinone) | Reversible myelosuppression (most commonly thrombocytopenia) after 2 weeks, neuropathies after 28 days | SSRI interaction | Hospital- and community-acquired pneumonia (good lung penetration); uncomplicated and complicated skin and soft tissue infections, including diabetic foot infections without osteomyelitis; and vancomycin-resistant *Enterococcus* infections | $$$ |
| Tedizolid (oxazolidinone) | Nausea, headache, diarrhea | Patients taking SSRIs were excluded from clinical trials | ABSSSI caused by susceptible gram-positive organisms (methicillin-sensitive and resistant *S. aureus*, linezolid-resistant *S. aureus*, *S. pyogenes*, *S. agalactiae*, *S. anginosus* group, *Streptococcus intermedius*, *Streptococcus constellatus*, *Enterococcus faecalis*) | $$ |
| Telavancin (glycolipopeptide) | Nephrotoxicity | Interaction with coagulation tests, decreased efficacy in preexisting chronic kidney disease (estimated glomerular filtration rate <90 mL/min per 1.73 m$^2$) | Complicated skin and soft tissue infections caused by susceptible organisms and *S. aureus* (including MRSA) hospital-acquired pneumonia | $$$ |
| Tigecycline (glycylcycline) | Diarrhea, nausea, vomiting | Black box warning (2013): increased risk for death; should be used only in situations in which alternative treatments are not available | Complicated skin and soft tissue infections, complicated intra-abdominal infections, community-acquired bacterial pneumonia caused by susceptible organisms | $$$ |

ABSSSI = acute bacterial skin and skin structure infections; IV = intravenous; MRSA = methicillin-resistant *Staphylococcus aureus*; SSRI = selective serotonin reuptake inhibitor; UTI = urinary tract infection.

**H CONT.**

*Enterobacter* species, and *Nocardia* infections. TMP-SMX has come into wider use with the emergence of community-associated MRSA. It has broad aerobic, gram-positive (including MRSA), and gram-negative (excluding *P. aeruginosa*) activity. The most common adverse reactions associated with TMP-SMX are urticaria and rash. Hyperkalemia is an adverse effect of treatment, regardless of dosage. Reversible decreases in creatinine clearance also occur, and TMP-SMX may interfere with accurate measurement of creatinine, leading to falsely elevated levels. **H**

**KEY POINT**

- Trimethoprim-sulfamethoxazole has broad aerobic, gram-positive, and gram-negative activity and is active against community-associated methicillin-resistant *Staphylococcus aureus*.

## Polymyxins

Colistin (polymyxin E), a bactericidal agent used to treat multi-drug- and pan-resistant, aerobic, gram-negative infections, is active against many aerobic gram-negative bacteria, including *P. aeruginosa*, *K. pneumoniae*, *A. baumannii*, and carbapenem-resistant Enterobacteriaceae species. *Burkholderia cepacia* and *Proteus*, *Providencia*, and *Serratia* species are resistant. Colistin, usually formulated as colistimethate sodium, can be administered by nebulized aerosol to treat pan-resistant, gram-negative pneumonia or intraventricularly for multidrug-resistant, gram-negative meningitis (usually hospital acquired). Kidney function should be monitored because of colistin's dose-dependent nephrotoxic effects (mainly acute tubular necrosis) and used with caution in patients with preexisting kidney insufficiency. Transient neurologic dysfunction may be alleviated by decreasing the dose.

> **KEY POINT**
> - When colistin is used, kidney function should be monitored because of its dose-dependent nephrotoxic effects; it should be used with caution in patients with preexisting kidney insufficiency.

## Fosfomycin

Fosfomycin is a bactericidal agent available as an oral formulation that has gram-negative and gram-positive activity (including against MRSA and VRE). It has 30% to 37% bioavailability with good distribution into the kidneys, bladder, and prostate, achieving high urine levels for up to 48 hours after a single dose. It is an option for treating lower urinary tract infections caused by VRE and other multidrug-resistant uropathogens. Because of rapid clearance from serum, fosfomycin should not be used in bacteremia; because it does not achieve adequate levels in kidney tissue, it should not be used to treat pyelonephritis.

> **KEY POINT**
> - Fosfomycin can be used to treat lower urinary tract infections caused by vancomycin-resistant *Enterococcus faecium* and other multidrug-resistant uropathogens but should not be used to treat bacteremia or pyelonephritis.

## Aminoglycosides

Aminoglycosides, rapidly bactericidal agents with aerobic gram-negative activity, are generally not used alone because other antimicrobial options are easier to use and do not require monitoring of serum levels to avoid associated nephrotoxicity and ototoxicity. Aminoglycosides may be used to broaden empiric antimicrobial coverage or for synergy to enhance bactericidal activity in the treatment of some gram-positive infections (enterococcal endocarditis). Aminoglycosides remain active against some problem pathogens (*A. baumannii*, *P. aeruginosa*, carbapenem-resistant Enterobacteriaceae species). Extended-interval dosing is associated with less nephrotoxicity

and has replaced traditional aminoglycoside dosing in many clinical situations.

> **KEY POINT**
> - Aminoglycosides require monitoring of serum levels to avoid associated nephrotoxicity and ototoxicity, but extended-interval dosing creates less nephrotoxicity and has replaced traditional dosing in many clinical situations.

## Rifamycins

Rifamycins include rifampin (most common), rifapentine, and rifabutin. Rifampin is a bactericidal agent used against staphylococci, including MRSA, but is not used as monotherapy because resistance develops. Rifampin may be used with other antimicrobial agents, especially to treat prosthetic or indwelling foreign-body staphylococcal infections. Rifampin has excellent bioavailability and distributes widely in body tissues and fluids, including cerebrospinal fluid. Rifampin induces hepatic microsomal enzymes, causing multiple drug-drug interactions, and other medication doses should be adjusted as necessary. Hepatitis is the most serious potential adverse effect related to rifampin.

> **KEY POINT**
> - Rifampin, the most commonly used rifamycin, is not used as monotherapy because resistance develops; it may be used with other antimicrobial agents and has excellent bioavailability, distributing widely through body tissues and fluids, including cerebrospinal fluid.

# Antimicrobial Stewardship

Suboptimal use of antimicrobial agents drives the emergence of antimicrobial resistance, leads to poor outcomes, and increases adverse events (5% risk per patient) and costs. Suboptimal use may include inappropriate use of antimicrobial agents when not indicated and incorrect antimicrobial choice, dose, route of administration, or duration of therapy. Antimicrobial stewardship programs promote responsible antimicrobial use by monitoring and giving advice on high-risk, high-cost agents; combination therapy; intravenous-to-oral conversion; streamlining; de-escalation; and duration of therapy.

Combination therapy has not been clinically shown to minimize the emergence of resistance but may be used as empiric therapy to broaden the spectrum of activity, provide coverage for potential antimicrobial-resistant organisms pending culture and in vitro susceptibility results, or for synergy (more rapid killing) in specific situations such as enterococcal endocarditis. Conversion from an intravenous to an oral antimicrobial agent should be considered whenever possible to limit the need for intravenous catheter access and the risk for a catheter-related bloodstream infection. Considerations include a temperature less than 38.0 °C

(100.4 °F) or clinical improvement over 24 hours, an improving leukocyte count, improving signs and symptoms related to infection with the patient clinically stable, a functional gastrointestinal tract with the ability to swallow medications (or having a nasogastric tube in place), no diagnostic indication for intravenous therapy (such as endocarditis, central nervous system infection, *S. aureus* bacteremia), and having a suitable oral alternative available with good oral bioavailability (including fluoroquinolones, oxazolidinones, metronidazole, clindamycin, trimethoprim-sulfamethoxazole, fluconazole, and voriconazole). **H**

**KEY POINT**

HVC
- Suboptimal use of antimicrobial agents drives the emergence of antimicrobial resistance, leads to poor outcomes, and increases adverse events and costs.

# Outpatient Parenteral Antimicrobial Therapy

Outpatient parenteral antimicrobial therapy (OPAT) allows patients to complete intravenous antimicrobial treatment safely and effectively in an outpatient setting. Common infections considered for OPAT include cellulitis and soft tissue infections, bone and joint infections, infective endocarditis (after an initial period of hospital care and clinical stabilization), antimicrobial-resistant infections in which parenteral therapy is the only option (such as urinary tract infection), and central nervous system infections (including meningitis, brain abscess, encephalitis after initial hospital care and clinical stabilization). In choosing an OPAT regimen, it may be necessary to consider an agent other than the one being used in the hospital to minimize the number of daily doses needed (by choosing agents with a long half-life to maximize the required dosing interval), required monitoring, and the potential for adverse effects that would require closer observation. All patients receiving OPAT should be followed closely by a physician to ensure the appropriate therapy is received, the monitoring plan (antibiotic levels, complete blood count, creatinine level, liver function tests, coagulation tests as appropriate for the antibiotic) is being followed, and the antibiotic dose and timing are adjusted as needed or stopped if adverse effects are encountered. Additionally, patient education regarding signs and symptoms of early intravenous line infection and how to report such concerns is important. OPAT is not appropriate if the patient's medical needs would be better met in the hospital. It is being increasingly used without initial hospitalization, which makes a thorough medical assessment even more important. **H**

**KEY POINT**

HVC
- Outpatient parenteral antimicrobial therapy provides appropriately selected patients the ability to complete antimicrobial treatment in an outpatient setting.

## Bibliography

### Central Nervous System Infections

Armangue T, Leypoldt F, Málaga I, et al. Herpes Simplex Virus Encephalitis is a Trigger of Brain Autoimmunity. Ann Neurol. 2014 Feb;75(2):317-23. [PMID: 24318406]

Helweg-Larsen J, Astradsson A, Richhall H, Erdal J, Laursen A, Brennum J. Pyogenic brain abscess, a 15 year survey. BMC Infect Dis. 2012 Nov 30;12:332. [PMID: 23193986]

Pahud BA, Glaser CA, Dekker CL, et al. Varicella zoster disease of the central nervous system: epidemiological, clinical, and laboratory features 10 years after the introduction of the varicella vaccine. J Infect Dis. 2011 Feb 1;203(3):316-23. [PMID: 21177308]

Petersen LR, Brault AC, Nasci RS. West Nile virus: review of the literature JAMA 2013 Jul 17;310(3):308-15. [PMID: 23860989]

Solomon T, Michael BD, Smith PE, et al. Management of suspected viral encephalitis in adults–Association of British Neurologists and British Infection Association National Guidelines. J Infect. 2012 Apr;64(4):347-73. [PMID: 22120595]

Thigpen MC, Whitney CG, Messonnier NE, Zell ER, Lynfield R, Hadler JL, Harrison LH, Farley MM, Reingold A, Bennett NM, Craig AS, Schaffner W, Thomas A, Lewis MM, Scallan E, Schuchat A, Emerging Infections Programs Network. Bacterial meningitis in the United States, 1998-2007. N Engl J Med. 2011 May 26;364(21):2016-25. [PMID: 21612470]

Titulaer MJ, McCracken L, Gabilondo I, et al. Treatment and prognostic factors for long-term outcome in patients with anti-NMDA receptor encephalitis: an observational cohort study. Lancet Neurol. 2013 Feb;12(2):157-65. [PMID: 23290630]

Tunkel AR, Glaser CA, Bloch KC, et al. The management of encephalitis: clinical practice guidelines by the Infectious Diseases Society of America. Clin infect Dis. 2008 Aug 1;47(3):303-327. [PMID: 18582201]

van de Beek D, Drake JM, Tunkel AR. Nosocomial bacterial meningitis. N Engl J Med. 2010 Jan 14;362(2):146-54. [PMID: 20071704]

Venkatesan A, Geocadin RG. Diagnosis and management of acute encephalitis: A practical approach. Neurol Clin Pract. 2014 Jun;4(3):206-215. [PMID: 25110619]

### Prion Diseases of the Central Nervous System

Imran M, Mahmood S. An overview of human prion diseases. Virol J. 2011 Dec 24;8:599. [PMID: 22196171]

Ironside JW. Variant Creutzfeldt-Jakob disease: an update. Folia Neuropathol. 2012;50(1)50-6. [PMID: 22505363]

Sikorska B, Liberski PP. Human prion diseases: from Kuru to variant Creutzfeldt-Jakob disease. Subscell Biochem. 2012;65:457-96. [PMID: 23225013]

### Skin and Soft Tissue Infections

Hirschmann JV, Raugi GJ. Lower limb cellulitis and its mimics: part II. Conditions that simulate lower limb cellulitis. J Am Acad Dermatol. 2012 Aug;67(2):177.e1-9. [PMID: 22794816]

Lipsky BA, Berendt AR, Cornia PB, et al; Infectious Diseases Society of America. Executive summary: 2012 Infectious Diseases Society of America clinical practice guideline for the diagnosis and treatment of diabetic foot infections. Clin Infect Dis. 2012 Jun;54(12):1679-84. [PMID: 22619239]

Liu C, Bayer A, Cosgrove SE, et al; Infectious Diseases Society of America. Clinical practice guidelines by the Infectious Diseases Society of America for the treatment of methicillin-resistant *Staphylococcus aureus* infections in adults and children [erratum in: Clin Infect Dis. 2011 Aug 1;53(3):319]. Clin Infect Dis. 2011 Feb 1;52(3):e18-55. [PMID: 21208910]

Oehler RL, Velez AP, Mizrachi M, Lamarche J, Gompf S. Bite-related and septic syndromes caused by cats and dogs [erratum in: Lancet Infect Dis. 2009 Sep;9(9):536]. Lancet Infect Dis. 2009 Jul;9(7):439-47. [PMID: 19555903]

Singer AJ, Talan DA. Management of skin abscesses in the era of methicillin-resistant *Staphylococcus aureus*. N Engl J Med. 2014 Mar 13;370(11):1039-47. [PMID: 24620867]

Stevens DL, Bisno AL, Chambers, HF, et al. Practice guidelines for the diagnosis and management of skin and soft tissue infections: 2014 update by the Infectious Diseases Society of America. Clin Infect Dis. 2014;59(2):147-59. [PMID: 24947530]

Stevens DL, Eron LL. Cellulitis and soft-tissue infections. Ann Intern Med. 2009 Jan 6;150(1):ITC11. [PMID: 19124814]

Wong CH, Khin LW, Heng KS, Tan KC, Low CO. The LRINEC (Laboratory Risk Indicator for Necrotizing Fasciitis) score: a tool for distinguishing necrotizing fasciitis from other soft tissue infections. Crit Care Med. 2004 Jul;32(7):1535-41. [PMID: 15241098]

**Community-Acquired Pneumonia**

Baron EJ, Miller JM, Weinstein MP, et al. A guide to utilization of the microbiology laboratory for diagnosis of infectious diseases: 2013 recommendations by the Infectious Diseases Society of America (IDSA) and the American Society for Microbiology (ASM)(a). Clin Infect Dis. 2013 Aug;57(4):e22-e121. [PMID: 23845951]

Bartlett JG, Dowell SF, Mandell LA, File Jr TM, Musher DM, Fine MJ. Practice guidelines for the management of community-acquired pneumonia in adults. Infectious Diseases Society of America. Clin Infect Dis. 2000 Aug;31(2):347-82. [PMID: 10987697]

Christ-Crain M, Stolz D, Bingisser R, et al. Procalcitonin guidance of antibiotic therapy in community-acquired pneumonia: a randomized trial. Am J Respir Crit Care Med. 2006 Jul 1;174(1):84-93. [PMID: 16603606]

Falguera M, Trujillano J, Caro S, et al; NAC-CALIDAD (Proyecto Integrado de Investigación de la Sociedad Española de Patología del Aparato Respiratorio sobre Infecciones Respiratorias de Vías Bajas) Study Group. A prediction rule for estimating the risk of bacteremia in patients with community-acquired pneumonia. Clin Infect Dis. 2009 Aug 1;49(3):409-16. [PMID: 19555286]

File TM Jr, Marrie TJ. Burden of community-acquired pneumonia in North American adults. Postgrad Med. 2010 Mar;122(2):130-41. [PMID: 20203464]

Lim WS, Baudouin SV, George RC, et al. Pneumonia Guidelines Committee of the BTS Standards of Care Committee. BTS guidelines for the management of community acquired pneumonia in adults: update 2009. Thorax. 2009 Oct; 64(Suppl 3):iii1-55. [PMID: 19783532]

Liu C, Bayer A, Cosgrove SE, et al; Infectious Diseases Society of America. Clinical practice guidelines by the Infectious Diseases Society of America for the treatment of methicillin-resistant Staphylococcus aureus infections in adults and children [erratum in: Clin Infect Dis. 2011 Aug 1;53(3):319]. Clin Infect Dis. 2011Feb 1;52(3):e18-55. [PMID: 21208910]

Mandell LA, Wunderink RG, Anzueto A, et al; Infectious Diseases Society of America; American Thoracic Society. Infectious Diseases Society of America; American Thoracic Society consensus guidelines on the management of community-acquired pneumonia in adults. Clin Infect Dis. 2007 Mar;44 Suppl 2:S27-72. [PMID: 17278083]

**Tick-Borne Diseases**

Chapman AS, Bakken JS, Folk SM, et al; Tickborne Rickettsial Diseases Working Group; CDC. Diagnosis and management of tickborne rickettsial diseases: Rocky Mountain spotted fever, ehrlichiosis, and anaplasmosis–United States: a practical guide for physicians and other health-care and public health professionals. MMWR Recomm Rep. 2006 Mar 31;55(RR-4):1-27. [PMID: 16572105]

Hu LT. In the clinic. Lyme disease. Ann Intern Med. 2012 Aug 7;157(3):ITC2-2-16. [PMID: 22868858]

Ismail N, Bloch KC, McBride JW. Human ehrlichiosis and anaplasmosis. Clin Lab Med. 2010 Mar;30(1):261-92. [PMID: 20513551]

Nadelman RB, Hanincová K, Mukherjee P, et al. Differentiation of reinfection from relapse in recurrent Lyme disease. N Engl J Med. 2012 Nov 15;367(20):1883-90. [PMID: 23150958]

Vannier E, Krause PJ. Human babesiosis. N Engl J Med. 2012 Jun 21;366(25):2397-407. [PMID: 22716978]

Wormser GP, Dattwyler RJ, Shapiro ED, et al. The clinical assessment, treatment, and prevention of lyme disease, human granulocytic anaplasmosis, and babesiosis: clinical practice guidelines by the Infectious Diseases Society of America [erratum in: Clin Infect Dis. 2007 Oct 1;45(7):941]. Clin Infect Dis. 2006 Nov 1;43(9):1089-134. [PMID: 17029130]

**Urinary Tract Infections**

Brede CM, Shoskes DA. The etiology and management of acute prostatitis. Nat Rev Urol. 2011 Apr;8(4);207-12. [PMID 21403661]

Dielubanza EJ, Mazur DJ, Schaeffer AJ. Management of non-catheter-associated complicated urinary tract infection. Infect Dis Clin North Am. 2014 Mar;28(1);121-34. [PMID: 24484579]

Foxman B. Urinary tract infection syndromes: occurrence, bacteriology, risk factors, and disease burden. Infect Dis Clin North Am. 2014 Mar;28(1);1-13. [PMID: 24484571]

Geerlings SE, Beerepoot MA, Prins JM. Prevention of recurrent urinary tract infections in women: antimicrobial and nonantimicrobial strategies. Infect Dis Clin North Am. 2014 Mar;28(1);135-47. [PMID: 24484580]

Gupta K, Hooton TM, Naber KG, et al; Infectious Diseases Society of America; European Society for Microbiology and Infectious Diseases. International clinical practice guidelines for the treatment of acute uncomplicated cystitis and pyelonephritis in women: A 2010 update by the Infectious Diseases Society of America and the European Society for Microbiology and Infectious Diseases. Clin Infect Dis. 2011 Mar 1;52(5);e103-20. [PMID: 21292654]

Hooton TM. Clinical practice. Uncomplicated urinary tract infection. N Engl J Med. 2012 Mar 15;366(11);1028-37. [PMID: 22417256]

Trautner BW, Grigoryan L. Approach to a positive urine culture in a patient without urinary symptoms. Infec Dis Clin North Am. 2014 Mar;28(1);15-31. [PMID: 24484572]

***Mycobacterium tuberculosis* Infection**

American Thoracic Society, CDC, Infectious Diseases Society of America. Treatment of tuberculosis [erratum in: MMWR Recomm Rep. 2005 Jan 7;53(51):1203]. MMWR Recomm Rep. 2003 Jun 20;52(RR-11):1-77. [PMID: 12836625]

Centers for Disease Control and Prevention (CDC). Availability of an assay for detecting *Mycobacterium tuberculosis*, including rifampin-resistant strains, and considerations for its use–United States, 2013 [erratum in: MMWR Morb Mortal Wkly Rep. 2013 Nov 15;62(45):906]. MMWR Morb Mortal Wkly Rep. 2013 Oct 18;62(41): 821-7. [PMID: 24141407]

Centers for Disease Control and Prevention (CDC). Reported tuberculosis in the United States, 2013. Atlanta, GA: U.S. Department of Health and Human Services, CDC, September 2014. www.cdc.gov/tb/statistics/reports/2013/default.htm. Updated October 6, 2014. Accessed October 8, 2014.

Mazurek GH, Jereb J, Vernon A, LoBue P, Goldberg S, Castro K. Centers for Disease Control and Prevention (CDC). Updated guidelines for using interferon gamma release assays to detect *Mycobacterium tuberculosis* infection–United States, 2010. MMWR Recomm Rep. 2010 Jun 25;59(RR-5):1-25. [PMID: 20577159]

Rowland R, McShane H. Tuberculosis vaccines in clinical trials. Expert Rev Vaccines. 2011 May;10(5):645-58. [PMID: 21604985]

World Health Organization. Global tuberculosis report 2014. www.who.int/tb/publications/global_report/en/. Accessed June 6, 2014.

**Nontuberculous Mycobacterial Infections**

Griffith DE, Aksamit T, Brown-Elliott BA, et al. An official ATS/IDSA statement: Diagnosis, treatment, and prevention of nontuberculous mycobacterial diseases [erratum in: Am J Respir Crit Care Med. 2007 Apr 1;175(7):744-5]. Am J Respir Crit Care Med. 2007 Feb 15;(4)175:367-416. [PMID: 17277290]

Runyon EH. Anonymous mycobacteria in pulmonary disease. Med Clin North Am. 1959 Jan;43(1):273-290. [PMID: 13612432]

Wentworth AB, Drage LA, Wengenack NL, Wilson JW, Lohse CM. Increased incidence of cutaneous nontuberculous mycobacterial infection, 1980 to 2009: a population-based study. Mayo Clin Proc. 2013 Jan;88(1):38-45. [PMID: 23218797]

**Fungal Infections**

Chiller TM, Nguyen D, Guh A, et al. Clinical findings for fungal infections caused by methylprednisolone injections. N Engl J Med. 2013 Oct 24;369(17):1610-9. [PMID: 24152260]

Hage CA, Knox KS, Wheat LJ. Endemic mycoses: overlooked causes of community acquired pneumonia. Respir Med 2012 Jun;106(6):769-76. [PMID: 22386326]

Ibrahim AS, Kontoyiannis DP. Update on mucormycosis pathogenesis. Curr Opin Infect Dis. 2013 Dec;26(6):508-15. [PMID: 24126718]

La Hoz, RM, Pappas PG. Cryptococcal infections: changing epidemiology and implications for therapy. Drugs. 2013 May;73(6):495-504. [PMID: 23575940]

Leroux S, Ullmann AJ. Management and diagnostic guidelines for fungal diseases in infectious diseases and clinical microbiology: critical appraisal. Clin Microbiol Infect. 2013 Dec;19(12):1115-21. [PMID: 24118188]

López-Martínez R, Méndez-Tovar LJ. Blastomycosis. Clin Dermatol. 2012 Nov-Dec;30(6):565-72. [PMID: 23068144]

McKinsey DS, McKinsey JP. Pulmonary histoplasmosis. Semin Respir Crit Care Med. 2011 Dec;32(6):735-44. [PMID: 22167401]

Pappas PG, Kauffman CA, Andes D, et al. Clinical practice guidelines for the management of candidiasis: 2009 update by the Infectious Diseases Society of America. Clin Infect Dis. 2009 Mar 1;48(5):503-35. [PMID: 19191635]

Perfect JR. Fungal diagnosis: how do we do it and can we do it better? Curr Med Res Opin. 2013 Apr;29 Suppl 4:3-11. [PMID: 23621588]

Welsh O, Vera-Cabrera L, Rendon A, et al. Coccidioidomycosis. Clin Dermatol. 2012 Nov-Dec;30(6):573-91. [PMID: 23068145]

**Sexually Transmitted Infections**

Ganschow PS, Jacobs EA, Mackinnon J, Charney P. Update in women's health. J Gen Intern Med. 2009 Jun;24(6):765-70. [PMID: 19259751]

Kirkcaldy RD, Kidd S, Weinstock HS, Papp JR, Bolan GA. Trends in antimicrobial resistance in Neisseria gonorrhoeae in the USA: the Gonococcal Isolate Surveillance Project (GISP), January 2006-June 2012. Sex Transm Infect. 2013 Dec;89-Suppl 4:iv5-10. [PMID: 24243881]

Martin-Iguacel R, Llibre JM, Nielsen H, et al. Lymphogranuloma venereum proctocolitis: a silent endemic disease in men who have sex with men in industrialised countries. Eur J Clin Microbiol Infect Dis. 2010 Aug;29(8):917-25. [PMID: 20509036]

U.S. Preventive Services Task Force. Screening for chlamydial infection: U.S. Preventive Services Task Force recommendation statement. Ann Intern Med. 2007 Jul 17;147(2):128-34. [PMID: 17576996]

Workowski KA, Berman S; Centers for Disease Control and Prevention (CDC). Sexually transmitted diseases treatment guidelines, 2010 [erratum in: MMWR Recomm Rep. 2011 Jan 14;60(1):18]. MMWR Recomm Rep. 2010 Dec 17;59(RR-12):1-110. [PMID: 21160459]

Workowski K. In the clinic. Chlamydia and gonorrhea [erratum in: Ann Intern Med. 2013 Mar 19;158(6):504]. Ann Intern Med. 2013 Feb 5;158(3):ITC2-1. [PMID: 23381058]

**Osteomyelitis**

Conterno LO, Turchi MD. Antibiotics for treating chronic osteomyelitis in adults. Cochrane Database Syst Rev. 2013;Sep 6(9):CD008344. [PMID: 24014191]

Fridman R, Bar-David T, Kamen S, et al. Imaging diabetic foot infections. Clin Podiatr Med Surg. 2014 Jan;31(1):43-56. [PMID: 24296017]

Hatzenbuehler J, Pulling TJ. Diagnosis and management of osteomyelitis. Am Fam Physician. 2011 Nov 1;84(9):1027-1033. [PMID: 22046943]

Lipsky BA, Berendt AR, Cornia PB, et al. 2012 Infectious Diseases Society of America clinical practice guideline for the diagnosis and treatment of diabetic foot infections. Clin Infect Dis. 2012 Jun;54(12):1679-1684. [PMID: 22619239]

Liu R, Li L, Yang M, et al. Systematic review of the effectiveness of hyperbaric oxygenation therapy in the management of chronic diabetic foot ulcers. Mayo Clin Proc. 2013 Feb;88(2):166-175. [PMID: 23374620]

Peters EJ, Lipsky BA. Diagnosis and management of infection in the diabetic foot. Med Clin North Am. 2013; Sept;97(5):911-946. [PMID: 23992901]

Rao N, Ziran BH, Lipsky BA. Treating osteomyelitis: antibiotics and surgery. Plast Reconstr Surg. 2011 Jan;127 Suppl 1:177S-187S. [PMID: 21200289]

Sanders J, Mauffrey C. Long bone osteomyelitis in adults: fundamental concepts and current techniques [erratum in: Orthopedics. 2014 Jan;37(1):16]. Orthopedics. 2013 May;36(5):368-375. [PMID: 23672894]

Weissman S, Parker RD, Siddiqui W, et al. Vertebral osteomyelitis: Retrospective review of 11 years of experience. Scand J Infect Dis. 2014 Mar;46(3):193-199. [PMID: 24450841]

**Fever of Unknown Origin**

Hayakawa K, Ramasamy B, Chandrasekar PH. Fever of unknown origin: an evidence-based review. Am J Med Sci. 2012 Oct;344(4):307-16. [PMID: 22475734]

**Primary Immunodeficiencies**

Abolhassani H, Sagvand BT, Shokuhfar T, Mirminachi B, Rezaei N, Aghamohammadi A. A review on guidelines for management and treatment of common variable immunodeficiency. Expert Rev Clin Immunol. 2013 June;9(6):561-74. [PMID: 23730886]

Hampson FA, Chandra A, Screaton NJ, et al. Respiratory disease in common variable immunodeficiency and other primary immunodeficiency disorders. Clin Radiol. 2012 Jun;67(6):587-95. [PMID: 22226567]

Uzzaman A, Fuleihan RL. Approach to primary immunodeficiency. Allergy Asthma Proc. 2012 May-Jun;33(Suppl 1):S91-5. [PMID: 22794700]

**Bioterrorism**

Breman JG, Henderson DA. Diagnosis and management of smallpox. N Engl J Med. 2002 Apr 25; 346(17):1300-1308. [PMID: 11923491]

Bush LM, Perez MT. The anthrax attacks 10 years later. Ann Intern Med. 2012 Jan 3; 156(1 PT 1):41-44. [PMID: 21969275]

Christian MD. Biowarfare and bioterrorism. Crit Care Clin. 2013 Jul; 29(3):717-756. [PMID: 23830660]

Hendricks KA, Wright ME, Shadomy SV, et al. Centers for disease control and prevention expert panel meetings on prevention and treatment of anthrax in adults. Emerg Infec Dis. 2014 Feb;20(2). [PMID: 24447897]

Inglesby TV, O'Toole T, Henderson DA, et al. Anthrax as a biological weapon, 2002: updated recommendations for management [erratum in: JAMA 2002 Oct 16;288(15):1849]. JAMA. 2002 May 1; 287(-17):2236-2252. [PMID: 11980524]

McFee RB. Viral hemorrhagic fever viruses. Dis Mon. 2013; 59(12):410-425. [PMID: 24314803]

Thomas LD, Schaffner W. Tularemia pneumonia. Infec Dis Clin North Am. 2010 Mar; 24(1):43-55. [PMID: 20171544]

Zhang JC, Sun L, Nie QH. Botulism, where are we now? Clin Toxicol (Phila). 2010 Nov; 48(9):867-879. [PMID: 21171845]

**Travel Medicine**

Feder HM Jr, Mansilla-Rivera K. Fever in returning travelers: a case-based approach. Am Fam Physician. 2013 Oct 15;88(8):524-30. [PMID: 24364573]

Genton B, D'Acremont V. Malaria prevention in travelers. Infec Dis Clin North Am. 2012 Sep;26(3):637-54. [PMID: 22963775]

Herman JS, Hill DR. Vaccine-preventable diseases and their prophylaxis. Infect Dis Clin North Am. 2012 Sep;26(3):595-608. [PMID: 22963772]

Malcom TR, Chin-Hong PV. Endemic mycoses in immunocompromised hosts. Curr Infect Dis Rep. 2013 Dec;15(6):536-43. [PMID: 24197921]

Matheny SC, Kingery JE. Hepatitis A. Am Fam Physician. 2012 Dec 1;86(11):1027-34. [PMID: 23198670]

Nair D. Travelers' diarrhea: prevention, treatment, and post-trip evaluation [erratum in: J Fam Pract. 2013 Sep;62(9):464]. J Fam Pract. 2013 Jul;62(7):356-61. [PMID: 23957028]

Parola P, Paddock CD, Socolovschi C, et al. Update on tick-borne rickettsioses around the world: a geographic approach [erratum in: Clin Microbiol Rev. 2014 Jan;27(1):166]. Clin Microbiol Rev. 2013 Oct;26(4):657-702. [PMID: 24092850]

Simmons CP, Farrar JJ, Nguyen VV, Wills B. Dengue. N Engl J Med. 2012 Apr 12;366(15):1423-32. [PMID: 22494122]

Steffen R, Hill DR, DuPont HL. Traveler's diarrhea: a clinical review. JAMA. 2015 Jan 6;313(1):71-80. [PMID: 25562268]

White NJ, Pukrittayakamee S, Hien TT, Faiz MA, Mokuolu OA, Dondorp AM. Malaria. Lancet. 2014 Feb 22;383(9918):723-35. [PMID: 23953767]

**Infectious Gastrointestinal Syndromes**

Alasmari F, Seiler SM, Hink T, Burnham CA, Dubberke ER. Prevalence and risk factors for asymptomatic Clostridium difficile carriage. Clin Infect Dis. 2014 Jul 15;59(2):216-22. [PMID: 24755858]

Centers for Disease Control and Prevention (CDC). Vital signs: preventing *Clostridium difficile* infections. MMWR Morb Mortal Wkly Rep. 2012 Mar 9;61(9):157-62. [PMID: 22398844]

Christopher PR, David KV, John SM, Sankarapandian V. Antibiotic therapy for Shigella dysentery. Cochrane Database Syst Rev. 2010 Aug 4;(8):CD006784. [PMID: 20687081]

Dupont HL. Approach to the patient with infectious colitis. Curr Opin Gastroenterol. 2012 Jan;28(1):39-46. [PMID: 22080825]

Dupont HL. Diagnosis and management of *Clostridium difficile* infection. Clin Gastroenterol Hepatol. 2013 Oct;11(10):1216-23. [PMID: 23542332]

Leffler DA, Lamont JT. Clostridium difficile infection. N Engl J Med. 2015 Apr 16;372(16):1539-48. [PMID: 25875259]

Onwuezobe IA, Oshun PO, Odigwe CC. Antimicrobials for treating symptomatic non-typhoidal *Salmonella* infection. Cochrane Database Syst Rev. 2012 Nov 14;11:CD001167. [PMID: 23152205]

Page AV, Liles WC. Enterohemorrhagic *Escherichia coli* infections and hemolytic-uremic syndrome. Med Clin North Am. 2013 Jul;97(4):681-95. [PMID: 23809720]

Ross AG, Olds GR, Cripps AW, Farrar JJ, McManus DP. Enteropathogens and chronic illness in returning travelers. N Engl J Med. 2013 May 9;368(19):1817-25. [PMID: 23656647]

Wright SG. Protozoan infections of the gastrointestinal tract. Infect Dis Clin North Amer. 2012 Jun;26(2):323-39. [PMID: 22632642]

**Infections in Transplant Recipients**

Cervera C, Fernández-Ruiz M, Valledor A, et al. Epidemiology and risk factors for late infection in solid organ transplant recipients. Transplant Infect Dis. 2011 Dec;13(6):598-607. [PMID: 21535336]

Danziger-Isakov L, Kumar D; AST Infectious Diseases Community of Practice. Vaccination in solid organ transplantation. Am J Transplant. 2013 Mar;13(Suppl 4):311-7. [PMID: 23465023]

Fishman JA. Infections in immunocompromised hosts and organ transplant recipients: essentials. Liver Transpl. 2011 Nov;17(Suppl 3):S34-7. [PMID: 21748845]

Grim SA, Clark NM. Management of infectious complications in solid-organ transplant recipients. Clin Pharmacol Ther. 2011 Aug;90(2):333-42. [PMID: 21716270]

Hodson EM, Ladhani M, Webster AC, Stripoli GF, Craig JC. Antiviral medications for preventing cytomegalovirus disease in solid organ transplant recipients. Cochrane Database Syst Rev. 2013 Feb 28;2:CD003774. [PMID: 23450543]

Majhail NS, Rizzo JD, Lee SJ, et al; Center for International Blood and Marrow Transplant Research (CIBMTR); American Society for Blood and Marrow Transplantation (ASBMT); European Group for Blood and Marrow Transplantation (EBMT); Asia-Pacific Blood and Marrow Transplantation

Group (APBMT); Bone Marrow Transplant Society of Australia and New Zealand (BMTSANZ); East Mediterranean Blood and Marrow Transplantation Group (EMBMT); Sociedade Brasileira de Transplante de Medula Ossea (SBTMO). Recommended screening and preventive practices for long-term survivors after hematopoietic cell transplantation. Biol Blood Marrow Transplant. 2012 Mar;18(3):348-71. [PMID: 22178693]

Trofe-Clark J, Lemonovich TL; AST Infectious Diseases Community of Practice. Interactions between anti-infective agents and immunosuppressants in solid organ transplantation. Am J Transplant. 2013 Mar;13(Suppl 4):318-26. [PMID: 23465024]

Weigt SS, Gregson AL, Deng JC, Lynch JP 3rd, Belperio JA. Respiratory viral infections in hematopoietic stem cell and solid organ transplant recipients. Semen Respire Crit Care Med. 2011 Aug;32(4):471-93. [PMID: 21858751]

## Health Care–Associated Infections

Anderson DJ, Podgorny K, Berríos-Torres SI, et al. Strategies to prevent surgical site infections in acute care hospitals: 2014 update. Infect Control Hosp Epidemiol. 2014 Sep;35 Suppl 2:S66-88. [PMID: 25376070]

Chenoweth CE, Gould CV, Saint S. Diagnosis, management and prevention of catheter-associated urinary tract infections. Infect Dis Clin North Am. 2014 Mar;28(1):105-19. [PMID: 24484578]

de Mestral C, Nathens AB. Prevention, diagnosis, and management of surgical site infections: relevant considerations for critical care medicine. Crit Care Clin. 2013 Oct;29(4):887-94. [PMID: 24094383]

Klompas M, Branson R, Eichenwald EC, et al; Society for Healthcare Epidemiology of America (SHEA). Strategies to prevent ventilator-associated pneumonia in acute care hospitals: 2014 update. Infect Control Hosp Epidemiol. 2014 Aug;35(8):915-36. [PMID: 25026607]

Marschall J, Mermel LA, Fakih M, et al; Society for Healthcare Epidemiology of America. Strategies to prevent central line-associated bloodstream infections in acute care hospitals: 2014 update. Infect Control Hosp Epidemiol. 2014 Jul;35(7):753-71. [PMID: 24915204]

Sievert DM, Ricks P, Edwards JR, et al; National Healthcare Safety Network (NHSN) Team and Participating NHSN Facilities. Antimicrobial-resistant pathogens associated with healthcare-associated infections: summary of data reported to the National Healthcare Safety Network at the Centers of Disease Control and Prevention, 2009-2010. Infect Control Hosp Epidemiol. 2013 Jan;34(1):1-14. [PMID: 23221186]

Sydnor ER, Perl TM. Hospital epidemiology and infection control in acute-care settings. Clin Microbiol Rev. 2011 Jan;24(1):141-73. [PMID: 21233510]

Thwaites GE, Edgeworth JD, Gkrania-Klotsas E, et al; UK Clinical Infection Research Group. Clinical management of *Staphylococcus aureus* bacteremia. Lancet Infect Dis. 2011 Mar;11(3):208-22. [PMID: 21371655]

van Hal SJ, Fowler VG Jr. Is it time to replace vancomycin in the treatment of methicillin-resistant *Staphylococcus aureus* infections? Clin Infect Dis. 2013 Jun;56(12):1779-88. [PMID: 23511300]

## HIV/AIDS

Aberg JA, Gallant JE, Ghanem KG, et al. Primary care guidelines for the management of persons infected with HIV: 2013 update by the HIV Medicine Association of the Infectious Diseases Society of America. Clin Infect Dis 2014 Jan;58:1-10. [PMID: 24343580]

Centers for Disease Control and Prevention, Association of Public Health Laboratories; Laboratory testing for the diagnosis of HIV infection: updated recommendations. http://stacks.cdc.gov/view/cdc/23447. Published June 27, 2014. Accessed July 14, 2015.

Kuhar DT, Henderson DK, Struble KA, et al. Updated US Public Health Service guidelines for the management of occupational exposures to human immunodeficiency virus and recommendations for postexposure prophylaxis [erratum in: Infect Control Hosp Epidemiol. 2013 Nov;34(11):1238]. Infect Control Hosp Epidemiol 2013 Sept;34(9):875-92. [PMID: 23917901]

Lichterfeld M, Rosenberg ES. Acute HIV-1 infection: a call to action. Ann Intern Med. 2013 Sept 17;159(6):425-7. [PMID: 24042369]

Marrazzo JM, del Rio C, Holtgrave DR, et al. HIV prevention in clinical care settings: 2014 recommendations of the International Antiviral Society-USA Panel [errata in: JAMA. 2014 Jul 23-30;312(4):403. JAMA. 2014 Aug 13;312(6):652]. JAMA. 2014 Jul 23-30;312(4):390-409. [PMID: 25038358]

Moyer VA, US Preventive Services Task Force. Screening for HIV: U.S. Preventive Services Task Force recommendation statement. Ann Intern Med. 2013 Jul 2;159:51-60. [PMID: 23698354]

Panel on Antiretroviral Guidelines for Adults and Adolescents. Guidelines for the use of antiretroviral agents in HIV-1-infected adults and adolescents. Department of Health and Human Services. http://aidsinfo.nih.gov/contentfiles/lvguidelines/AdultandAdolescentGL.pdf. Updated April 8, 2015. Accessed July 14, 2015.

Panel on Opportunistic Infections in HIV-Infected Adults and Adolescents. Guidelines for the prevention and treatment of opportunistic infections in HIV-infected adults and adolescents: recommendations from the Centers for Disease Control and Prevention, the National Institutes of Health, and the HIV Medicine Association of the Infectious Diseases Society of America. http://aidsinfo.nih.gov/contentfiles/lvguidelines/adult_oi.pdf. Updated April 16, 2015. Accessed July 14, 2015.

Panel on Treatment of HIV-Infected Pregnant Women and Prevention of Perinatal Transmission. Recommendations for use of antiretroviral drugs in pregnant HIV-1 infected women for maternal health and interventions to reduce perinatal HIV transmission in the United States. http://aidsinfo.nih.gov/contentfiles/lvguidelines/PerinatalGL.pdf. Updated March 28, 2014. Accessed July 14, 2015.

Rubin LG, Levin MJ, Ljungman P, et al. 2013 IDSA clinical practice guideline for vaccination of the immunocompromised host [erratum in: Clin Infect Dis. 2014 Jul 1;59(1):144]. Clin Infect Dis. 2014 Feb;58(3):309-18. [PMID: 24421306]

## Viral Infections

Arabi YM, Arifi AA, Balky HH, et al. Clinical course and outcomes of critically ill patients with middle east respiratory syndrome coronavirus infection. Ann Intern Med. 2014 Mar 18;160(6):389-397. [PMID: 24474051]

Cernik C, Gallina K, Brodell RT. The treatment of herpes simplex infections: an evidence-based review. Arch Intern Med. 2008 Jun 9;168(11):1137-44. [PMID: 1854120]

Christian MD, Poutanen SM, Loutfy MR, et al. Severe acute respiratory syndrome. Clin Infec Dis. 2004 May 15;38(10):1420-1427. [PMID: 15156481]

Cohen JI. Herpes zoster. N Engl J Med. 2013;369:255-263. [PMID: 24171531]

Fatahzadeh M, Schwartz RA. Human herpes simplex virus infections: epidemiology, pathogenesis, symptomatology, diagnosis, and management. J Am Acad Dermatol. 2007 Nov;57(5):737-763. [PMID: 17939933]

Gershon AA, Gershon MD. Pathogenesis and current approaches to control of varicella-zoster virus infections. Clin Micriobiol Rev. 2013 Oct;26(4):728-743. [PMID: 24092852]

Harper SA, Bradley JS, Englund JA, et al. Seasonal influenza in adults and children– Diagnosis, treatment, chemoprophylaxis, and institutional outbreak management: Clinical practice guidelines of the Infectious Diseases Society of America. Clin Infect Dis. 2009 Apr 15; 48(8):1003-1032. [PMID: 19281331]

Hui DS, Memish ZA, Zumla A. Severe acute respiratory syndrome vs. the Middle East respiratory syndrome. Curr Opin Pulm Med. 2014 May;20(3):233-241. [PMID: 24626235]

Kidd M. Influenza viruses: update of epidemiology, clinical; features, treatment and vaccination. Curr Opin Pulm Med. 2014 May; 20(3):242-6. [PMID: 24637227]

## New Topics in Anti-infective Therapy

Chapman AL. Outpatient Parenteral Antimicrobial Therapy. BMJ 2013;346:f1585. [PMID: 23532865]

Damodaran SE, Madhan S. Telavancin: A novel lipoglycopeptide antibiotic. J Pharmacol Pharmacother. 2011 Apr;2(2):135-137. [PMID: 21772784]

Falagas ME, Kasiakou SK. Colistin: the revival of polymyxins for the management of multidrug-resistant gram-negative bacterial infections [erratum in: Clin Infect Dis. 2006 Jun 15;42(12):1819]. Clin Infect Dis. 2005 May 1;40(9):1333-1341. [PMID: 15825037]

Petrosillo N, Giannella M, Lewis R, Viale P. Treatment of carbapenem-resistant Klebsiella pneumoniae: the state of the art. Expert Rev Anti Infect Ther. 2013 Feb;11(2):159-177. [PMID: 23409822]

Pogue JM, Marchaim D, Kaye D, Kaye KS. Revisiting "older" antimicrobials in the era of multidrug resistance. Pharmacotherapy. 2011 Sept;31(9):912-921. [PMID: 21923592]

Seaton RA, Barr DA. Outpatient Parenteral Antibiotic Therapy: Principles and Practice. Eur J Intern Med. 2013 Oct;24(7):617-623. [PMID: 23602223]

Society for Healthcare Epidemiology of America; Infectious Diseases Society of America; Pediatric Infectious Diseases Society. Policy Statement on Antimicrobial Stewardship by the Society for Healthcare Epidemiology of America (SHEA), the Infectious Diseases Society of America (IDSA), and the Pediatric Infectious Diseases Society (PIDS). Infect Control Hosp Epidemiol. 2012 Apr;33(4):322-327. [PMID: 22418625]

Tamma PD, Cosgrove SE, Maragakis LL. Combination Therapy for Treatment of Infections with Gram-Negative Bacteria. Clin Microbiol Rev. 2012 Jul;25(3):450-470. [PMID: 22763634]

Tice AD, Rehm SJ, Dalovisio JR, et al. Practice Guidelines for Outpatient Parenteral Antimicrobial Therapy. Clin Infect Dis. 2004 Jun 15;38(12):1651-1672. [PMID: 15227610]

Vidaillac C, Rybak MJ. Ceftobiprole: First Cephalosporin with Activity against Methicillin-resistant Staphylocccus aureus. Pharmacotherapy. 2009 May;29(5):511-525. [PMID: 19397461]

# Infectious Disease Self-Assessment Test

This self-assessment test contains one-best-answer multiple-choice questions. Please read these directions carefully before answering the questions. Answers, critiques, and bibliographies immediately follow these multiple-choice questions. The American College of Physicians is accredited by the Accreditation Council for Continuing Medical Education (ACCME) to provide continuing medical education for physicians.

The American College of Physicians designates MKSAP 17 **Infectious Disease** for a maximum of **19** *AMA PRA Category 1 Credits*™. Physicians should claim only the credit commensurate with the extent of their participation in the activity.

## *Earn "Instantaneous" CME Credits Online*

Print subscribers can enter their answers online to earn CME credits instantaneously. You can submit your answers using online answer sheets that are provided at mksap.acponline.org, where a record of your MKSAP 17 credits will be available. To earn CME credits, you need to answer all of the questions in a test and earn a score of at least 50% correct (number of correct answers divided by the total number of questions). Take any of the following approaches:

➤ Use the printed answer sheet at the back of this book to record your answers. Go to mksap.acponline.org, access the appropriate online answer sheet, transcribe your answers, and submit your test for instantaneous CME credits. There is no additional fee for this service.

➤ Go to mksap.acponline.org, access the appropriate online answer sheet, directly enter your answers, and submit your test for instantaneous CME credits. There is no additional fee for this service.

➤ Pay a $15 processing fee per answer sheet and submit the printed answer sheet at the back of this book by mail or fax, as instructed on the answer sheet. Make sure you calculate your score and fax the answer sheet to 215-351-2799 or mail the answer sheet to Member and Customer Service, American College of Physicians, 190 N. Independence Mall West, Philadelphia, PA 19106-1572, using the courtesy envelope provided in your MKSAP 17 slipcase. You will need your 10-digit order number and 8-digit ACP ID number, which are printed on your packing slip. Please allow 4 to 6 weeks for your score report to be emailed back to you. Be sure to include your email address for a response.

If you do not have a 10-digit order number and 8-digit ACP ID number or if you need help creating a username and password to access the MKSAP 17 online answer sheets, go to mksap.acponline.org or email custserv@acponline.org.

CME credit is available from the publication date of December 31, 2015, until December 31, 2018. You may submit your answer sheets at any time during this period.

*Each of the numbered items is followed by lettered answers. Select the **ONE** lettered answer that is **BEST** in each case.*

## Item 1

A 33-year-old woman is evaluated in the emergency department for a 2-month history of fever, lethargy, weight loss, and headache. She moved to the United States from India 4 years ago. Her father died of tuberculosis 20 years ago. Medical history is otherwise unremarkable, and she takes no medications.

On physical examination, temperature is 38.6 °C (101.5 °F), blood pressure is 114/70 mm Hg, pulse rate is 94/min, and respiration rate is 18/min. BMI is 20. Except for lethargy, neurologic examination is unremarkable. No abnormalities are noted on ophthalmologic, cardiac, or pulmonary examinations or in the remainder of the physical examination.

**Cerebrospinal fluid (CSF) studies:**

| | |
|---|---|
| Leukocyte count | 275/µL (275 × 10⁶), with 98% lymphocytes |
| Glucose | 30 mg/dL (1.7 mmol/L) |
| Protein | 250 mg/dL (2500 mg/L) |
| CSF opening pressure | 150 mm H₂O |

The remainder of a complete blood count and comprehensive metabolic panel are normal. Acid-fast bacilli smear of CSF is negative, but polymerase chain reaction is positive for *Mycobacterium tuberculosis*.

Minimal basilar meningeal enhancement is seen on CT scan of the head without any evidence of cisternal or ventricular abnormalities, midline shift, or mass lesion.

**In addition to four-drug antituberculous therapy, which of the following is the most appropriate additional treatment?**

(A) Acetazolamide
(B) Dexamethasone
(C) Furosemide
(D) Ventriculoperitoneal shunt

## Item 2

A 33-year-old man is admitted to the hospital after experiencing a generalized tonic-clonic seizure. He has also had increasing weakness of the left hand and arm, headaches, and fever of 1 week's duration. Medical history is significant for AIDS, without opportunistic infections in the past several years. His last clinic visit was more than 2 years ago, and his family reports that he has been taking his antiretroviral therapy (ART) only intermittently since around that time.

On physical examination, temperature is 37.3 °C (99.1 °C), blood pressure is 142/92 mm Hg, pulse rate is 96/min, and respiration rate is 14/min. He is somnolent and slightly confused. His general medical examination is normal. On neurologic examination, there is no nuchal rigidity. Left upper extremity weakness is noted, but the examination is otherwise unremarkable.

**Laboratory studies:**

| | |
|---|---|
| CD4 cell count | 66/µL |
| Leukocyte count | 4400/µL (4.4 × 10⁹/L) (differential: 80% polymorphonuclear cells, 12% lymphocytes, 5% eosinophils, 3% monocytes) |
| Cryptococcal antigen, serum | Negative |
| *Toxoplasma gondii* | IgG positive, IgM negative |

Noncontrast head CT shows a single lesion in the right parietal area. Brain MRI with contrast confirms this lesion with additional smaller lesions in the left frontal, basal ganglia, and cerebellar areas; all show a small surrounding area of enhancement without edema. No meningeal enhancement is seen.

**Which of the following is the most likely diagnosis?**

(A) Central nervous system lymphoma
(B) Cryptococcosis
(C) Progressive multifocal leukoencephalopathy
(D) Toxoplasmosis

## Item 3

A 59-year-old man is evaluated in the ICU for fever and leukocytosis. He was admitted to the ICU 13 days ago with respiratory failure resulting from Guillain-Barré syndrome and was intubated and mechanically ventilated. On hospital day 9, he developed fever without an increase in secretions or change in oxygenation. A new left lower-lobe infiltrate was seen on chest radiograph, and his leukocyte count was 17,500/µL (17.5 × 10⁹/L). Sputum culture grew methicillin-sensitive *Staphylococcus aureus*. Nafcillin was started, with temporary resolution of the fever within 48 hours. Medical history is otherwise unremarkable. Medications are nafcillin and intravenous immune globulin.

On physical examination, temperature is 38.2 °C (100.8 °F), blood pressure is 132/84 mm Hg, pulse rate is 94/min, and respiration rate is 18/min. Pulmonary examination reveals decreased breath sounds in the left lower lung field. The remainder of the examination is noncontributory.

Laboratory studies show a leukocyte count of 17,300/µL (17.3 × 10⁹/L). Sputum Gram stain reveals 1+ leukocytes and 1+ gram-positive cocci in clusters.

A new moderate left pleural effusion, but no increase in the left lower lobe infiltrate, is seen on chest radiograph. CT scan shows left lower lobe consolidation with air bronchograms and a moderate left pleural effusion.

**Which of the following is the most appropriate next step in management?**

(A) Add gram-negative antimicrobial coverage
(B) Change nafcillin to vancomycin
(C) Perform bronchoscopy with bronchoalveolar lavage
(D) Perform thoracentesis

## Item 4

A 42-year-old woman undergoes evaluation after being admitted to the hospital 2 days ago with fever; chills; and redness, pain, and swelling over the left mid-anterior shin to just below the knee. She reports falling 5 days before admission and abrading her shin. Empiric vancomycin was started on admission. Medical history is notable for type 2 diabetes mellitus controlled by diet. She takes no other medications.

On physical examination, temperature is 38.7 °C (101.7 °F), blood pressure is 112/74, pulse rate is 110/min, and respiration rate is 20/min. On cardiopulmonary examination, the lungs are clear, and no murmur is heard. A large area of erythema, tense edema, and diffuse tenderness is observed over the left anterior shin without signs of lymphangitic spread.

Laboratory studies show a leukocyte count of 14,500/μL (14.5 × 10⁹/L) and serum vancomycin trough level of 17 μg/mL. Blood cultures obtained at admission grow methicillin-resistant *Staphylococcus aureus* with a vancomycin minimum inhibitory concentration of 4 μg/mL.

**Which of the following is the most appropriate management of this patient's antimicrobial regimen?**

(A)  Add rifampin

(B)  Continue current vancomycin dose

(C)  Increase vancomycin dose

(D)  Switch vancomycin to daptomycin

## Item 5

A 40-year-old woman is evaluated for a 1-month history of cough, fever, night sweats, and weight loss. Pulmonary tuberculosis is strongly suspected, and the community has no reported cases of drug-resistant tuberculosis. She takes no medications.

On physical examination, temperature is 37.9 °C (100.2 °F), blood pressure is 130/70 mm Hg, pulse rate is 95/min, and respiration rate is 15/min. BMI is 21. Crackles are heard in the lung apices bilaterally.

Chest radiograph shows bilateral apical fibrocavitary disease.

A sputum smear reveals acid-fast bacilli.

The initial phase of four-drug tuberculosis therapy with isoniazid, rifampin, pyrazinamide, and ethambutol is planned.

**In addition to liver function testing, which of the following baseline studies should be obtained in this patient as part of monitoring for potential adverse drug effects?**

(A)  Audiogram

(B)  CD4 cell count

(C)  Vestibular testing

(D)  Visual acuity and color vision

## Item 6

A 19-year-old woman is hospitalized for a 3-day history of fever. She has removed several embedded ticks from her skin in the last month. One day before admission, she noted onset of a bilateral temporal headache. On the day of admission, she noted neck stiffness, photophobia, and a new skin eruption.

On physical examination, temperature is 39.4 °C (102.9 °F), blood pressure is 130/58 mm Hg, pulse rate is 115/min, and respiration rate is 24/min. She is ill-appearing and resists passive flexion of the neck. Findings on neurologic examination are normal.

A typical representation of the skin rash on the trunk and extremities, including the palms and soles of her feet, is shown.

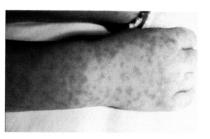

**Laboratory studies:**

| | |
|---|---|
| Leukocyte count | 14,900/μL (14.9 × 10⁹/L) |
| Platelet count | 36,000/μL (36 × 10⁹/L) |
| Alanine aminotransferase | 95 U/L |
| Aspartate aminotransferase | 116 U/L |
| Cerebrospinal fluid (CSF) leukocyte count | 173 (173 × 10⁶/L) (45% polymorphonucleocytes, 52% lymphocytes, 3% eosinophils) |
| CSF Gram stain | Negative for organisms |
| Urine pregnancy test | Negative |

Dexamethasone, ceftriaxone, vancomycin, and doxycycline are initiated. Within 48 hours, her fever has resolved, and her platelet count has normalized. Laboratory tests sent at admission reveal no growth on CSF bacterial cultures, and results on serologic testing for Rocky Mountain spotted fever are negative.

**Which of the following is the most likely diagnosis?**

(A)  Enterovirus

(B)  Heartland virus

(C)  Lyme disease

(D)  Rocky Mountain spotted fever

(E)  West Nile virus

## Item 7

A 52-year-old woman admitted 5 days ago with severe community-acquired pneumonia is evaluated for new onset of acute diarrhea. She has been treated with empiric antibiotic therapy, consisting of ceftriaxone and azithromycin. She has had five liquid bowel movements in the last 24 hours.

On physical examination, temperature is 37.9 °C (100.2 °F), blood pressure is 122/64 mm Hg, pulse rate is 90/min, and respiration rate is 18/min. There are crackles at the right lung base. Abdominal examination reveals normal bowel sounds and no tenderness to palpation.

Leukocyte count is 10,300/μL (10.3 × 10⁹/L). The result of *Clostridium difficile* toxin polymerase chain reaction assay on stool sample is negative.

**CONT.**
Which of the following is the most appropriate management?

(A) Order stool bacterial cultures
(B) Prescribe an antimotility agent
(C) Prescribe metronidazole
(D) Repeat stool *Clostridium difficile* toxin polymerase chain reaction test

## Item 8

A 40-year-old woman is admitted to the hospital for a 1-month history of diffuse abdominal pain, fever, sweats, fatigue, and weight loss. She reports no swallowing or other focal symptoms. Medical history is significant for AIDS, for which she began antiretroviral therapy and opportunistic infection prophylaxis 2 months ago. At that time, CD4 cell count was 23/µL and HIV viral load was 320,875 copies/mL. Medications are abacavir-lamivudine, ritonavir, darunavir, azithromycin, and trimethoprim-sulfamethoxazole.

On physical examination, temperature is 37.9 °C (100.2 °F), blood pressure is 122/76 mm Hg, pulse rate is 88/min, and respiration rate is 14/min. BMI is 22. The oropharynx is clear. Cervical, axillary, and inguinal 1-cm lymph nodes are palpated bilaterally. Lungs are clear. Heart examination is normal. The liver edge extends 2 cm below the right costal margin, and the spleen tip is palpable. No rash is noted, and the neurologic examination is normal.

**Laboratory studies:**

| | |
|---|---|
| CD4 cell count | 56/µL |
| HIV viral load | 5140 copies/mL |
| Hemoglobin | 9.2 g/dL (92 g/L) |
| Leukocyte count | 3600/µL ($3.6 \times 10^9$/L) |
| Alkaline phosphatase | 349 U/L |

Serum aminotransferases, bilirubin, and kidney function are normal.

Chest radiograph is normal. Abdominal CT shows retroperitoneal lymphadenopathy; diffuse hepatic and splenic enlargement without focal lesions; and normal stomach, small and large bowel, and kidneys.

**Which of the following is the most likely diagnosis?**

(A) Cytomegalovirus infection
(B) Disseminated candidal infection
(C) Disseminated *Mycobacterium avium* complex infection
(D) Medication toxicity

## Item 9

A 28-year-old woman is admitted to the hospital with fever, vomiting, and change in mental status over the past 2 days. Her family reports that she has reported a headache for the past 4 weeks and that her symptoms have been progressively worsening. Medical history is significant for type 1 diabetes mellitus. Her only medication is insulin. She does not smoke, drink, or use drugs. She resides in Arizona.

On physical examination, temperature is 38.9 °C (102.0 °F), blood pressure is 110/80 mm Hg, pulse rate is 100/min, and respiration rate is 18/min. BMI is 22. Oxygen saturation breathing ambient air is 97%. She is oriented to person but not place or time. The general medical examination is unremarkable. On neurologic examination, nuchal rigidity is noted, but no additional focal findings are present.

Laboratory studies show a cerebrospinal fluid (CSF) leukocyte count of 1500/µL ($1500 \times 10^6$/L) with a predominant lymphocytosis but also presence of eosinophils, glucose level of 30 mg/dL (1.7 mmol/L), and protein level of 90 mg/dL (900 mg/L). CSF IgG complement fixation is positive for *Coccidioides immitis*.

MRI of the brain shows generalized leptomeningeal enhancement.

**Which of the following is the most appropriate treatment?**

(A) Caspofungin
(B) Fluconazole
(C) Intrathecal amphotericin B
(D) Itraconazole

## Item 10

A 74-year-old woman is evaluated for positive syphilis serologic results. She is being evaluated for progressive difficulty with memory. She reports no known history of syphilis but lists several risk factors for possible infection in the past. Medical history is significant for hypertension and type 2 diabetes mellitus. Medications are enalapril, amlodipine, and metformin.

On physical examination, vital signs are normal. The general physical examination is normal, and her neurologic examination is unremarkable.

Cognitive testing is notable for a score of 19/30 on the Mini–Mental State Examination. Findings on serum rapid plasma reagin testing are positive, with a titer of 1:4. Results of confirmatory fluorescent treponemal antibody absorption testing are positive.

**Which of the following is the most appropriate next step in management?**

(A) Cerebrospinal fluid analysis
(B) Intramuscular benzathine penicillin
(C) Intravenous penicillin
(D) Serum VDRL test

## Item 11

A 47-year-old man is evaluated in follow-up for a diagnosis of pulmonary tuberculosis 2 months ago. He is now completing the initial 2-month treatment phase consisting of rifampin, isoniazid, and ethambutol. Pyrazinamide was withheld owing to acute gouty arthritis at initial presentation. His isolate of *Mycobacterium tuberculosis* is susceptible to all first-line antituberculous agents. Medical history is remarkable for hypertension and gout, including recurrent acute gouty attacks and chronic tophaceous gout. Other medications are lisinopril and allopurinol.

On physical examination, vital signs are normal. The knees and several joints on the hands bilaterally show gouty changes, and tophi are noted at the elbows. The remainder of the examination is normal.

Chest radiography reveals no cavitary lesions. Current sputum acid-fast smears are negative.

**Which of the following is the most appropriate duration for the continuation phase of this patient's tuberculosis treatment with isoniazid and rifampin?**

(A) 4 months
(B) 7 months
(C) 10 months
(D) 12 months

## Item 12

A 33-year-old man is seen to establish ongoing care. He underwent kidney transplantation 3 years ago and has been stable since then, with no episodes of rejection or infection. A review of his immunizations indicates he received the scheduled childhood vaccinations, and his pretransplantation immunizations included the hepatitis A and B and the pneumococcal conjugate and polysaccharide vaccines. He has never received the varicella vaccine, and he was last administered a diphtheria-tetanus immunization following an accidental laceration 8 months ago. Medical history is significant for postinfectious glomerulonephritis as a child resulting in end-stage kidney disease requiring transplantation. Medications are cyclosporine, prednisone, and mycophenolate mofetil.

On physical examination, vital signs are normal. A well-healed abdominal incision is noted, but the examination is otherwise unremarkable.

**Which of the following immunizations should be given now?**

(A) 13-Valent pneumococcal conjugate vaccine
(B) 23-Valent pneumococcal polysaccharide vaccine
(C) Tetanus-diphtheria-acellular pertussis vaccine
(D) Varicella vaccine

## Item 13

A 28-year-old man is evaluated after being informed his roommate at a homeless shelter was diagnosed with pulmonary tuberculosis. He reports no fever, cough, night sweats, or weight loss. Medical history is significant for injection drug use, most recently 2 weeks ago, although he reports no known infectious complications in the past. Medical history is otherwise unremarkable, and he takes no medications.

On physical examination, vital signs are normal. BMI is 22. Track marks secondary to injection drug use are present bilaterally on the antecubital fossa, without tenderness, warmth, erythema, or fluctuance. Cardiopulmonary examination and all other examination findings are normal.

A tuberculin skin test induces 7-mm induration.
Chest radiograph is normal.

**Which of the following is the most appropriate next step in the management of this patient?**

(A) Chest CT
(B) Isoniazid
(C) Isoniazid, rifampin, pyrazinamide, and ethambutol
(D) No further intervention

## Item 14

A 30-year-old woman is evaluated for a 2-day history of increasing pain in the right antecubital fossa and biceps. She reports daily injection drug use. Medical history is otherwise unremarkable, and she takes no prescription medications.

On physical examination, temperature is 39.7 °C (103.5 °F), blood pressure is 90/56 mm Hg, pulse rate is 120/min, and respiration rate is 28/min. BMI is 28. She appears ill. No lymphangitis or right axillary or epitrochlear lymphadenopathy is evident. The right biceps area is extremely tender and warm, with multiple track marks, woody induration, edema, and overlying ecchymotic bullous lesions.

**Laboratory studies:**

| | |
|---|---|
| Leukocyte count | 23,000/µL ($23 \times 10^9$/L) (80% neutrophils, 12% band forms, 8% lymphocytes) |
| Aspartate aminotransferase | 55 U/L |
| Bilirubin, total | 2.0 mg/dL (34.2 µmol/L) |
| Creatinine | 1.7 mg/dL (150 µmol/L) |
| Electrolytes: | |
| Sodium | 135 mEq/L (135 mmol/L) |
| Potassium | 4.2 mEq/L (4.2 mmol/L) |
| Chloride | 95 mEq/L (95 mmol/L) |
| Bicarbonate | 16 mEq/L (16 mmol/L) |

No gas or foreign body is seen on plain radiographs of the right arm and shoulder.

**In addition to emergent surgical evaluation, which of the following is the most appropriate empiric treatment?**

(A) Ceftriaxone plus metronidazole
(B) Doxycycline plus ciprofloxacin
(C) Penicillin plus clindamycin
(D) Vancomycin plus piperacillin-tazobactam

## Item 15

A 50-year-old woman is evaluated in the hospital for persistent fever and flank pain. She was admitted 3 days ago for treatment of pyelonephritis because of nausea and vomiting. Her fever is persistent after 72 hours of treatment. Medical history is unremarkable. Her only medication is intravenous ceftriaxone.

On physical examination, temperature is 39.0 °C (102.2 °F), blood pressure is 110/60 mm Hg, pulse rate is 110/min, and respiration rate is 18/min. BMI is 26. Right costovertebral angle tenderness is noted on abdominal examination. The remainder of the examination is noncontributory.

Urinalysis and culture on admission revealed greater than 100,000 colony-forming units/mL of *Escherichia coli* susceptible to ceftriaxone. Blood culture is negative.

**Which of the following is the most appropriate management?**

(A) Kidney imaging
(B) Repeat urine culture
(C) Switch to gentamicin
(D) Continued observation

## Item 16

A 35-year-old man undergoes consultation for concerns of a possible HIV exposure. He reports that the condom broke the previous night during receptive anal intercourse with a partner who has HIV. He states that his partner is reliably taking antiretroviral therapy and is healthy. Medical history is notable for a negative HIV test result 6 months ago. He takes no medications.

On physical examination, vital signs are normal, as is the remainder of the physical examination.

An HIV antigen/antibody combination immunoassay is ordered.

**Which of the following is the most appropriate next step in management?**

(A)  Determine partner's viral load
(B)  Start combination tenofovir-emtricitabine
(C)  Start combination tenofovir-emtricitabine and raltegravir
(D)  Await results of HIV testing

## Item 17

A 65-year-old woman is hospitalized for fever and altered mental status. Four days ago, she experienced headaches and had a temperature of 39.0 °C (102.2 °F). Today she developed aphasia, prompting hospital admission. Her medical history is otherwise noncontributory, and she takes no medications.

On physical examination, temperature is 39.3 °C (102.7 °F), blood pressure is 122/64 mm Hg, pulse rate is 98/min, and respiration rate is 18/min. The patient is unresponsive and grimaces to sternal rub. The neck is resistant to passive flexion. All extremities move spontaneously. There is no rash.

**Cerebrospinal fluid (CSF) studies:**

| | |
|---|---|
| Leukocyte count | 150/µL (150 × 10$^6$/L); 38% lymphocytes, 34% neutrophils, 28% monocytes |
| Erythrocyte count | 0/µL (0 × 10$^6$/L) |
| Glucose | 54 mg/dL (3.0 mmol/L) |
| Protein | 137 mg/dL (1370 mg/L) |
| Pressure (opening) | 150 mm H$_2$O |
| Gram stain | No organisms |

Brain MRI shows no focal abnormality or hydrocephalus. The patient is administered empiric therapy with dexamethasone, vancomycin, ceftriaxone, ampicillin, and acyclovir pending additional test results.

**Which of the following is the most appropriate next step in management?**

(A)  Monitor intracranial pressure
(B)  Perform transcranial Doppler ultrasonography
(C)  Perform electroencephalography
(D)  Start mannitol

## Item 18

A 22-year-old man is admitted to the hospital for a 1-day history of severe headache, photophobia, and neck stiffness.

He had noted fever starting 2 days before admission. Medical history is significant for an episode of meningococcal meningitis 5 years ago but is otherwise unremarkable. He takes no medications.

On physical examination, temperature is 38.8 °C (101.8 °F), blood pressure is 100/60 mm Hg, pulse rate is 110/min, and respiration rate is 18/min. BMI is 20. Nuchal rigidity is noted. Extraocular movements are intact, and the eye examination is unremarkable with no papilledema or retinal findings. The general medical examination is otherwise normal except for a petechial rash across the trunk and lower extremities.

Cerebrospinal fluid Gram stain is positive for gram-negative diplococci.

Ceftriaxone is started.

**Which of the following is the most likely diagnosis?**

(A)  Selective IgA deficiency
(B)  Common variable immunodeficiency
(C)  Late complement component deficiency
(D)  Classical complement pathway deficiency

## Item 19

A 42-year-old woman is evaluated for headache of 4 days' duration. The headache is nonlocalizing and without apparent triggers. She reports no recurrent headaches and has no history of migraine. She has had untreated dental caries for 2 months and has noticed jaw swelling in the left mandibular region for the past 3 days. She takes no medications.

On physical examination, the patient is awake, alert, and oriented but appears uncomfortable. Vital signs, including temperature, are normal. Neck stiffness is present. Oral examination reveals several broken teeth and generally poor dentition, with the left upper molars showing evidence of dental caries. Neurologic examination reveals impaired extraocular movements, but mental status is normal. The remainder of the physical examination is unremarkable.

A CT scan of the head shows a small ring-enhancing lesion in left temporoparietal junction, approximately 1 cm in diameter.

CT-guided stereotactic aspiration of the abscess is planned.

**Which of the following is the most appropriate empiric antibiotic to administer intravenously?**

(A)  Meropenem
(B)  Penicillin and metronidazole
(C)  Trimethoprim-sulfamethoxazole
(D)  Vancomycin

## Item 20

A 31-year-old woman is evaluated for a 5-day history of a nonpainful cutaneous lesion on the back of her left hand. She works as a packer in a parcel distribution center. She does not recall injury to this area and reports no unusual employment or recreational exposures. She has not had fever, cough, shortness of breath, headache, chest discomfort, or gastrointestinal symptoms. Yesterday, two coworkers were evaluated for similar lesions. Her husband has recently been prescribed an antibiotic after being diagnosed with a "boil" from which methicillin-resistant *Staphylococcus aureus* was cultured. Her only medication is an oral contraceptive pill.

On physical examination, vital signs are normal. Other than the lesion on the proximal dorsal surface of her left hand, the physical examination is normal.

The hand lesion is shown.

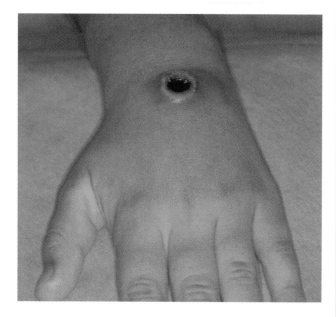

**Which of the following is the most appropriate management?**

(A) Begin doxycycline, imipenem, and rifampin

(B) Begin ciprofloxacin

(C) Begin trimethoprim-sulfamethoxazole

(D) Obtain biopsy and culture prior to initiating therapy

## Item 21

A 22-year-old woman is evaluated during a routine office visit. She is pregnant at 38 weeks' gestation. She reports no dysuria, urgency, fever, or chills. Medical history is unremarkable. Her only medication is a prenatal vitamin.

On physical examination, temperature is 37.0 °C (98.6 °F), blood pressure is 100/70 mm Hg, pulse rate is 80/min, and respiration rate is 16/min. Abdominal examination is consistent with her stage of pregnancy; no costovertebral angle tenderness is noted. The remainder of the examination is unremarkable.

Urine dipstick is positive for nitrites and leukocyte esterase. Urine culture grows greater than 100,000 colony-forming units/mL of *Escherichia coli* susceptible to ampicillin, nitrofurantoin, and trimethoprim-sulfamethoxazole.

**Which of the following is the most appropriate treatment?**

(A) Amoxicillin

(B) Nitrofurantoin

(C) Trimethoprim-sulfamethoxazole

(D) No treatment

## Item 22

A 30-year-old woman is requesting HIV testing. She is asymptomatic and reports no known exposure to a person with HIV. She has had multiple lifetime sexual partners, all of whom are men, and none of whom were men known to have sex with other men. She reports no intravenous drug use by a sexual partner or herself. She does not use condoms and has been in a monogamous relationship for the past 6 months. Medical history is negative for any opportunistic infections or sexually transmitted infections. Her only medication is an oral contraceptive pill.

On physical examination, vital signs are normal. BMI is 23. The remainder of the evaluation is normal.

The HIV-1/2 antigen/antibody combination immunoassay is reactive. Result on a subsequent HIV-1/HIV-2 antibody differentiation immunoassay is negative, as is result on an HIV-1 nucleic acid amplification test.

**Which of the following is the most appropriate next step in management?**

(A) Repeat HIV-1/2 antigen/antibody combination immunoassay in 6 weeks

(B) T-cell subset testing

(C) Western blot HIV-1 antibody testing

(D) No further testing

## Item 23

A 31-year-old man is evaluated for a recent exposure to chickenpox. He visited his sister's home last week. His nephew was subsequently developed a rash and was diagnosed with chickenpox 1 day after he left. He has no symptoms and states that he feels well. He never had chickenpox as a child and has not been immunized against varicella. Medical history is notable for psoriatic arthritis. His only medication is etanercept.

On physical examination, vital signs are normal. No skin rash is present. The remainder of the examination is normal.

The result of a serologic assay for antibodies against varicella-zoster virus is negative.

**Which of the following is the most appropriate management?**

(A) Acyclovir therapy

(B) Varicella vaccine

(C) Varicella-zoster immune globulin

(D) Varicella vaccine and varicella-zoster immune globulin

(E) Observation for 21 days after exposure

## Item 24

A 34-year-old woman is evaluated following elective cholecystectomy 2 weeks ago. She notes mild pain, redness, and swelling at the incision site with some "cloudy" drainage that started 3 days ago. She reports no fever or chills. Medical history is otherwise unremarkable, and she takes no medications.

On physical examination, temperature is 36.7 °C (98.1 °F), blood pressure is 110/72 mm Hg, pulse rate is 76/min, and respiration rate is 14/min. BMI is 30. She has erythema and mild tenderness around the incision site with a small amount of pinkish drainage. The remainder of the examination is noncontributory.

Laboratory studies show a leukocyte count of 6700/μL ($6.7 \times 10^9$/L).

**Which of the following is the most appropriate diagnostic test to perform next?**

(A) Blood cultures

(B) Gram stain and culture of fluid drainage

(C) Opening of incision site for tissue Gram stain and culture

(D) Ultrasonography of incision site

## Item 25

A 57-year-old woman is evaluated in the emergency department for a 2-day history of severe headache. She also reports nausea without vomiting and difficulty tolerating bright lights. Medical history is unremarkable, and she takes no medications.

On physical examination, temperature is 38.5 °C (101.3 °F), blood pressure is 136/86 mm Hg, pulse rate is 110/min, and respiration rate is 14/min. BMI is 24. The general medical examination is unremarkable. On neurologic examination, she shows photophobia, and a nondilated funduscopic examination shows no papilledema. The remainder of the examination is nonfocal.

A lumbar puncture is performed.

**Cerebrospinal fluid (CSF) profile:**

| | |
|---|---|
| Leukocyte count | 2235/μL ($2235 \times 10^6$/L) with neutrophilic predominance |
| Glucose | 24 mg/dL (1.3 mmol/L) |
| Pressure (opening) | 410 mm H$_2$O |
| Protein | 468 mg/dL (4680 mg/L) |

CSF Gram stain and culture results are pending.

**In addition to dexamethasone, which of the following is the most appropriate intravenous empiric antibiotic treatment?**

(A) Ampicillin, ceftriaxone, and vancomycin

(B) Ceftazidime and vancomycin

(C) Meropenem

(D) Moxifloxacin

## Item 26

A 22-year-old woman is evaluated for a 4-day history of vaginal discharge. The discharge is thick and yellow. She has no abdominal pain. She is sexually active. Medical history is unremarkable, with no drug allergies.

On physical examination, vital signs are normal. Pelvic examination reveals an inflamed and friable cervix. Mucopurulent discharge is noted from the cervical os. No cervical motion, adnexal, or uterine tenderness is noted. The vaginal mucosa and vulvar area are normal in appearance. Wet mount shows only numerous leukocytes. The pH of the vaginal secretions is 5. Result of the whiff test is negative, and no fungal elements are seen on examination of the potassium hydroxide preparation.

**Which of the following is the most appropriate treatment?**

(A) Cefotetan and doxycycline

(B) Ceftriaxone and azithromycin

(C) Fluconazole

(D) Metronidazole

## Item 27

A 27-year-old man is hospitalized for a 2-day history of fever and headaches and a 1-day history of left lower-extremity weakness. Ten days earlier he had returned from a 1-week trip to Idaho, which involved rafting and sleeping outdoors. He reports no known tick bite.

On physical examination, temperature is 39.1 °C (102.4 °F), blood pressure is 122/72 mm Hg, pulse rate is 118/min, and respiration rate is 28/min. The patient is oriented to person, place, and time. He has mild nuchal rigidity limiting neck flexion. He has left lower-extremity weakness with inability to flex or extend the knee or ankle. Deep tendon reflexes are absent. Sensation is intact. No rash is present.

**Cerebrospinal fluid (CSF) studies:**

| | |
|---|---|
| Erythrocyte count | 17/μL ($17 \times 10^6$/L) |
| Leukocyte count | 256/μL ($256 \times 10^6$/L) |
| Glucose | 55 mg/dL (3.1 mmol/L) |
| Protein | 299 mg/dL (2990 mg/L) |

MRI of the brain shows no focal abnormalities.

**Which of the following is the most appropriate CSF laboratory test to perform next?**

(A) Eastern equine encephalitis virus antibody

(B) La Crosse encephalitis virus antibody

(C) Powassan virus antibody

(D) West Nile virus antibody

## Item 28

A 63-year-old woman is evaluated in the hospital for decompensated heart failure. She presented to the emergency department with increased shortness of breath and pedal edema yesterday. An indwelling urinary catheter was placed, intravenous diuretics were given, and she was admitted for further treatment. Medical history is notable for hypertension, type 2 diabetes mellitus, and chronic kidney disease. Medications are aspirin, carvedilol, insulin, lisinopril, rosuvastatin, spironolactone, and as-needed furosemide.

On physical examination, temperature is 36.8 °C (98.2°F), blood pressure is 124/72 mm Hg, pulse rate is

100/min, and respiration rate is 18/min. Bibasilar crackles are heard on pulmonary examination, and cardiac examination is significant for an S$_3$. Bilateral lower-extremity edema to the mid-calf is noted. The urinary catheter is draining clear urine.

Laboratory study results show a serum creatinine level of 2.8 mg/dL (248 µmol/L) (baseline, 2.2 mg/dL [194 µmol/L]).

**Which of the following is the most appropriate management of this patient's urinary catheter?**

(A) Change catheter after 3 days
(B) Change catheter now
(C) Remove catheter now
(D) Remove catheter when kidney function returns to baseline

## Item 29

A 57-year-old woman is evaluated for blood cultures growing yeast during long-term intravenous antibiotic therapy. She has completed 4 weeks of a planned 6-week course of intravenous antibiotics for methicillin-sensitive *Staphylococcus aureus* infective endocarditis. A peripherally inserted central venous catheter (PICC) was placed at the beginning of her treatment. She developed a high fever 3 days ago, and blood cultures drawn peripherally and through the catheter at that time grew *Candida* species; further identification is pending. Medical history is otherwise negative, and her only medication is nafcillin.

On physical examination, temperature is 37.8 °C (100.0 °F), blood pressure is 126/80 mm Hg, pulse rate is 82/min, and respiration rate is 16/min. The eye grounds are clear. Chest examination is unremarkable. Cardiac auscultation reveals a grade 2/6 crescendo-decrescendo murmur at the right upper sternal border. She has no spinal tenderness. The right brachial PICC site is without erythema, drainage, or tenderness.

**In addition to continuing intravenous antibiotic therapy, which of the following is the most appropriate management?**

(A) Continue PICC use
(B) Continue PICC use and add antifungal therapy
(C) Remove PICC
(D) Remove PICC and add antifungal therapy

## Item 30

A 23-year-old man is evaluated in the emergency department for a 5-day history of malaise and an erythematous macular and papular rash that began on the chest and spread to involve the extremities. The rash is not pruritic. The patient is sexually active with men; he has a new sexual partner and does not use condoms. He takes no medications and has no known allergies.

On physical examination, temperature is 37.6 °C (99.7 °F), blood pressure is 110/65 mm Hg, pulse rate is 90/min, and respiration rate is 12/min. A generalized rash is noted. Cervical, axillary, and inguinal lymph nodes are freely movable and nontender on palpation. No genital or mucosal lesions are present.

Rash of the palm is shown.

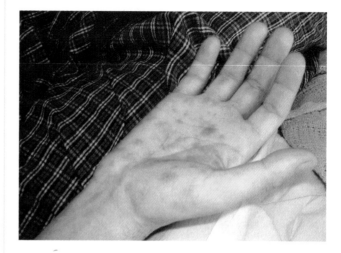

**Which of the following is the most appropriate treatment?**

(A) Azithromycin
(B) Benzathine penicillin
(C) Ceftriaxone
(D) Methylprednisolone

## Item 31

**H**

A 46-year-old woman is admitted to the hospital with abdominal pain, worsening diarrhea, and intermittent low-grade fever of 1 week's duration. She reports no nausea, vomiting, or swallowing symptoms; no melena or hematochezia; and no rash. She underwent kidney transplantation 4 months ago. She is cytomegalovirus seropositive and received an organ from a cytomegalovirus-seronegative donor; she received valganciclovir for 3 months after transplantation with no clinical or laboratory evidence of cytomegalovirus disease. Medical history is significant for autosomal-dominant polycystic kidney disease. Medications are tacrolimus, prednisone, mycophenolate mofetil, and trimethoprim-sulfamethoxazole.

On physical examination, temperature is 37.3 °C (99.1 °F), blood pressure is 144/90 mm Hg, pulse rate is 104/min, and respiration rate is 16/min. BMI is 23. Mucous membranes are dry. The abdomen is soft with mild tenderness in lower quadrants, bowel sounds are normal, and no rebound or guarding is noted. No skin rash is noted, and the remainder of the examination is unremarkable.

Stool culture is positive for *Candida albicans*. Results on *Clostridium difficile* toxin nucleic acid testing are negative.

Plain radiograph of the abdomen is unremarkable and shows a normal bowel gas pattern without free air.

**Which of the following is the most likely cause for the patient's diarrhea?**

(A) *Candida albicans*
(B) *Clostridium difficile*
(C) Cytomegalovirus
(D) Mycophenolate toxicity
(E) Polyoma BK virus

## Item 32

A 78-year old man is evaluated in the emergency department for confusion. He is a retiree living in an assisted-living facility. Five weeks ago, he underwent outpatient debridement of a right foot plantar bunion. He ambulates with the assistance of a walker because of poor balance following a cerebral vascular accident. Medical history is also significant for type 2 diabetes mellitus, hypertension, remote smoking history, and amputation of the left great toe because of infection. Medications are insulin, lisinopril, simvastatin, hydrochlorothiazide, and aspirin.

On physical examination, temperature is 38.8 °C (101.8 °F), blood pressure is 106/66 mm Hg, pulse rate is 98/min, and respiration rate is 14/min. BMI is 25. The patient is lethargic and confused. His right foot is edematous and erythematous, with a palpable dorsalis pedis pulse. A 2.5- × 3.1-cm ulceration is located beneath the fifth metatarsal-phalangeal joint with malodorous drainage. Metal probe detects bone. The proximal leg is unremarkable.

Laboratory studies reveal a leukocyte count of 17,400/μL (17.4 × 10⁹/L) with 15% band forms, a serum creatinine level of 1.5 mg/dL (132.6 μmol/L), normal electrolytes, and serum glucose level of 249 mg/dL (13.8 mmol/L).

Plain radiography of the foot reveals edema over the fifth metatarsal-phalangeal joint but no gas or obvious osteoarticular destruction.

**Which of the following is the most appropriate management?**

(A) Cefazolin and metronidazole

(B) Clindamycin and gentamicin

(C) Vancomycin and piperacillin-tazobactam

(D) Hold antibiotic therapy pending bone biopsy

## Item 33

A 54-year-old man is hospitalized for a 5-day history of fever, frontal headache, back pain, and rash. He recently returned from a 10-day vacation on the Caribbean island of Martinique. Six days after returning, he suddenly developed fever; generalized body, lower back, and joint achiness; and a headache localized behind his eyes. Yesterday he developed a rash on his chest and inner arms.

On physical examination, temperature is 39.6 °C (103.3 °F), blood pressure is 112/68 mm Hg, pulse rate is 118/min, and respiration rate is 16/min. BMI is 31. A maculopapular rash is present on the flexor surfaces of the arms and chest wall. He has discomfort of wrists, elbows, and knees with passive flexion and extension. The remainder of the examination is normal.

**Laboratory studies:**

| | |
|---|---|
| Hemoglobin | 15.2 g/dL (152 g/L) |
| Leukocyte count | 3210/μL (3.2 × 10⁹/L); 38% polymorphonuclear cells, 58% lymphocytes, 4% monocytes |
| Platelet count | 87,000/μL (87 × 10⁹/L) |
| Alanine aminotransferase | 226 U/L |
| Aspartate aminotransferase | 138 U/L |
| Bilirubin, total | 0.7 mg/dL (12.0 μmol/L) |

Peripheral blood smear is normal.

**Which of the following is the most likely diagnosis?**

(A) Anaplasmosis

(B) Chikungunya

(C) Dengue fever

(D) Leptospirosis

## Item 34

A 68-year-old man was admitted to the hospital 4 days ago for community-acquired pneumonia. He has COPD and presented with a 2-week history of fever and increasing shortness of breath, but no increase in his baseline cough. He was hypoxic, and a chest radiograph showed new patchy infiltrates in addition to his underlying interstitial changes but no pleural effusions. Empiric antibiotics were initiated, and blood and sputum cultures have shown no growth. His dyspnea and oxygenation have not improved significantly since admission. Medical history is otherwise unremarkable. He has a 45-pack-year smoking history and continues to smoke. Medications are tiotropium, fluticasone-salmeterol, and as-needed albuterol metered dose inhalers and intravenous cefotaxime and azithromycin.

On physical examination, temperature is 38.6 °C (101.5 °F), blood pressure is 128/55 mm Hg, heart rate is 97/min, and respiration rate is 33/min. Oxygen saturation is 92% with the patient breathing 6 L/min of oxygen by nasal cannula. BMI is 28. Pulmonary examination shows decreased air movement and scattered rhonchi throughout both lung fields, unchanged from admission. Cardiac and abdominal examinations are unremarkable, and no lower extremity edema is present.

Laboratory studies show a leukocyte count of 13,500/μL (13.5 × 10⁹/L) (14,700/μL [14.7 × 10⁹/L] on admission). Metabolic studies are normal.

Chest radiograph continues to show multilobar, patchy infiltrates and increased interstitial markings without pleural effusions, unchanged from admission.

**Which of the following is the most appropriate next step in management?**

(A) Bronchoscopy

(B) Chest CT

(C) Chest ultrasonography

(D) Thoracoscopic lung biopsy

## Item 35

An 82-year-old man is evaluated for a 2-month history of progressive fatigue and midline lower back pain that has increased in severity. He reports no trauma to the area. Medical history is significant for elective coronary artery bypass surgery 3 months ago. While hospitalized, he developed a central line–associated bloodstream infection with *Staphylococcus aureus* and a catheter-associated urinary tract infection with *Proteus mirabilis*. Medications are aspirin, metoprolol, and simvastatin. He is allergic to penicillin.

On physical examination, temperature is 36.8 °C (98.2 °F), blood pressure is 110/72 mm Hg, pulse rate is 68/min, and respiration rate is 14/min. BMI is 26. Cardiopulmonary examination is normal. He has moderate point tenderness over the third lumbar vertebrae. Lower-extremity evaluation reveals normal motor strength and sensation with symmetrical patellar deep tendon reflexes.

Laboratory studies reveal an erythrocyte sedimentation rate of 110 mm/h, leukocyte count of 10,200/µL (10.2 × 10⁹/L), and serum creatinine of 1.2 mg/dL (106.1 µmol/L). A blood culture is positive for *Corynebacterium* species, but subsequent cultures are negative.

Findings of MRI of the lumbar spine, with contrast, are consistent with osteomyelitis of the L4 and adjacent L5 vertebral bodies, abnormality in the intervening disc space, and no evidence of an epidural collection.

**Which of the following is the most appropriate management?**

(A) Antimicrobial therapy with vancomycin and ciprofloxacin
(B) CT-guided biopsy of the lumbar disc space
(C) Echocardiography
(D) Three-phase nuclear bone scan

## Item 36

A 30-year-old woman is evaluated in follow-up after being recently diagnosed with HIV infection. She is asymptomatic. Medical history is unremarkable, and she takes no medications; she has not yet started antiretroviral therapy. She received all scheduled childhood immunizations.

On physical examination, vital signs are normal. She has shotty cervical lymphadenopathy, but the examination is otherwise unremarkable.

**Laboratory studies:**

| | |
|---|---|
| Absolute CD4 cell count | 461/µL |
| HIV viral load | 44,874 copies/mL |
| Hepatitis A IgG antibody | Negative |
| Hepatitis B surface antibody | Positive |
| Hepatitis B surface antigen | Negative |
| Hepatitis C antibody | Negative |

**Which of the following immunizations should this patient receive today?**

(A) Hepatitis A vaccine
(B) Hepatitis B vaccine
(C) Human papillomavirus vaccine
(D) Pneumococcal conjugate vaccine
(E) Pneumococcal polysaccharide vaccine

## Item 37

A 62-year-old woman is admitted to the hospital for management of varicella-zoster infection. She developed pain and tingling over the right posterior flank area 3 days ago, followed by the development of vesicular lesions. She reports fever without chills and no cough. She is undergoing immunosuppressive chemotherapy for breast cancer and received her last dose 10 days ago. Medical history is otherwise unremarkable, and her only medication is valacyclovir.

On physical examination, temperature is 38.0 °C (100.4 °F), blood pressure is 126/84 mm Hg, pulse rate is 88/min, and respiration rate is 16/min. A vesicular rash is present over the right flank that does not cross the midline, with vesicles in various stages of development with no crusting and no purulent drainage.

**Which of the following is the most appropriate in-hospital precaution for preventing spread of infection?**

(A) Airborne
(B) Airborne and contact
(C) Contact
(D) Contact and droplet
(E) Droplet

## Item 38

A 25-year-old woman e-mails her internist from Mexico with a report of diarrhea for 2 days. She is travelling and reports three to four loose bowel movements per day. She has been dining in the hotel restaurants but has also consumed foods and bottled soft drinks served with ice from local food vendors. She feels urgency to move her bowels but no tenesmus. She has mild abdominal cramping without pain, vomiting, or fever. Stools are described as watery without mucus or blood. Although she is uncomfortable, she has not had to alter her travel plans. Medical history is unremarkable and she takes no medications. She was given levofloxacin and loperamide to take with her on her trip.

**In addition to encouraging oral hydration, which of the following is the most appropriate treatment recommendation for this patient?**

(A) Begin levofloxacin and loperamide now
(B) Begin levofloxacin now and start loperamide 24 hours later
(C) Begin loperamide now
(D) No further treatment unless symptoms worsen

## Item 39

A 55-year-old man is evaluated in the hospital for pulmonary tuberculosis. He was admitted 10 days ago with cough, fever, and night sweats. A chest radiograph showed bilateral, apical fibronodular disease without cavities. Findings on sputum evaluation were positive for *Mycobacterium tuberculosis*. Because drug-resistant tuberculosis had not been reported in the community, a four-drug antituberculous regimen was started. Since the patient began therapy, his initial symptoms have resolved. Medical history is otherwise unremarkable. Medications are isoniazid, rifampin, pyrazinamide, and ethambutol.

On physical examination, vital signs are normal. Lungs are clear to auscultation. The remainder of the examination is otherwise unremarkable.

His three most recent acid-fast bacilli sputum smears have been negative.

Which of the following additional criteria is required for this patient to be considered noncontagious?

(A) Absence of a cavity on initial chest radiograph

(B) Adequate tuberculosis treatment for at least 2 weeks

(C) Negative tuberculin skin test result

(D) Normal leukocyte count

## Item 40

A 72-year-old man is admitted to the hospital with fever and chills of 2 days' duration. He underwent left hemicolectomy 12 days ago for diverticular disease, which was complicated by methicillin-resistant *Staphylococcus aureus* bacteremia. A planned, 14-day course of vancomycin was started through a central venous catheter, and he was afebrile with negative blood cultures and normal leukocyte count at the time of hospital discharge 1 week ago. Medical history is otherwise significant for hypertension, diabetes mellitus, and chronic kidney disease. Medications are vancomycin, losartan, and insulin.

On physical examination, temperature is 39.2 °C (102.6 °F), blood pressure is 130/70 mm Hg, pulse rate is 100/min and regular, and respiration rate is 16/min. The patient has a right subclavian central venous catheter. His abdominal surgical site is clean and dry. The remainder of the examination is normal.

Laboratory studies reveal a leukocyte count of 16,000/µL (16×10⁹/L); a serum creatinine level of 2.1 mg/dL (186 µmol/L), which is unchanged from his baseline; and a therapeutic vancomycin level. Two sets of blood cultures are positive for budding yeast.

The central venous catheter is removed.

**Which of the following is the most appropriate treatment?**

(A) Amphotericin B deoxycholate

(B) Fluconazole

(C) Liposomal amphotericin B

(D) Micafungin

## Item 41

A 42-year-old man is admitted to the hospital for a 1-month history of high fever and 6.8-kg (15-lb) weight loss. Medical history is significant for AIDS diagnosed 10 years ago after an episode of pneumocystis pneumonia. He recently immigrated to the United States from Central America. Medical history is otherwise unremarkable. He is taking no antiretroviral or prophylactic therapy.

On physical examination, temperature is 39.9 °C (103.8 °F), blood pressure is 90/60 mm Hg, pulse rate is 120/min, and respiration rate is 18/min. Diffuse crackles are heard in the lungs. Abdominal examination reveals hepatosplenomegaly. No skin rash is present.

**Laboratory studies:**

| | |
|---|---|
| Hemoglobin | 8 g/dL (80 g/L) |
| Leukocyte count | 1800/µL (1.8×10⁹/L) |
| Platelet count | 90,000/µL (90×10⁹/L) |
| CD4 cell count | 5/µL (0.005×10⁹/L) |

Small yeast forms within neutrophils are seen on a peripheral blood smear.

A chest radiograph shows a diffuse reticular pattern.

**Which of the following is the most likely diagnosis?**

(A) Blastomycosis

(B) Candidiasis

(C) Coccidioidomycosis

(D) Histoplasmosis

## Item 42

A 28-year-old woman was admitted to the hospital 3 days ago with fever, chills, dysuria, flank pain, and nausea. Empiric ceftriaxone was initiated for pyelonephritis. She reports her nausea is improved, and she has no vomiting. Medical history is unremarkable, and she takes no other medications.

On physical examination, temperature is 37.6 °C (99.7 °F), blood pressure is 106/70 mm Hg, pulse rate is 78/min, and respiration rate is 16/min. She has minimal left costovertebral angle tenderness. Bowel sounds are normal.

Laboratory studies show a leukocyte count of 9300/µL (9.3 × 10⁹/L) and serum creatinine level of 0.7 mg/dL (61.9 µmol/L). Urine and blood cultures grow *Escherichia coli* sensitive to ampicillin, ceftriaxone, trimethoprim-sulfamethoxazole, and ciprofloxacin. The organism was also sensitive to nitrofurantoin on the urine panel.

**Which of the following is the most appropriate treatment for this patient at this time?**

(A) Intravenous ciprofloxacin

(B) Oral nitrofurantoin

(C) Oral trimethoprim-sulfamethoxazole

(D) Intravenous ceftriaxone

## Item 43

A 30-year-old woman is evaluated for a reactive tuberculin skin test (TST). She developed 6-mm induration 48 hours after the test was performed. She has no fever, weight loss, or cough, and cannot recall any exposure to tuberculosis. Medical history is notable for psoriasis diagnosed 10 years ago. Her only medication is infliximab. A TST result was negative before initiation of therapy.

On physical examination, vital signs are normal. Stable plaque psoriasis is noted. The lungs are clear, and the remainder of the examination is normal.

**Which of the following is the most appropriate next step in the management of this patient?**

(A) Chest radiography

(B) Interferon-γ release assay

(C) Rifampin, isoniazid, pyrazinamide, and ethambutol

(D) No further intervention

## Item 44

A 27-year-old woman is evaluated for a 4-day history of painful vulvar lesions accompanied by fatigue and malaise. The patient reports dysuria but no urgency or frequency and no vaginal discharge. She has been sexually active with a single male partner for the past 2 years. She has no history of genital lesions or sexually transmitted infections.

On physical examination, temperature is 38.1 °C (100.6 °F), blood pressure is 120/70 mm Hg, pulse rate is 90/min, and respiration rate is 12/min. Multiple shallow ulcers on an erythematous base are located over the labia majora and minora, consistent with herpes simplex virus infection. Palpation reveals bilateral inguinal lymphadenopathy.

**Which of the following is the most appropriate diagnostic test to perform next?**

(A) Direct fluorescent antibody testing of lesion specimen
(B) Polymerase chain reaction of lesion specimen
(C) Type-specific serum antibody testing
(D) Tzanck smear of lesion specimen

## Item 45

A 27-year-old male park ranger is evaluated for a 3-week history of diarrhea and weight loss. He notes four to seven pale, greasy, and foul-smelling bowel movements per day, with an oily sheen. He reports no visible blood or mucus. He has no fever but does have abdominal bloating and increased flatulence. He states he has lost 10 pounds since the onset of symptoms. In the last 2 months, he has been clearing trails in the backcountry and camping in primitive sites. He admits to drinking from freshwater streams but uses chlorine water purification tablets for disinfection.

On physical examination, temperature is 37.0 °C (98.6 °F), blood pressure is 132/68 mm Hg, pulse rate is 56/min, and respiration rate is 18/min. The patient has a mildly bloated abdomen with tenderness to palpation but no peritoneal signs.

Laboratory studies show a leukocyte count of 7400/μL ($7.4 \times 10^9$/L). The stool is negative for occult blood and fecal leukocytes.

**Which of the following is the most appropriate diagnostic stool test?**

(A) *Entamoeba* antigen testing
(B) *Giardia* antigen testing
(C) Microscopy for ova and parasites
(D) Modified acid-fast staining

## Item 46

A 33-year-old woman is evaluated during tuberculosis screening. She reports no cough, weight loss, or any other symptoms. She uses heroin daily and is transiently homeless. Medical history is otherwise unremarkable, and she takes no medications.

On physical examination, vital signs are normal. BMI is 20. Other than needle marks without evidence of infection, the examination is normal.

**Which of the following is the preferred method of tuberculosis screening in this patient?**

(A) Chest radiography
(B) Induced sputum examination
(C) Interferon-γ release assay
(D) Tuberculin skin test

## Item 47

A 44-year-old man is evaluated after a new diagnosis of HIV infection. He is asymptomatic and reports no fever, chills, sweats, weight loss, cough, chest pain, dyspnea on exertion, diarrhea, or difficulty swallowing. He reports no history of opportunistic infections, and he has had no known exposure to tuberculosis. Medical history is otherwise unremarkable. He has just started taking tenofovir-emtricitabine and raltegravir.

On physical examination, vital signs are normal. He has erythematous, scaly patches on his face consistent with seborrheic dermatitis. No thrush or oral lesions are observed. Mild lymphadenopathy is noted in cervical, axillary, and inguinal areas. The lungs are clear throughout. No hepatosplenomegaly, masses, or tenderness is noted on abdominal examination.

**Laboratory studies:**

| | |
|---|---|
| Absolute CD4 cell count | 41/μL |
| HIV viral load | 108,522 copies/mL |
| Cytomegalovirus IgG antibody | Positive |
| *Toxoplasma* IgG antibody | Positive |
| Tuberculosis interferon-γ release assay | Indeterminate |

**In addition to trimethoprim-sulfamethoxazole, which of the following should be started now?**

(A) Azithromycin
(B) Fluconazole
(C) Isoniazid and vitamin B$_6$
(D) Pyrimethamine and leucovorin
(E) Valganciclovir

## Item 48

A 44-year-old man is evaluated for acute rejection of a transplanted kidney. Medical history is significant for autosomal-dominant polycystic kidney disease requiring transplantation 18 months ago. He and his donor were both seronegative for cytomegalovirus, and the patient received standard prophylaxis. His posttransplantation course has been remarkable for previous episodes of rejection, the last of which was approximately 6 months ago. He also has hypertension. Current medications are amlodipine, tacrolimus, prednisone, and mycophenolate mofetil. He is scheduled to have his level of immunosuppression increased significantly for the current episode of rejection.

Physical examination findings are unremarkable.

Laboratory studies show a leukocyte count of 4500/μL ($4.5 \times 10^9$/L) with 88% polymorphonuclear cells and 8% lymphocytes and a serum creatinine level of 1.8 mg/dL (159 μmol/L).

**For which infection should this patient receive prophylaxis at this time?**

(A) Aspergillus
(B) Cytomegalovirus
(C) *Pneumocystis jirovecii*
(D) *Mycobacterium avium* complex

## Item 49

A 61-year-old woman is evaluated for immunization before traveling. She plans to travel to Cambodia in 2 weeks and will spend 4 weeks in rural areas. Medical history is significant for controlled rheumatoid arthritis. She has been provided all adult immunizations recommended by the Advisory Committee on Immunization Practices but has not previously received any hepatitis A immunization. Medications are infliximab and methotrexate.

On physical examination, vital signs are normal. No active inflammatory joint disease is evident, and the remainder of the examination is unremarkable.

**Which of the following is the most appropriate hepatitis A prophylaxis regimen for this patient?**

(A) Hepatitis A vaccine now
(B) Hepatitis A vaccine and immune globulin now
(C) Immune globulin now
(D) Immune globulin now and hepatitis A vaccine upon return

## Item 50

A 77-year-old woman is evaluated for a 5-day history of diarrhea. She has been diagnosed with *Clostridium difficile* colitis twice in the last 3 months and both times was successfully treated with metronidazole. This is her third episode. She has four to six liquid bowel movements per day. She reports no fevers, abdominal pain, nausea, or vomiting.

On physical examination, the patient is afebrile, blood pressure is 150/82 mm Hg, pulse rate is 106/min, and respiration rate is 18/min. The patient's abdomen is soft and nontender with positive bowel sounds.

Laboratory studies reveal a leukocyte count of 8800/µL ($8.8\times10^9$/L) and serum creatinine of 0.8 mg/dL (70.7 µmol/L). Stool polymerase chain reaction assay is positive for *C. difficile* toxin.

**Which of the following is the most appropriate oral treatment?**

(A) Metronidazole for 14 days
(B) Metronidazole for 6 weeks
(C) Rifaximin for 14 days
(D) Vancomycin for 14 days
(E) Vancomycin for 6 weeks

## Item 51

A 74-year-old man was admitted to the hospital 3 days ago for treatment of community-acquired pneumonia. Supplemental oxygen and empiric intravenous ceftriaxone and azithromycin were initiated; blood and sputum cultures showed no growth. He reports feeling much better, with decreased shortness of breath and cough; he has been afebrile since the second hospital day. Medical history is unremarkable. Medications are intravenous ceftriaxone and azithromycin.

On physical examination, temperature is 37.7 °C (99.9 °F), blood pressure is 120/75 mm Hg, pulse rate is 92/min, and respiration rate is 18/min. Oxygen saturation is 94% breathing ambient air. He is breathing comfortably. Pulmonary examination reveals decreased breath sounds at both lung bases but no dullness to percussion. Cardiac and abdominal examinations are unremarkable, and no lower extremity edema is present.

Laboratory studies show a leukocyte count of 13,500/µL ($13.5\times10^9$/L) (18,300/µL [$18.3\times10^9$/L] on admission) and an otherwise normal complete blood count. A comprehensive metabolic profile, including kidney function, is normal.

**Which of the following is the most appropriate management of this patient's antibiotic therapy?**

(A) Continue current intravenous antibiotic therapy
(B) Switch to oral antibiotic and discharge
(C) Switch to oral antibiotic and observe for 24 hours
(D) Switch to oral antibiotic and overlap with intravenous therapy for 24 hours

## Item 52 H

A 40-year-old woman is admitted to the hospital for significant hypoxemia. She reports a 3-day history of fever, fatigue, headache, dry cough, and pleuritic chest pain. She also notes several tender, raised soft tissue "lumps" on her legs. Four weeks before symptom onset, she traveled to Arizona to participate in an outdoor art convention. Medical history is significant for well-controlled Crohn disease, and results of surveillance testing for *Mycobacterium tuberculosis* have been negative. Her only medication is infliximab.

On physical examination, temperature is 38.7 °C (101.7 °F), blood pressure is 102/82 mm Hg, pulse rate is 98/min, and respiration rate is 22/min. BMI is 26. Oxygen saturation is 96% with 5 L/min of oxygen via nasal cannula. No lymphadenopathy is palpable. Coarse crackles and scattered rhonchi are heard in all lung fields with dullness to percussion at the bases. Cardiac examination reveals no murmurs. No hepatosplenomegaly is noted. She has four to five discrete, tender, 1- to 2-cm erythematous nodules on both anterior lower extremities.

Laboratory studies show a leukocyte count of 4500/µL ($4.5\times10^9$/L) (40% polymorphonuclear cells, 50% lymphocytes, 4% monocytes, 6% eosinophils). Results of pneumococcal and *Legionella* urine antigen assays are negative, and a serum mycoplasma IgM antibody assay is reactive.

Chest radiography shows bilateral airspace opacities, small bilateral pleural effusions, and enlarged right-sided hilar lymphadenopathy.

**Which of the following is the most likely diagnosis?**

(A) Blastomycosis
(B) Coccidioidomycosis
(C) Histoplasmosis
(D) *Mycoplasma* pneumonia

## Item 53 H

An 85-year-old man is being treated in the ICU for bacteremia secondary to a urinary tract infection. He was evaluated 2 days ago for intermittent confusion, weakness, bladder pain, and hematuria. Because of hemodynamic instability, he was admitted to the ICU. Intravenous fluids were given, and empiric meropenem was started, with resolution of his hypotension and fever. Medical history is otherwise noncontributory. He takes no other medications.

On physical examination, temperature is 37.7 °C (99.9 °F), blood pressure is 118/84 mm Hg, pulse rate is 96/min, and respiration rate is 18/min. Cardiac examination is normal. He has no flank or abdominal tenderness.

Urine culture is now reported to be growing more than $10^5$ colony-forming units of *Enterococcus faecalis*. Blood culture grows *E. faecalis* sensitive to ampicillin, vancomycin, and gentamicin.

**Which of the following is the most appropriate treatment?**

(A) Switch to ampicillin
(B) Switch to ampicillin and gentamicin
(C) Switch to vancomycin
(D) Switch to vancomycin and gentamicin
(E) Continue meropenem

## Item 54

A 52-year-old man is admitted to the hospital for a 2-day history of right maxillary sinus pain and exophthalmos of the right eye with fever. Empiric cefepime is initiated. Medical history is significant for acute myelogenous leukemia, for which he recently completed induction chemotherapy.

On physical examination, temperature is 38.8 °C (101.8 °F), blood pressure is 100/70 mm Hg, pulse rate is 100/min, and respiration rate is 18/min. Exophthalmos of the right eye is noted, with ecchymosis around the eye and right nostril and bloody nasal discharge. The remainder of the examination is unremarkable.

Laboratory studies show an absolute neutrophil count of 100/µL ($0.1 \times 10^9$/L). The result of a serum galactomannan antigen immunoassay is positive.

Septate hyphae with acute angle branching are noted in tissue from sinus debridement.

CT of the head and sinuses reveals right maxillary sinusitis, right ethmoid sinusitis, and right eye retro-orbital inflammation.

**Which of the following is the most likely diagnosis?**

(A) *Aspergillus* rhinosinusitis
(B) *Candida* rhinosinusitis
(C) Cryptococcal rhinosinusitis
(D) *Pseudomonas* rhinosinusitis

## Item 55

A 35-year-old woman is evaluated for intermittent fever, sweats, fatigue, and dull midchest pain of 2 weeks' duration. Medical history is significant for liver transplantation 6 months ago for primary biliary cirrhosis; she was seronegative for cytomegalovirus and Epstein-Barr virus, and her donor was positive for both. Results of pretransplant testing for tuberculosis were negative. She received valganciclovir prophylaxis for 3 months after transplantation.

Medications are tacrolimus, prednisone, mycophenolate mofetil, and trimethoprim-sulfamethoxazole.

On physical examination, temperature is 37.7 °C (99.9 °F), blood pressure is 142/88 mm Hg, pulse rate is 92/min, and respiration rate is 14/min. Oropharynx has whitish plaques on the palate and buccal mucosa. No enlarged lymph nodes are palpable. Cardiopulmonary examination is normal. Abdomen is soft and nontender without hepatosplenomegaly. Extremities are without edema. No skin lesions are noted.

Laboratory studies are significant for a leukocyte count of 5200/µL ($5.2 \times 10^9$/L) and hematocrit of 33%. Liver and kidney function are normal. Bacterial and fungal blood cultures show no growth.

Chest radiograph shows clear lung fields but left hilar enlargement. Chest CT confirms an enlarged, 3-cm left hilar lymph node; the liver and spleen are unremarkable.

**Which of the following is the most likely cause of her clinical findings?**

(A) Cytomegalovirus infection
(B) Invasive candidal infection
(C) Posttransplant lymphoproliferative disease
(D) Reactivation tuberculosis

## Item 56

A 22-year-old woman is evaluated for a dog bite to the right arm. The dog is reported to be up to date on all vaccinations. Medical history is notable for Crohn disease, and she is up to date on all immunizations, with a tetanus-diphtheria-acellular pertussis vaccine administered 3 years ago. Her only medication is infliximab.

On physical examination, vital signs are normal. No epitrochlear or axillary lymphadenopathy is noted. The right forearm has several minor punctures and tears, with a small amount of erythema and minimal tenderness. No warmth, edema, or purulence is present.

Plain radiograph of the right forearm shows no evidence of fracture, gas, or foreign body.

**Which of the following is the most appropriate next step in the management of this patient?**

(A) Amoxicillin-clavulanate
(B) Metronidazole
(C) Tetanus immunization
(D) No additional evaluation or therapy

## Item 57

A 48-year-old woman is evaluated for a skin rash located on her left buttock. She describes the rash as irritating but not painful or associated with any systemic symptoms. She has had a similar rash approximately four times over the past year in the same area. She reports that when the rash has occurred before, the lesions last approximately 6 days, then crust over and resolve. On multiple occasions, she noticed a severe headache lasting 2 to 3 days when she had the rash. Medical history is unremarkable, and she takes no medications. She is married, and her husband has not had any similar symptoms. Her only medication is naproxen for menstrual cramps.

On physical examination, temperature is 36.9 °C (98.4 °F), blood pressure is 126/68 mm Hg, pulse rate is 72/min, and respiration rate is 12/min. BMI is 22. She appears well. Pelvic examination is unremarkable.

The rash, located at the mid-lower sacral area lateral to the gluteal crease, is shown.

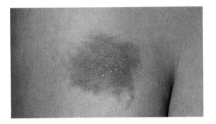

**Which of the following is the most likely cause of this patient's rash?**

(A) Dermatitis herpetiformis
(B) Fixed drug eruption
(C) Herpes simplex virus 2 infection
(D) Localized herpes zoster

## Item 58

A 29-year-old woman is evaluated for a 1-day history of diarrhea. She notes liquid stools with no mucus or visible blood. She has mild abdominal cramping relieved by defecation. She reports no nausea or vomiting. Three days ago, she ate almond butter from a manufacturer that posted a voluntary recall of the product due to contamination with *Salmonella braenderup.*

On physical examination, temperature is 37.9 °C (100.2 °F), blood pressure is 116/52 mm Hg, pulse rate is 90/min, and respiration rate is 18/min. The patient's abdomen is soft and mildly tender, with hyperactive bowel sounds.

Laboratory studies reveal a leukocyte count of 9700/µL $(9.7 \times 10^9/L)$.

**Which of the following is the most appropriate treatment?**

(A) Azithromycin
(B) Ciprofloxacin
(C) Loperamide
(D) Probiotics
(E) No therapy

## Item 59

A 46-year-old man is evaluated for fever, dysuria, and urinary frequency of 1 day's duration. He also notes a sensation of deep pelvic pain near the rectum. He has no urethral discharge or testicular pain. He states that he felt well before the current illness and has no other symptoms. Medical history is unremarkable. He is not sexually active. He takes no medications.

On physical examination, temperature is 38.8 °C (101.8 °F), blood pressure is 130/80 mm Hg, pulse rate is 100/min, and respiration rate is 16/min. Rectal examination reveals a tender and tense prostate.

Blood and urine cultures are pending. Urine dipstick is positive for leukocyte esterase and nitrites.

**Which of the following is the most appropriate treatment?**

(A) Ampicillin
(B) Ceftriaxone (single dose) and doxycycline
(C) Ciprofloxacin
(D) Meropenem

## Item 60

A 58-year-old man is evaluated in January during a recent outbreak of influenza virus in the assisted-living facility, where he works as a patient care aide. He reports declining influenza immunization offered in the autumn months because his sister told him that a friend developed a neurologic illness after receiving the vaccine. He is worried about possibly becoming ill and cannot afford to miss work. Medical history is significant for asthma, and his only medication is inhaled albuterol as needed.

On physical examination, vital signs are normal. The remainder of the examination is unremarkable.

**Which of the following is the most appropriate influenza prophylaxis regimen to recommend to this patient?**

(A) Amantadine chemoprophylaxis
(B) Oseltamivir chemoprophylaxis
(C) Oseltamivir chemoprophylaxis and inactivated influenza vaccine
(D) Oseltamivir chemoprophylaxis and live-attenuated influenza vaccine

## Item 61

A 73-year-old woman is hospitalized for a 1-day history of altered mental status and fever. Her family notes that yesterday she seemed confused and had trouble getting dressed. This morning, she was unable to be roused, and she was transported to the hospital by ambulance.

On physical examination, temperature is 39.1 °C (102.4 °F), blood pressure is 122/82 mm Hg, pulse rate is 110/min, and respiration rate is 24/min. The patient responds to deep stimulation with a grimace. No rash is present.

**Cerebrospinal fluid (CSF) studies:**

| | |
|---|---|
| Erythrocyte count | 3/µL $(3 \times 10^6/L)$ |
| Leukocyte count | 11/µL $(11 \times 10^6/L)$ |
| Glucose | 66 mg/dL (3.7 mmol/L) |
| Protein | 76 mg/dL (760 mg/L) |
| Gram stain | No organisms |

MRI of the brain is shown (top of next page).

Empiric treatment with intravenous dexamethasone, vancomycin, ceftriaxone, ampicillin, and acyclovir is begun. The next day, herpes simplex virus polymerase chain reaction assay of the CSF returns a negative result.

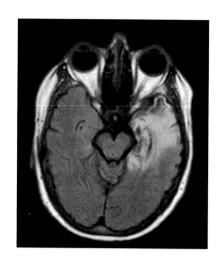

**Which of the following is the most likely diagnosis?**

(A) Enteroviral meningoencephalitis

(B) Herpes simplex encephalitis

(C) Pneumococcal meningitis

(D) West Nile neuroinvasive disease

## Item 62

A 25-year-old woman is admitted to the hospital for a 3-day history of severe headache localizing to the back of the head. She recently had an episode of sinusitis and has a history of sinus infections. Medical history is otherwise unremarkable, and she takes no medications.

On physical examination, temperature is 38.9 °C (102.0 °F), blood pressure is 134/82 mm Hg, pulse rate is 95/min, and respiration rate is 13/min. The general medical examination is unremarkable except for mild, bilateral maxillary sinus tenderness. On neurologic examination, she is awake and alert but reports photophobia. There are no focal findings.

Lumbar puncture is performed.

**Cerebrospinal fluid (CSF) profile:**

| | |
|---|---|
| Leukocyte count | 1200/μL (1200 × 10⁶/L) with 60% neutrophils and 40% lymphocytes |
| Glucose | 30 mg/dL (1.7 mmol/L) |
| Pressure (opening) | 2200 mm H₂O |
| Protein | 350 mg/dL (3500 mg/L) |

Gram stain of a CSF specimen shows gram-positive cocci in chains.

**In addition to appropriate empiric antibiotics, which of the following additional interventions is most likely to improve outcomes?**

(A) Dexamethasone

(B) Diuresis

(C) Maintaining head of the bed at greater than 30 degrees

(D) Mannitol

## Item 63

A 23-year-old woman is evaluated in the ICU. She was in a motor vehicle accident 7 days ago and has required mechanical ventilation since admission. She now has fever, an increased oxygen requirement, and increased respiratory secretions requiring suctioning every hour. Three other patients in the ICU are colonized or infected with extended-spectrum β-lactamase (ESBL)–producing *Klebsiella pneumoniae*. Medical history is unremarkable.

On physical examination, temperature is 39.0 °C (102.2 °F), blood pressure is 105/70 mm Hg, pulse rate is 110/min, and respiration rate is 16/min. Pulmonary examination reveals scattered rhonchi. On cardiac examination, the heart is hyperdynamic but otherwise normal. Her trauma sites are clean and dry.

Laboratory studies show a leukocyte count of 19,300/μL (19.3 × 10⁹/L). Sputum Gram stain reveals 2+ leukocytes and 3+ gram-negative rods; sputum culture is pending. Blood cultures return no growth.

Chest radiograph shows a new right lower-lobe infiltrate.

**Which of the following is the most appropriate empiric antimicrobial treatment?**

(A) Cefepime

(B) Ceftazidime

(C) Meropenem

(D) Piperacillin-tazobactam

## Item 64

A 26-year-old man is evaluated in follow-up after starting antiretroviral therapy 1 month ago. He reports no adverse effects of the medications. Medical history is notable for chronic active hepatitis B virus infection. His only medication is once-daily combination tenofovir-emtricitabine-cobicistat-elvitegravir initiated last month.

On physical examination, temperature is 36.6 °C (97.9 °F), blood pressure is 122/76 mm Hg, pulse rate is 68/min, and respiration rate is 12/min. The lungs are clear. No edema or rash is present.

Laboratory studies are significant for an increase in his serum creatinine from his pretreatment baseline of 1.2 mg/dL (106 μmol/L) to 1.5 mg/dL (133 μmol/L). Serum electrolytes are normal. Urinalysis is dipstick negative for blood or protein, and microscopic examination shows no cells or casts. The HIV viral load is undetectable.

**Which of the following is the most appropriate management?**

(A) Change antiretroviral therapy to an abacavir-lamivudine–based regimen

(B) Hold antiretroviral therapy and reassess kidney function in 4 weeks

(C) Kidney biopsy

(D) Continue current antiretroviral regimen

## Item 65

A 37-year-old man is hospitalized for diabetic foot infection with sepsis of the right lower extremity. He is treated with piperacillin-tazobactam and vancomycin and symptoms improve. However, 4 days later he develops a fever and diarrhea, described as four to five liquid bowel movements over the last 24 hours. Medical history is significant for type 2 diabetes mellitus with a baseline creatinine of 1.0 mg/dL (88.4 µmol/L). Medications are piperacillin-tazobactam, vancomycin, and metformin.

On physical examination, temperature is 38.7 °C (101.7 °F), blood pressure is 150/72 mm Hg, pulse rate is 106/min, and respiration rate is 18/min. The patient's abdomen is soft and mildly tender with positive bowel sounds.

Laboratory studies reveal leukocyte count is 18,800/µL (18.8 × 10⁹/L) and serum creatinine level is 1.6 mg/dL (141 µmol/L). Result of stool polymerase chain reaction assay is positive for *Clostridium difficile* toxin.

**Which of the following is the most appropriate treatment?**

(A) Oral metronidazole
(B) Oral vancomycin
(C) Oral vancomycin plus intravenous metronidazole
(D) Oral vancomycin plus intravenous vancomycin
(E) Oral vancomycin plus oral metronidazole

## Item 66

A 60-year-old woman is admitted to the hospital for a 2-week history of confusion and change in personality. Her symptoms began acutely and have progressed steadily since onset. She is no longer able to maintain activities of daily living. She has had an ataxic gait for 2 days. She has no history of travel outside the United States and no known infectious exposures. Medical history is unremarkable, and she takes no medications.

On physical examination, temperature is 36.8 °C (98.2 °F), blood pressure is 140/70 mm Hg, pulse rate is 88/min and regular, and respiration rate is 14/min. She is oriented to person only and has difficulty finding words. The general medical examination is unremarkable. On neurologic examination, the cranial nerves are intact. She has preserved motor strength throughout, although myoclonus is present.

Laboratory studies demonstrate a normal metabolic profile, kidney and liver function, and complete blood count. On lumbar puncture, the opening pressure is normal. The cerebrospinal fluid is clear with a leukocyte count of 1/µL (1 × 10⁶/L) and an erythrocyte count of 0/µL. The glucose level is normal, and the 14-3-3 protein is elevated.

MRI of the brain reveals focal cortical hyperintensity.

**Which of the following is the most likely diagnosis?**

(A) Alzheimer disease
(B) Kuru
(C) Neurosyphilis
(D) Sporadic Creutzfeldt-Jakob disease

## Item 67

A 32-year-old man is evaluated in the emergency department for a 2-day history of fever, rash, severe headache, back pain, sore throat, and vomiting. He is employed as an international emergency aid worker and recently returned to the United States after an extended overseas assignment. The rash began a few days after the onset of fever, beginning first on the inside of the mouth and then spreading to his face, hands, and eventually both arms and legs. The initial lesions were flat and red but later became raised and blistered. Other members of his work team have also fallen ill. He does not recall his complete vaccination history but believes that he received all of his scheduled immunizations and that he was exposed as a young child to chickenpox when his sister had it. Medical history is unremarkable, and he takes no medications.

On physical examination, the patient appears very ill. Temperature is 39.3 °C (102.7 °F), blood pressure is 114/70 mm Hg, pulse rate is 110/min, and respiration rate is 16/min. BMI is 28. He has multiple clusters of pus-filled vesicles dispersed on the face, arms, and legs. Bilateral conjunctivitis is present. Pulmonary examination reveals mild bilateral lower lung field crackles. No meningeal signs are found.

**Which of the following is the most likely infection in this patient?**

(A) Measles
(B) Rickettsial pox
(C) Smallpox
(D) Varicella

## Item 68

A 32-year-old man is evaluated in the emergency department for a severe occipital headache. He reports flulike symptoms for the past 2 to 3 weeks, with fever, malaise, fatigue, neck stiffness, generalized achiness, sore throat, and mild nausea. He also notes having "swollen glands" in his neck and neck stiffness but no vomiting, abdominal pain, diarrhea, or cough. He indicates that he had a reddish skin rash located across his chest and upper abdomen that first appeared several days after onset of his fevers and other symptoms and began to fade several days ago; the rash was present for approximately 1 week. Medical history is unremarkable, and he takes no medications. The patient thinks he had all standard childhood vaccinations. He is sexually active with both men and women, with intermittent condom use.

On physical examination, the patient appears uncomfortable. Temperature is 38.3 °C (100.9 °F), and other vital signs are normal. No abnormalities are seen on nondilated funduscopic examination. Cervical lymphadenopathy and pharyngeal erythema are noted. A faint maculopapular rash is present on the trunk. The remainder of the examination is unremarkable.

A lumbar puncture is performed.

**Cerebrospinal fluid (CSF) profile:**

| | |
|---|---|
| Leukocyte count | 55/µL (55 × 10⁶/L), with lymphocytic predominance |
| Glucose | 70 mg/dL (3.9 mmol/L) |
| Pressure (opening) | 80 mm H₂O |
| Protein | 149 mg/dL (1490 mg/L) |

CSF Gram stain is negative, and culture results are pending.

**H** **CONT.** Which of the following studies is most likely to confirm the diagnosis in this patient?

(A) CSF enterovirus polymerase chain reaction assay
(B) HIV antigen/antibody combination immunoassay
(C) Lyme serologic testing
(D) Mumps IgM serologic testing

**H** ## Item 69

A 59-year-old man is evaluated in the emergency department after sustaining a puncture wound to the right foot 12 days ago. He is a construction worker. He stepped on a metallic object that punctured through his leather work boots into the plantar aspect of his foot. He reports pain on walking and notes swelling, warmth, and erythema on the top of his foot above the site of injury. He reports no fever or chills and has noted no drainage from the area of injury. Medical history is significant only for a fracture of the fourth and fifth metatarsal bones of the right foot 27 years ago treated with an internal fixation plate. His only medication is as-needed acetaminophen.

On physical examination, temperature is 38.1 °C (100.6 °F), blood pressure is 146/76 mm Hg, pulse rate is 89/min, and respiration rate is 16/min. BMI is 31. Examination is unremarkable except for the right foot, which is edematous, warm, and erythematous on the dorsal surface with a closed puncture wound on the plantar aspect of the foot directly beneath the first metatarsal-phalangeal area. The foot is tender to palpation but displays no drainage or fluctuance. The proximal leg is unremarkable, and no lymphadenopathy is detected.

Laboratory studies reveal a leukocyte count of 12,300/μL (12.3 × 10$^9$/L) and serum creatinine level of 1.0 mg/dL (88.4 μmol/L).

Plain radiograph of the right foot shows diffuse soft tissue swelling and metallic fixation plate. No gas is detectable in the soft tissues.

Which of the following is the most appropriate diagnostic test to perform next?

(A) CT with contrast
(B) MRI with gadolinium
(C) Tagged leukocyte nuclear scanning
(D) Three-phase nuclear bone scanning

## Item 70

A 29-year-old woman is evaluated for a 5-day history of nodules over her lower extremities. She reports that she regularly visits a local spa that uses whirlpool footbaths during her pedicure procedures; she always shaves her legs with a razor before these visits. Medical history is unremarkable, and she takes no medications.

On physical examination, temperature is 37.0 °C (98.6 °F), blood pressure is 120/70 mm Hg, pulse rate is 70/min, and respiration rate is 14/min. BMI is 22. No inguinal lymphadenopathy is apparent. Several mildly tender, erythematous nodules and papules are noted over the distal lower extremities bilaterally; several lesions appear furuncular with associated ulceration. The remainder of the examination is normal.

Punch biopsy of a lesion reveals a necrotizing granulomatous dermatitis, and tissue culture grows a mycobacterial species within 4 days.

Which of the following is the most likely cause of infection?

(A) *Mycobacterium fortuitum*
(B) *Mycobacterium gordonae*
(C) *Mycobacterium kansasii*
(D) *Mycobacterium marinum*

## Item 71

**H**

A 46-year-old man is evaluated in the emergency department for fever and altered mental status. Five days ago he underwent replacement of a ventriculoperitoneal shunt used to manage congenital hydrocephalus. The procedure was unremarkable, and he did well postoperatively until the rapid onset of confusion and fever over the past several hours. Medical history is otherwise unremarkable, and he takes no medications.

On physical examination, the patient is confused and mildly agitated. Temperature is 39.7 °C (103.5 °F), blood pressure is 142/87 mm Hg, pulse rate is 110/min, and respiration rate is 16/min. The general medical examination shows healing surgical incisions on the scalp, neck, and upper abdomen that are clean and dry. Marked nuchal rigidity is noted. Neurologic examination reveals altered sensorium but is otherwise nonfocal.

Head CT shows the ventriculoperitoneal shunt in proper position and no hydrocephalus or other focal lesions.

Laboratory evaluation of the cerebrospinal fluid shows a leukocyte count of 4660/μL (4660 × 10$^6$/L) with neutrophilic predominance, glucose level of 15 mg/dL (0.8 mmol/L), and protein level of 480 mg/dL (4800 mg/L). Gram stain and culture results are pending.

Which of the following is the most appropriate empiric antibiotic treatment?

(A) Ampicillin, vancomycin, and ceftriaxone
(B) Meropenem and vancomycin
(C) Moxifloxacin
(D) Vancomycin and ceftriaxone

## Item 72

A 22-year-old man is evaluated in follow-up for a recent diagnosis of HIV infection. He has sex with other men and is careful about selection of partners; because of this, he expresses disbelief at the diagnosis. He is asymptomatic and has no history of opportunistic infections. Medical history is otherwise unremarkable. He uses marijuana and cocaine recreationally but reports no injection drug use.

Oh physical examination, vital signs are normal. BMI is 22. Oral, genitourinary, and anal examinations are without lesions. No lymphadenopathy or rash is present. The remainder of the examination is normal.

Laboratory study results include an absolute CD4 cell count of 680/μL and HIV viral load of 3285 copies/mL; complete blood count is normal, as are kidney and liver function studies. HIV genotypic testing demonstrates resistance to efavirenz and nevirapine.

Counseling on HIV transmission prevention is provided.

**Which of the following is the most appropriate next step in management?**

(A) Begin antiretroviral therapy today

(B) Begin trimethoprim-sulfamethoxazole

(C) Defer therapy pending further discussion of HIV treatment

(D) Initiate antiretroviral therapy when CD4 cell count is less than 350/µL

## Item 73

A 36-year-old woman is evaluated in the ICU for a possible urinary tract infection. She was admitted for management of injuries sustained in a motor vehicle accident and has undergone multiple orthopedic surgical procedures. Yesterday, her temperature was elevated to 38.1 °C (100.6 °F) and a urinalysis with culture was ordered. She has no urinary symptoms. Medical history is otherwise unremarkable. Her only medication is vancomycin.

On physical examination, temperature is 36.8 °C (98.2 °F), blood pressure is 110/70 mm Hg, pulse rate is 88/min, and respiration rate is 16/min. BMI is 22. The general medical examination is unremarkable except for multiple contusions and surgical incision sites on the left upper extremity and bilateral lower extremities that are clean and dry. An indwelling urinary catheter is in place.

Urinalysis reveals 25 to 30 leukocytes/hpf and more than $10^5$ colony-forming units of yeast identified as *Candida albicans*.

**Which of the following is the most appropriate management?**

(A) Amphotericin B bladder irrigation

(B) Caspofungin

(C) Fluconazole

(D) Voriconazole

(E) No antifungal therapy

## Item 74

A 46-year-old man is diagnosed with methicillin-sensitive *Staphylococcus aureus* osteomyelitis of the L2 and L3 vertebrae during a recent hospitalization. He is discharged home to complete 6 weeks of nafcillin therapy. Medical history is otherwise unremarkable, and he takes no other medications.

**Which of the following tests should be completed weekly in monitoring this patient?**

(A) Complete blood count, liver enzyme tests, and serum potassium level

(B) Serum creatinine level and complete blood count

(C) Serum creatinine level, complete blood count, and liver enzyme tests

(D) Serum creatinine level, liver enzyme tests, and serum potassium level

## Item 75

A 40-year-old man is evaluated for a 2-day history of cough and progressive dyspnea. He notes that the cough is minimally productive of a small amount of whitish sputum. He reports receiving his influenza vaccination this season. Medical history is notable only for cellulitis 2 months ago treated with a brief course of cephalexin. He does not smoke cigarettes or consume alcohol. He takes no medications.

On physical examination, temperature is 37.7 °C (99.9 °F), blood pressure is 127/78 mm Hg, heart rate is 87/min, and respiration rate is 20/min. Oxygen saturation is 99% breathing ambient air. Pulmonary examination reveals decreased breath sounds at the right lung base with no wheezes, crackles, or rhonchi auscultated. The remainder of the examination is unremarkable.

Chest radiograph shows a right lower lobe infiltrate.

**Which of the following is the most appropriate empiric antibiotic therapy for this patient?**

(A) Amoxicillin-clavulanate

(B) Azithromycin

(C) Doxycycline

(D) Moxifloxacin

## Item 76

A 22-year-old man is evaluated in the emergency department for a 1-day history of fever and headache. One week ago, he presented to his internist with a skin eruption on his abdomen, which was diagnosed as erythema migrans. A 14-day course of amoxicillin was initiated. The skin eruption has since resolved.

On physical examination, temperature is 39.1 °C (102.4 °F), blood pressure is 122/64 mm Hg, pulse rate is 104/min, and respiration rate is 22/min. The patient is ill-appearing. No skin lesions are noted.

**Laboratory studies:**

| | |
|---|---|
| Haptoglobin | 125 mg/dL (1250 mg/L) |
| Hematocrit | 45% |
| Leukocyte count | 2300/µL ($2.3 \times 10^9$/L) |
| Platelet count | 96,000/µL ($96 \times 10^9$/L) |
| Alanine aminotransferase | 74 U/L |
| Aspartate aminotransferase | 88 U/L |
| Bilirubin, total | 1.0 mg/dL (17.1 µmol/L) |
| Lactate dehydrogenase | 95 U/L |

**Which of the following is the most likely diagnosis?**

(A) Infection with *Anaplasma phagocytophilum*

(B) Infection with *Babesia microti*

(C) Infection with Powassan virus

(D) Relapsed Lyme disease

## Item 77

An 82-year-old woman is evaluated for a 1-week history of urinary incontinence with lower abdominal discomfort. She reports no dysuria, fever, or back pain. Medical history is significant for hypertension and allergic reaction to sulfa drugs, which cause a generalized rash. Her only medication is hydrochlorothiazide.

On physical examination, temperature is 36.8 °C (98.2 °F), blood pressure is 150/90 mm Hg, pulse rate is 72/min, and respiration rate is 16/min. Mild suprapubic tenderness but no costovertebral angle tenderness are noted on abdominal examination. The remainder of the examination is noncontributory.

Urine dipstick is positive for leukocyte esterase and nitrites.

**Which of the following is the most appropriate management?**

(A) Levofloxacin

(B) Nitrofurantoin

(C) Urine culture

(D) Clinical observation

### Item 78

A 25-year-old man is admitted to the hospital for chills and fever of 3 days' duration. He reports that he injects heroin daily. Medical history is notable for multiple methicillin-resistant *Staphylococcus aureus*–associated skin and soft tissue infections and for vancomycin hypersensitivity, which causes respiratory failure and hypotension. He takes no medications.

On physical examination, temperature is 39.4 °C (102.9 °F), blood pressure is 104/65 mm Hg, pulse rate is 110/min, and respiration rate is 20/min. A recent injection site in the antecubital fossa is noted, with erythema, tenderness to palpation, and warmth. He has no mucosal lesions or lymphadenopathy. Cardiopulmonary examination is normal. The remainder of the examination is normal.

Laboratory studies show a leukocyte count of 19,000/μL (19 × 10⁹/L) with 95% neutrophils.

Multiple blood cultures reveal gram-positive cocci in clusters. Findings on chest imaging and electrocardiography are normal.

**Which of the following is the most appropriate empiric antibiotic treatment for this patient?**

(A) Ceftriaxone

(B) Daptomycin

(C) Imipenem

(D) Nafcillin

### Item 79

A 19-year-old man is evaluated for a 4-day history of dysuria and pruritus in the area of the meatus. Scant urethral discharge is noted. He has recently become sexually active with a new female partner. He takes no medications and has no known allergies.

On physical examination, vital signs are normal. The remainder of the physical examination is unremarkable.

The results of a nucleic acid amplification test on first voided urine are positive for *Chlamydia trachomatis* and negative for *Neisseria gonorrhoeae*. Urine culture reveals fewer than 10,000 CFU/mL of *Escherichia coli*.

**Which of the following is the most appropriate treatment?**

(A) Amoxicillin

(B) Azithromycin

(C) Cefixime

(D) Ceftriaxone plus azithromycin

### Item 80

A 36-year-old woman is evaluated for fever and right flank pain of 1 day's duration and dysuria of 3 days' duration. Medical history is unremarkable, and she takes no medications.

On physical examination, temperature is 38.9 °C (102.0 °F), blood pressure is 100/70 mm Hg, pulse rate is 100/min, and respiration rate is 16/min. Right costovertebral angle tenderness is noted. The remainder of the examination is noncontributory.

Urinalysis is positive for leukocyte esterase and nitrites, with a leukocyte count greater than 10/hpf and with many bacteria present. Urine culture is pending.

**Which of the following is the most appropriate empiric therapy?**

(A) Ampicillin and gentamicin

(B) Ciprofloxacin

(C) Ertapenem

(D) Nitrofurantoin

### Item 81

A 45-year-old man is evaluated for a persistent intermittently draining wound. He sustained an open comminuted fracture of the left lower leg 4 years ago during a military deployment. Since that time, he has had a dry eschar over the original open wound that intermittently drains whitish-colored fluid. He reports no fever, chills, or fatigue and indicates only a dull ache around the injury site. He has had no previous evaluation or treatment for this condition. Medical history is significant for hypertension. His only medication is hydrochlorothiazide.

On physical examination, temperature is 37.3 °C (99.1 °F), blood pressure is 130/82 mm Hg, pulse rate is 78/min, and respiration rate is 13/min. Slight induration, hyperpigmentation, and an irregularly shaped 2.5- × 1.5-cm dry eschar are noted on the anteromedial aspect of the left lower leg. A sinus tract is noted after removal of the eschar with drainage of a scant amount of seropurulent fluid. The surrounding soft tissues are not warm, fluctuant, or crepitant.

Laboratory studies are significant for a leukocyte count of 7600/μL (7.6 × 10⁹/L) and erythrocyte sedimentation rate of 32 mm/h.

Plain radiography of the lower extremity demonstrates a healed tibial fracture site surrounded by a bone callus and an anterior soft tissue defect.

Gram stain of sinus tract drainage shows scant leukocytes and rare gram-positive cocci in pairs and clusters. Culture shows moderate growth of *Enterococcus faecalis* and light growth of *Staphylococcus epidermidis*.

**Which of the following is the most appropriate next step in management?**

(A) Bone biopsy and culture

(B) Intravenous vancomycin

(C) MRI

(D) Oral linezolid

## Item 82

A 65-year-old woman is evaluated for a 3-month history of right knee pain. She reports no previous injury to the joint. She lives in a rural area and has experienced frequent tick bites over the last several years but does not recall any tick attachments in the last 6 months. She has had no fever.

On physical examination, temperature is 37.0 °C (98.6 °F), blood pressure is 134/72 mm Hg, pulse rate is 86/min, and respiration rate is 16/min. The right knee is swollen but without warmth or erythema. Crepitus is present with passive flexion and extension. The patient has no skin lesions.

Arthrocentesis is performed, and synovial fluid analysis is compatible with inflammatory arthritis. On laboratory testing, result of Lyme antibody screen (enzyme immunoassay) is positive. Findings on subsequent Western blot IgM are positive, and Western blot IgG result is negative.

**Which of the following is the most appropriate management?**

(A) *Borrelia burgdorferi* polymerase chain reaction on synovial fluid

(B) Prescribe ceftriaxone

(C) Prescribe doxycycline

(D) No additional evaluation or treatment for Lyme disease

## Item 83

A 74-year-old man is evaluated in the emergency department for a 1-day history of grossly bloody diarrhea, abdominal cramps, and chills. Two days ago, he attended a church picnic where he ate coleslaw, corn, and oysters. Several other attendees also developed diarrhea. Medical history is significant for cirrhosis related to chronic hepatitis C.

On physical examination, temperature is 38.3 °C (100.9 °F), blood pressure is 148/82 mm Hg, pulse rate is 117/min, and respiration rate is 22/min. He is diaphoretic. He has gynecomastia and spider angiomata on the chest. Abdominal examination is unremarkable.

The patient's stool is liquid with bright red blood streaks.

**Which of the following is the most likely causative organism of this patient's dysentery?**

(A) *Clostridium difficile*

(B) *Norovirus*

(C) *Vibrio parahaemolyticus*

(D) *Yersinia enterocolitica*

## Item 84

A 20-year-old woman is evaluated in follow-up after an anaphylactic reaction associated with a blood transfusion given emergently following a motor vehicle accident; she has recovered completely from her injuries. Medical history is significant for systemic lupus erythematosus diagnosed 1 year ago and for recurrent sinus and respiratory tract infections since adolescence. Her only medication is hydroxychloroquine.

On physical examination, temperature is 36.8 °C (98.2 °F), blood pressure is 110/50 mm Hg, pulse rate is 86/min, and respiration rate is 14/min. BMI is 21. Examination of the nasal passages and upper airway is normal, and the remainder of the physical examination is unremarkable.

Laboratory studies show an undetectable serum IgA level.

**Which of the following is the most appropriate management?**

(A) Meningococcal conjugate vaccine

(B) Monthly intravenous IgA

(C) Monthly intravenous immune globulin

(D) Stem cell transplantation

(E) Clinical follow-up

## Item 85

A 47-year-old man is evaluated for a skin eruption. Approximately 2 weeks ago, his wife noted an erythematous macule on his back. Over the ensuing week, the site became progressively larger. He notes mild fatigue but no fevers. He recently returned from a vacation in Massachusetts, which included outdoor activities such as bike riding and walking to the beach. He reports no known tick attachment.

On physical examination, temperature is 37.2 °C (100.0 °F), blood pressure is 117/68 mm Hg, pulse rate is 52/min, and respiration rate is 18/min. The skin lesion is shown.

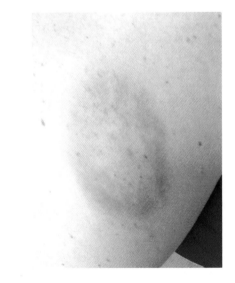

**Which of the following is the most appropriate management?**

(A) Prescribe doxycycline

(B) Prescribe levofloxacin

(C) Serologic testing for *Babesia microti*

(D) Serologic testing for *Borrelia burgdorferi*

## Item 86

A 23-year-old woman is hospitalized for a 2-day history of diarrhea. In the last 24 hours, there has been blood in the stools. She has had abdominal cramping but reports no fevers or chills. She eats only organically grown foods and drinks unpasteurized milk.

On physical examination, temperature is 36.8 °C (98.2 °F), blood pressure is 115/72 mm Hg, pulse rate is 86/min, and respiration rate is 18/min. She has mild abdominal pain diffusely on palpation.

The patient's stool shows visible bright red blood streaking.

**Which of the following is the most common complication associated with this patient's dysentery?**

(A) Aortitis

(B) Guillain-Barré syndrome

(C) Hemolytic uremic syndrome

(D) Mesenteric adenitis

(E) Reactive arthritis

## Item 87

A 45-year-old man is evaluated after notification that he received a blood transfusion from a donor who subsequently developed babesiosis. He received 2 units of packed red blood cells 2 months ago after trauma associated with a motor vehicle collision. Since hospital discharge, he has noted mild fatigue but reports no fevers, chills, weight loss, or myalgias.

On physical examination, temperature is 37.0 °C (98.6 °F), blood pressure is 134/72 mm Hg, pulse rate is 84/min, and respiration rate is 18/min. No jaundice, hepatomegaly, or splenomegaly is present.

**Laboratory studies:**

| | |
|---|---|
| Hematocrit | 45% |
| Leukocyte count | 7600/µL (7.6 × 10⁹/L) |
| Platelet count | 358,000/µL (358 × 10⁹/L) |
| Bilirubin, total | 1.4 mg/dL (23.9 µmol/L) |
| Reticulocyte count | 1% of erythrocytes |

Results of *Babesia* polymerase chain reaction of whole blood are positive.

**Which of the following is the most appropriate management?**

(A) Perform exchange transfusion

(B) Repeat polymerase chain reaction in 3 months

(C) Treat with atovaquone and azithromycin

(D) Treat with clindamycin and quinine

## Item 88

A 21-year-old woman is hospitalized for a 4-day history of progressively worsening right-lower-quadrant abdominal pain with dyspareunia, fever, and chills. On the day of admission, the patient developed nausea with several episodes of vomiting. She takes no medications and has no known allergies.

On physical examination, temperature is 38.8 °C (101.8 °F), blood pressure is 100/60 mm Hg, pulse rate is 110/min, and respiration rate is 12/min. Abdominal examination reveals positive bowel sounds with tenderness

in the right lower quadrant accompanied by localized rebound. On pelvic examination, the cervix is erythematous with a small amount of mucopurulent discharge. Cervical motion tenderness and tenderness in the right adnexal region are noted, without adnexal fullness or masses.

Result on a pregnancy test is negative, and pelvic ultrasonography shows fluid in the cul de sac with thickening of the right fallopian tube but no tubo-ovarian abscess.

**Which of the following is the most appropriate treatment?**

(A) Cefoxitin plus doxycycline

(B) Ceftriaxone plus azithromycin

(C) Ciprofloxacin

(D) Piperacillin-tazobactam

## Item 89

A 78-year-old man is admitted to the ICU with fever, malaise, weakness, and abdominal pain of 5 days' duration. He reports no nausea, vomiting, or diarrhea. Medical history is notable only for diverticulosis, and he takes no medications.

On physical examination, temperature is 38.6 °C (101.5 °F), blood pressure is 120/60 mm Hg, pulse rate is 112/min, and respiration rate is 18/min. Oxygen saturation is 92% breathing ambient air. Abdominal distention and moderate midabdominal tenderness are noted. Bowel sounds are normal. The remainder of the examination is noncontributory.

Laboratory studies show a leukocyte count of 21,000/µL (21 × 10⁹/L).

CT scan shows diverticulosis and a 3-cm × 4-cm enhancing fluid collection.

Percutaneous drainage and culture is pending.

**Which of the following is the most appropriate antimicrobial treatment?**

(A) Intravenous aztreonam and vancomycin

(B) Intravenous vancomycin and oral clindamycin

(C) Oral ampicillin and metronidazole

(D) Oral ciprofloxacin and metronidazole

## Item 90

A 25-year-old man is evaluated in follow-up after HIV testing. He states he has sex with other men and usually uses condoms. He had a negative HIV test result 1 year ago. He feels well today but reports having a flulike illness last week with mild fever, headache, myalgias, and fatigue; these symptoms have resolved. Medical history is unremarkable for sexually transmitted or other infections. Other than taking over-the-counter ibuprofen last week, he takes no medications.

On physical examination, he is afebrile and has small palpable anterior and posterior cervical, axillary, and inguinal lymph nodes. The remainder of the examination is normal.

HIV-1/2 antigen/antibody combination immunoassay is reactive. Result of an HIV-1/HIV-2 antibody differentiation immunoassay is negative for HIV-1 and HIV-2. Result of an HIV-1 nucleic acid amplification testing is positive, with 51,455 copies/mL.

Which of the following is the most appropriate next step in management?

(A) Repeat HIV-1/HIV-2 antibody differentiation immunoassay in 6 weeks

(B) Saliva rapid HIV testing

(C) T-cell subset testing

(D) Western blot HIV-1 antibody testing

Which of the following is the most appropriate management?

(A) Caspofungin

(B) Lumbar puncture

(C) Surgical removal of the nodule

(D) Clinical observation

## Item 91

A 65-year-old woman is evaluated for a 3-day history of diarrhea and fever. She reports no abdominal pain or vomiting. She notes mucus intermixed with the stool, but no visible blood. She is also experiencing fatigue and anorexia. She works as a nurse.

On physical examination, the patient appears uncomfortable but is in no acute distress. Temperature is 38.2 °C (100.8 °F), blood pressure is 148/66 mm Hg, pulse rate is 84/min, and respiration rate is 22/min. Abdominal examination reveals hyperactive bowel sounds and mild diffuse tenderness to palpation.

Laboratory studies reveal a leukocyte count of 11,400/µL (11.4 × 10⁹/L) and a positive result on a fecal occult blood test.

Empiric levofloxacin is started for presumed bacterial gastroenteritis, and a stool sample is sent for culture. Twenty-four hours later, the culture reveals *Campylobacter jejuni* resistant to levofloxacin. A call to the patient confirms she feels well, with resolution of diarrhea and fever.

Which of the following is the most appropriate management?

(A) Discontinue levofloxacin

(B) Perform blood culture testing

(C) Repeat stool culture

(D) Switch to azithromycin

(E) Switch to ciprofloxacin

## Item 92

A 45-year-old man is evaluated for right-sided chest discomfort and cough of 2 weeks' duration. His chest discomfort is described as a vague, painful sensation on the right. The cough occasionally produces a small amount of sputum; he reports no hemoptysis or shortness of breath. He has felt feverish with mild fatigue but has had no weight loss. He is a smoker with a 20-pack-year history. He takes no medications.

On physical examination, temperature is 37.6 °C (99.7 °F), blood pressure is 130/70 mm Hg, pulse rate is 86/min, and respiration rate is 18/min. BMI is 27. Oxygen saturation breathing ambient air is 98%. Chest examination is normal, and the remainder of the physical examination is unremarkable. No skin rash is present.

Chest radiograph shows a nodule in the right lower lung lobe, which CT of the chest confirms. CT-guided biopsy of the nodule is performed. Findings on histologic testing are positive for budding yeast, and culture indicates *Cryptococcus neoformans*.

An HIV test result is negative.

## Item 93

A 31-year-old man is evaluated in the emergency department for a 5-day history of abdominal discomfort, vomiting, and loose stools, accompanied by progressively increasing fever. He also has a moderate headache and a rash. He arrived from Sri Lanka 6 days ago.

On physical examination, temperature is 40 °C (104 °F), blood pressure is 102/70 mm Hg, pulse rate is 64/min, and respiration rate is 20/min. BMI is 26. The patient appears sick. There are blanching erythematous macules on the lower chest and upper abdominal wall. He has scleral icterus and injected conjunctivae. The pharynx is erythematous. Abdominal examination reveals tender hepatosplenomegaly. The remainder of the examination is normal.

**Laboratory studies:**

| | |
|---|---|
| Hemoglobin | 12.1 g/dL (121 g/L) |
| Leukocyte count | 4550/µL (4.55 × 10⁹/L); 68% polymorphonuclear cells, 10% band forms, 16% lymphocytes, 6% monocytes |
| Platelet count | 95,000/µL (95 × 10⁹/L) |
| Alanine aminotransferase | 250 U/L |
| Aspartate aminotransferase | 125 U/L |

Peripheral blood smear is normal. Two sets of aerobic blood cultures show gram-negative bacilli.

Which of the following is the most likely diagnosis?

(A) Brucellosis

(B) Lassa fever

(C) Leptospirosis

(D) Typhoid fever

## Item 94

A 24-year-old woman is hospitalized for a 1-month history of increasing paranoia and delusions according to her husband. On the day of admission, she had a tonic-clonic seizure with incontinence. Medical history is otherwise unremarkable, and she takes no medications.

On physical examination, temperature is 37.9 °C (100.2 °F), blood pressure is 107/48 mm Hg, pulse rate is 102/min, and respiration rate is 16/min. The patient is unresponsive but withdraws her extremities to painful stimuli. The neck is supple to passive flexion. Occasionally, choreoathetoid movements of the bilateral upper extremities are observed.

Lumbar puncture is performed.

**Cerebrospinal fluid (CSF) studies:**

| | |
|---|---|
| Leukocyte count | 57/µL (57 × 10⁶/L); 97% lymphocytes, 3% neutrophils |
| Erythrocyte count | 14/µL (14 × 10⁶/L) |
| Glucose | 57 mg/dL (3.2 mmol/L) |
| Protein | 142 mg/dL (1420 mg/L) |
| Gram stain | No organisms |

Results of herpes simplex virus polymerase chain reaction of the CSF are negative. HIV antibody serum test results are negative.

Brain MRI reveals no focal abnormality.

**Which of the following tests is most likely to confirm the diagnosis?**

(A) Anti–N-methyl-D-aspartate receptor (NMDAR) antibodies

(B) *Borrelia burgdorferi* (Lyme) antibody serology

(C) Nuchal skin biopsy

(D) VDRL test of CSF

## Item 95

A 75-year-old man is evaluated in the emergency department for fever, productive cough, and shortness of breath of 5 days' duration. Medical history is significant for type 2 diabetes mellitus. He has never smoked and does not drink alcohol. His only medication is metformin.

On physical examination, temperature is 39.2 °C (102.6 °F), blood pressure is 95/65 mm Hg, heart rate is 110/min, and respiration rate is 32/min. Oxygen saturation is 83% breathing ambient air and rises to 94% with 30% oxygen by face mask. BMI is 29. Pulmonary examination reveals decreased breath sounds and crackles at the left lung base. The remainder of the examination, including mental status, is normal.

Laboratory studies show a leukocyte count of 18,000/µL (18 × 10⁹/L). A basic metabolic panel is normal. Blood cultures are pending.

Chest radiograph shows left lower lobe consolidation.

The patient is transferred to the ICU, and empiric broad-spectrum antibiotics are ordered.

**Which of the following additional studies is most appropriate in this patient?**

(A) C-reactive protein level

(B) Chest CT

(C) Procalcitonin level

(D) Sputum cultures

## Item 96

A 29-year-old man is hospitalized for a 3-week history of fever, malaise, night sweats, and weight loss. Medical history is significant for HIV/AIDS infection, with an episode of *Pneumocystis jirovecii* pneumonia 2 years ago. He is nonadherent with all his HIV medications.

On physical examination, temperature is 39.2 °C (102.6 °F), blood pressure is 100/60 mm Hg, pulse rate is 100/min, and respiration rate is 18/min. BMI is 19. He appears cachectic. Abdominal palpation elicits mild pain without guarding or rebound and reveals hepatosplenomegaly. The remainder of the examination is normal.

Laboratory study results show a CD4+ cell count of 45/µL.

Blood cultures are positive for *Mycobacterium avium* complex.

**Which of the following is the most appropriate treatment?**

(A) Clarithromycin, ethambutol, and rifabutin

(B) Isoniazid and rifabutin

(C) Isoniazid, rifabutin, ethambutol

(D) Rifabutin, isoniazid, pyrazinamide, ethambutol

## Item 97

A 64-year-old man is evaluated for a 3-day history of fever, chills, and cough productive of yellow-green, but sometimes brownish, sputum. Although his breathing is comfortable at rest, he feels short of breath with minimal activity. He reports having received a flu shot this season. Medical history is significant for COPD, type 2 diabetes mellitus, and a 50-pack-year smoking history, although he quit 5 years ago. Medications are tiotropium and as-needed albuterol metered-dose inhalers and metformin.

On physical examination, temperature is 37.6 °C (99.7 °F), blood pressure is 130/90 mm Hg, pulse rate is 90/min, and respiration rate is 24/min. Oxygen saturation is 92% breathing ambient air. Pulmonary examination is notable for diffusely decreased breath sounds throughout and crackles at the right lung base; occasional mild expiratory wheezes are present. Cardiac and abdominal examinations are normal, and the remainder of the examination is unremarkable.

Chest radiograph shows a right lower lobe infiltrate.

**Which of the following is the most appropriate management?**

(A) Inpatient treatment with ampicillin-sulbactam and doxycycline

(B) Inpatient treatment with ceftriaxone and azithromycin

(C) Outpatient treatment with azithromycin

(D) Outpatient treatment with levofloxacin

## Item 98

A 53-year-old man is evaluated in the hospital for fever. He underwent elective coronary artery bypass graft surgery 2 days ago. An indwelling urinary catheter was inserted in the operating room. Medical history is unremarkable, and he takes no medications.

On physical examination, temperature is 38.4 °C (101.1 °F), blood pressure is 130/84 mm Hg, pulse rate is 88/min, and respiration rate is 18/min. Lungs are clear to auscultation. The sternotomy incision site is clean and dry. He has mild suprapubic tenderness but no costovertebral angle or flank tenderness.

Urinalysis reveals 10 to 20 leukocytes/hpf. Urine culture grows 10⁴ colony-forming units of gram-negative rods. Chest radiograph shows no infiltrate.

**In addition to removing the urinary catheter, which of the following is the most appropriate management?**

(A) Await antimicrobial sensitivities before beginning antimicrobial therapy

(B) Begin antimicrobial therapy now

(C) Repeat urinalysis and urine culture in 24 hours

(D) Provide no additional treatment

## Item 99

A 50-year-old man is admitted to the hospital for fever with increasing pain and redness of his left foot and leg. He stepped on a fishhook 2 days ago while wading through brackish water. He reports that only the foot was involved initially, but symptoms have spread up his leg to just below the knee. Medical history is significant for cirrhosis secondary to chronic hepatitis C. He is up to date on all immunizations. Medications are propranolol and as-needed furosemide.

On physical examination, temperature is 39.3 °C (102.7 °F), blood pressure is 90/60 mm Hg, pulse rate is 70/min, and respiration rate is 22/min. The left foot and leg up to the knee are edematous, exquisitely tender, and covered with several hemorrhagic bullae. The remainder of the examination is unremarkable.

Laboratory studies show a leukocyte count of 20,000/µL (20 × 10⁹/L), with 85% neutrophils, 10% immature band forms, and 5% lymphocytes.

Emergent surgical debridement shows necrotizing fasciitis. Gram stain of the intraoperative tissue specimen reveals curved gram-negative bacilli.

Empiric antimicrobial agents are initiated.

**Which of the following is the most likely infectious agent?**

(A) *Erysipelothrix rhusiopathiae*

(B) Methicillin-resistant *Staphylococcus aureus*

(C) *Mycobacterium marinum*

(D) *Vibrio vulnificus*

## Item 100

A 33-year-old man is evaluated in the emergency department in July for respiratory distress. He recently returned from an extended business trip through Guangdong Province of China, Saudi Arabia, and Liberia. Over the final 3 days of the trip, he noted feeling short of breath with exertion with dry cough, headache, nausea, and diarrhea. He is unaware of known exposure to ill contacts. Medical history is otherwise unremarkable, and he takes no medications. He has received all recommended travel-related immunizations.

On physical examination, temperature is 39.1 °C (102.4 °F), blood pressure is 110/72 mm Hg, pulse rate is 98/min, and respiration rate is 22/min. BMI is 28. Oxygen saturation is 91% breathing ambient air. No lymphadenopathy is detected. Pulmonary auscultation reveals diffuse bronchial breath sounds and rhonchi. He has no abdominal tenderness or hepatosplenomegaly, and no rash is present. The remainder of the examination is normal.

**Laboratory studies:**

| | |
|---|---|
| Hemoglobin | 10.9 g/dL (109 g/L) |
| Leukocyte count | 4750/µL (4.75 × 10⁹/L) (82% neutrophils, 10% lymphocytes, 8% monocytes) |
| Platelet count | 97,000/µL (97 × 10⁹/L) |
| Prothrombin time/INR | Normal |
| Alanine aminotransferase | 98 U/L |
| Blood urea nitrogen | 30 mg/dL (10.7 mmol/L) |
| Creatinine | 1.6 mg/dL (141 µmol/L) |
| Lactate dehydrogenase | 355 U/L |

Chest radiograph is shown.

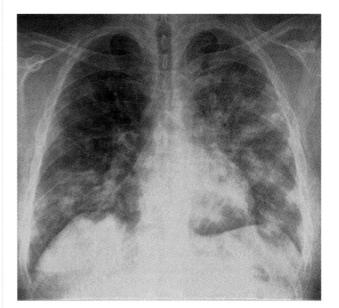

**Which is the following is the most likely diagnosis?**

(A) Ebola virus infection

(B) Influenza virus infection

(C) Middle East respiratory syndrome

(D) Respiratory syncytial virus infection

## Item 101

A 62-year-old man is evaluated in the hospital for fever and chills of 1 day's duration. He was admitted 3 days ago for lower gastrointestinal bleeding and hypotension, and a right internal jugular venous catheter was inserted for intravenous fluid hydration and blood transfusion. Blood cultures drawn through the central catheter and peripherally during initial evaluation of the fever were positive for gram-positive cocci in clusters. The central venous catheter was removed and vancomycin started. Medical history is otherwise unremarkable, and he takes no other medications.

On physical examination, temperature is 38.1 °C (100.6 °F), blood pressure is 118/74 mm Hg, pulse rate is 94/min, and respiration rate is 16/min. The previous intravenous catheter site is mildly tender to palpation, without erythema, drainage, or fluctuance. The remainder of the examination is unremarkable.

**CONT.**

The original blood cultures grew methicillin-sensitive *Staphylococcus aureus*, and repeat blood cultures 24 hours after the start of antibiotics are positive for gram-positive cocci. Transthoracic echocardiography shows no valvular vegetations.

**Which of the following is the most appropriate management?**

(A) Add rifampin

(B) Change vancomycin to nafcillin

(C) Obtain a serum vancomycin peak level

(D) Perform ultrasonography on the right internal jugular vein

**Item 102**

A 55-year-old woman is evaluated in the emergency department for fever, cough, decreased appetite, and night sweats of 2 weeks' duration. She has experienced a 4.5-kg (10 lb) weight loss over past 2 months. She lives in China and is visiting her daughter in the United States. Medical history is otherwise unremarkable, and she takes no medications

On physical examination, temperature is 38.3 °C (100.9 °F), blood pressure is 120/70 mm Hg, pulse rate is 90/min, and respiration rate is 19/min. BMI is 20. Egophony is heard in the upper lobes of both lungs.

Bilateral apical infiltrates are seen on chest radiograph.

**In addition to standard precautions, which of the following empiric infection control precautions should be instituted for this patient?**

(A) Airborne

(B) Contact

(C) Droplet

(D) No additional precautions

**Item 103**

An 18-year-old young man is evaluated for a tender skin lesion on the right leg, which appeared 2 days ago. He is a wrestler at his high school. Medical history is notable for a documented hypersensitivity allergy to trimethoprim–sulfamethoxazole. He takes no medications.

On physical examination, temperature is 36.9 °C (98.4 °F), blood pressure is 120/74 mm Hg, pulse rate is 80/min, and respiration rate is 13/min. BMI is 23. No lymphangitis or right inguinal lymphadenopathy is evident. A single 3-cm by 2-cm fluctuant, tender soft tissue lesion without erythema is noted over the right distal anterior thigh.

Complete blood count is normal.

**In addition to incision and drainage of the furuncle, which of the following is the most appropriate treatment?**

(A) Oral dicloxacillin

(B) Oral doxycycline

(C) Oral rifampin

(D) Clinical follow-up

**Item 104**

A 70-year-old woman is admitted to the hospital for a 1-week history of fever, productive cough, and worsening shortness of breath. Because of poor oxygenation and hypotension, she is admitted directly to the ICU. Medical history is significant for oxygen-dependent COPD and bronchiectasis with frequent exacerbations. She has a 55-pack-year smoking history and is a current smoker. Medications are tiotropium, fluticasone-salmeterol, and as-needed albuterol metered-dose inhalers; she recently completed a 10-day prednisone taper.

On physical examination, temperature is 38.3 °C (100.9 °F), blood pressure is 88/60 mm Hg, pulse rate is 105/min, and respiration rate is 30/min. Oxygen saturation is 82% breathing ambient air, which increases to 92% with 50% oxygen by face mask. Lung examination shows diffuse rhonchi. The remainder of the examination is unremarkable.

Laboratory studies are significant for a leukocyte count of 16,400/µL ($16.4 \times 10^9$/L), a normal metabolic profile, and normal kidney function. Sputum and blood cultures are pending.

Chest radiograph shows multilobar infiltrates.

**Which of the following is the most appropriate empiric antibiotic treatment for this patient?**

(A) Cefepime, levofloxacin, and gentamicin

(B) Ceftriaxone and azithromycin

(C) Levofloxacin and ceftriaxone

(D) Meropenem

**Item 105**

A 39-year-old man undergoes consultation about HIV prevention. He has a male sex partner with HIV infection. He reports they use condoms "most of the time." He asks about other options that can reduce his risk for acquiring HIV from his partner. He is asymptomatic. Medical history is noncontributory, although he has been vaccinated for hepatitis B. He takes no medications.

On physical examination, vital signs are normal, as is the remainder of the examination.

Results of testing for HIV are negative. Testing for hepatitis B surface antigen yields negative findings, and hepatitis B surface antibody results are positive.

**Which of the following is the most appropriate management?**

(A) Counsel that consistent condom use provides adequate protection

(B) Prescribe daily combination tenofovir-emtricitabine

(C) Prescribe daily combination tenofovir-emtricitabine and raltegravir

(D) Prescribe daily tenofovir

**Item 106**

A 45-year-old woman is seen for follow-up evaluation of daily fevers and fatigue of 1 month's duration. She reports measured temperatures as high as 38.3 °C (100.9 °F) but has no focal symptoms or weight loss. Medical history is unremarkable. She reports no travel or known infectious exposures. She takes no medications.

On physical examination, temperature is 38.2 °C (100.8 °F), blood pressure is 130/60 mm Hg, pulse rate is 90/min and regular, and respiration rate is 14/min. BMI is 27. The patient appears well, and the remainder of the physical examination is normal and unchanged from a clinic visit 3 weeks ago.

**Laboratory studies:**

| | |
|---|---|
| Erythrocyte sedimentation rate | <20 mm/h |
| Hemoglobin | 14.2 g/dL (142 g/L) |
| Leukocyte count | 6800/µL (6.8 × 10⁹/L) with normal differential |
| Platelet count | 223,000/µL (223 × 10⁹/L) |
| Alkaline phosphatase | 77 U/L |
| Aminotransferases | Normal |
| Urinalysis | 0-2 leukocytes/hpf |
| Complete metabolic profile and kidney function | Normal |

Results for antinuclear antibody are negative. Findings on HIV serologic testing, tuberculin skin test, and serum pregnancy test are negative. Three sets of blood cultures show no growth.

A chest radiograph and CT of the abdomen and pelvis with and without contrast are normal.

**Which of the following is the most appropriate next step in management?**

(A) Bone marrow aspirate and biopsy

(B) Empiric course of broad-spectrum antibiotics

(C) Empiric trial of systemic glucocorticoids

(D) Whole-body CT

(E) Clinical observation

## Item 107

A 68-year-old woman is admitted to the hospital for a 2-day history of fever, increasing dyspnea, and worsening cough. She was diagnosed with influenza pneumonia approximately 3 weeks ago. She had stayed home from work following her diagnosis and was beginning to recover when her current symptoms began. She started with fever and began to notice increasing shortness of breath. Her cough, which had almost resolved, returned and has been productive of moderate amounts of grey-colored sputum. Medical history is significant for hypertension. Her only medication is hydrochlorothiazide.

On physical examination, temperature is 38.1 °C (100.6 °F), blood pressure is 136/82 mm Hg, pulse rate is 89/min, and respiration rate is 28/min. Oxygen saturation is 90% breathing ambient air. Lung examination shows diffuse rhonchi. Cardiac and abdominal examinations are normal.

Chest radiograph shows bilateral cavitary infiltrates.

**Which of the following is the most likely causative pathogen in this patient?**

(A) *Legionella* species

(B) *Pseudomonas aeruginosa*

(C) *Staphylococcus aureus*

(D) *Streptococcus pneumoniae*

## Item 108

A 26-year-old woman is evaluated for recurrent episodes of cystitis. She has had four episodes within the previous 6 months but is currently asymptomatic. She has increased her fluid intake and voids after sexual intercourse. However, she continues to have episodes of infection. Medical history is unremarkable, and she takes no medications.

On physical examination, temperature is 37.0 °C (98.6 °F), blood pressure is 110/60 mm Hg, pulse rate is 60/min, and respiration rate is 14/min. BMI is 19. The remainder of the examination is normal.

**Which of the following is the most appropriate management?**

(A) Antimicrobial prophylaxis

(B) Daily methenamine hippurate

(C) Daily vitamin C

(D) Urethroscopy

# Answers and Critiques

## Item 1      Answer:  B

**Educational Objective: Treat a patient with tuberculous meningitis.**

This patient has tuberculous meningitis and should receive glucocorticoid therapy in addition to antituberculous therapy. Dexamethasone is recommended for adults with tuberculous meningitis because limited data show some mortality benefits. The recommended dose of dexamethasone is 12 mg/d for 3 weeks, with gradual tapering during the following 3 weeks. Some experts use prednisone instead of dexamethasone, and others recommend a slightly longer duration of glucocorticoid therapy (approximately 8 weeks). The recommendations for duration of treatment of extrapulmonary tuberculosis are generally the same as for pulmonary tuberculosis (6-9 months). However, the recommended treatment duration for tuberculous meningitis is longer (9-12 months), with the exact duration determined by response to therapy and antibiotic sensitivities of the isolate.

Diuretics—such as acetazolamide and furosemide, which decrease cerebrospinal fluid (CSF) production by the choroid plexus—have been used as temporizing measures for management of hydrocephalus in patients who are not stable enough to undergo surgical decompression. However, there is no indication for their use in this patient.

Patients with tuberculous meningitis can develop hydrocephalus, usually secondary to impaired CSF resorption. Ventriculoperitoneal shunts can be used to manage hydrocephalus. This patient has no evidence of hydrocephalus, which is typically associated with increased intracranial pressures and ventriculomegaly on brain imaging. Serial lumbar punctures after initiation of glucocorticoids and antituberculous medications can be attempted initially in patients with hydrocephalus before attempting surgical drainage with a shunt.

### KEY POINT

- Patients with tuberculous meningitis should receive a glucocorticoid in addition to antituberculous therapy.

### Bibliography

American Thoracic Society; CDC; Infectious Diseases Society of America. Treatment of tuberculosis [erratum in MMWR Recomm Rep. 2005 Jan 7;53(51):1203]. MMWR Recomm Rep. 2003 Jun 20;52(RR-11):1-77. [PMID: 12836625]

## Item 2      Answer:  D

**Educational Objective: Diagnose central nervous system toxoplasmosis.**

This patient most likely has central nervous system (CNS) *Toxoplasma gondii* infection. He has not been adherent to antiretroviral therapy, and his CD4 cell count has decreased to less than 100/µL, putting him at risk for opportunistic infection. Clinical presentation of CNS toxoplasmosis typically involves new headaches and focal neurologic deficits and may also include fever and seizures. The findings on this patient's MRI are classic for toxoplasmosis, with multiple ring-enhancing lesions. Because CNS toxoplasmosis in AIDS results from reactivation of earlier infection, patients usually have a positive result for IgG antibody but not IgM. He should be treated empirically and followed for clinical and radiographic response, which typically occurs within 1 to 2 weeks.

Primary CNS lymphoma generally requires a more severe degree of immunosuppression than most other AIDS-related complications, most commonly occurring when the CD4 cell count drops below 50/µL; the incidence has decreased with effective antiretroviral therapy. Although primary CNS lymphoma may present with more than one lesion on MRI, it most often presents with a single large lesion. Primary CNS lymphoma is strongly associated with Epstein-Barr virus infection, and polymerase chain reaction of cerebrospinal fluid to detect Epstein-Barr virus can facilitate the diagnosis. The prognosis remains poor.

Cryptococcal meningoencephalitis is another common CNS infection in AIDS but rarely results in focal mass lesions on imaging, more often presenting with mental status changes than focal deficits and seizure. The serum cryptococcal antigen and cerebrospinal fluid antigen are positive in 95% and 99% of cases, respectively; therefore, a negative antigen test result argues against this diagnosis.

Progressive multifocal leukoencephalopathy presents in AIDS with focal deficits and mental status changes. Onset usually occurs over several weeks, compared with several days for toxoplasmosis, and fever is uncommon. Furthermore, progressive multifocal leukoencephalopathy lesions on MRI are typically white-matter, noninflammatory lesions (unless accompanied by immune reconstitution inflammatory syndrome) with minimal enhancement and no mass effect.

### KEY POINT

- Central nervous system toxoplasmosis in AIDS results from reactivation of earlier infection, typically involves new focal neurologic deficits and headaches, and may also include fever and seizures.

### Bibliography

Panel on Opportunistic Infections in HIV-Infected Adults and Adolescents. Guidelines for the prevention and treatment of opportunistic infections in HIV-infected adults and adolescents: recommendations from the Centers for Disease Control and Prevention, the National Institutes of Health, and the HIV Medicine Association of the Infectious Diseases Society of America. http://aidsinfo.nih.gov/contentfiles/lvguidelines/adult_oi.pdf. Updated April 16, 2015. Accessed July 20, 2015.

## Item 3    Answer:    D

**Educational Objective: Manage nonresponse to antimicrobial therapy in a patient with ventilator-associated pneumonia.**

This patient should undergo thoracentesis to determine why he is not improving with treatment. Nonresponsive pneumonia is defined as an inadequate clinical response despite appropriate antimicrobial therapy. In most patients with ventilator-associated pneumonia (VAP), effective antimicrobial treatment usually results in defervescence and reduction in leukocyte count within 72 hours of beginning therapy, with improvement of oxygenation and decreased secretions, if hypoxia and excessive secretions were present. In patients who do not respond to appropriate antimicrobial treatment after 72 hours or who do not continue improving or worsen after an initial therapeutic response, it is imperative to search for another explanation for the patient's clinical findings (such as an infectious complication, another site of infection, or an alternate diagnosis). The possibility of a parapneumonic process should always be considered in the differential diagnosis of nonresponsive pneumonia. A new, or increasing, pleural effusion could represent a parapneumonic effusion, empyema, or a lung abscess. Thoracentesis and pleural fluid examination should be performed because the results could significantly alter management.

Suprainfections can occur, including suprainfection with gram-negative organisms, but the finding of only gram-positive cocci on Gram stain does not support this as a cause of nonresponse. Thus, broadening antimicrobial therapy to cover gram-negative organisms is not warranted.

With a new fever and no change in respiratory symptoms or oxygenation requirements, drug fever resulting from nafcillin therapy might be considered, especially if the chest radiograph was unchanged or showed improvement. Antimicrobial agents, particularly β-lactam agents, can cause drug fever but usually do not cause the level of leukocytosis seen in this patient. Because treatment for methicillin-sensitive *Staphylococcus aureus* VAP should continue for at least 7 days, the antibiotic should be changed to a different class if drug fever is suspected but not stopped altogether.

Evaluation of infectious complications or extrapulmonary sources of infection should occur before considering a bronchoscopy and bronchoalveolar lavage (BAL). BAL may be considered when there is a suspicion of antibiotic-resistant organisms not isolated from sputum culture.

### KEY POINT

- Patients with ventilator-associated pneumonia who do not improve within 72 hours of initiation of appropriate antimicrobial therapy should be evaluated for infectious complications, an alternate diagnosis, or another site of infection to explain the clinical picture.

### Bibliography

American Thoracic Society, Infectious Diseases Society of America. Guidelines for the management of adults with hospital-acquired, ventilator-associated, and healthcare associated pneumonia. Am J Respir Crit Care Med. 2005;171:388-416. [PMID: 15699079]

## Item 4    Answer:    D

**Educational Objective: Treat vancomycin-intermediate, methicillin-resistant *Staphylococcus aureus* bacteremia.**

This patient's vancomycin therapy should be discontinued, and treatment with an alternative agent, such as daptomycin, should be initiated. Although vancomycin is a reasonable choice for empiric therapy in patients suspected of having methicillin-resistant *Staphylococcus aureus* (MRSA) skin or soft tissue infection, it is only slowly bactericidal and generally less effective than agents more potently bactericidal against MRSA for treatment of bacteremia or infective endocarditis. The minimum inhibitory concentration (MIC) to vancomycin of the infecting organism is typically used to guide therapy. For isolates with a vancomycin MIC of 2 μg/mL or less, the patient's clinical response should determine whether to continue vancomycin or change to an alternative agent independent of the MIC. However, vancomycin is not recommended for bacteremia if the MIC to vancomycin is greater than 2 μg/mL. Therefore, continuing the current vancomycin dose in this patient would not be appropriate, and switching therapy to an alternative agent is indicated. If daptomycin is used, the MIC of the organism to daptomycin should also be verified to ensure susceptibility.

In patients in whom treatment with vancomycin for MRSA bacteremia is appropriate (vancomycin MIC of 2 μg/mL or less), the goal serum vancomycin trough level is 15 to 20 μg/mL. When the vancomycin trough level is within this range, as in this patient, increasing the vancomycin dose creates the risk of the trough level being higher than 20 μg/mL, which would increase the risks for adverse effects without providing additional clinical benefit. However, because the MIC of this organism to vancomycin is greater than 2 μg/mL, continuing dose-adjusted vancomycin would not be appropriate.

Adding rifampin to vancomycin has not been shown to improve clinical outcomes.

### KEY POINT

- Daptomycin is a better therapeutic option than vancomycin for treating methicillin-resistant *Staphylococcus aureus* with a vancomycin minimum inhibitory concentration greater than 2 μg/mL.

### Bibliography

Liu C, Bayer A, Cosgrove SE, et al; Infectious Diseases Society of America. Clinical practice guidelines by the Infectious Diseases Society of America for the treatment of methicillin-resistant *Staphylococcus aureus* infections in adults and children [erratum in Clin Infect Dis. 2011 Aug 1;53(3):319]. Clin Infect Dis. 2011;52:e18-55. [PMID: 21208910]

## Item 5    Answer:    D

**Educational Objective: Manage a patient receiving ethambutol for treatment of tuberculosis.**

This patient has strongly suspected pulmonary tuberculosis and will begin four-drug therapy with isoniazid, rifampin, pyrazinamide, and ethambutol. All patients starting antituberculous therapy should have baseline measurements of aminotransferases, bilirubin, alkaline phosphatase, serum creatinine, and a platelet count. Specific adverse effects of ethambutol include a retrobulbar neuritis manifesting as decreased green-red color discrimination or decreased visual acuity. Therefore, baseline testing of color discrimination and visual acuity with monthly questioning regarding any visual abnormalities is recommended for patients taking ethambutol, with monthly testing for patients taking the drug for more than 2 months, patients with kidney disease, and patients receiving more than 15 to 25 mg/kg of ethambutol. Rash and peripheral neuritis are also reported with ethambutol use. Adverse effects of isoniazid use include peripheral neuropathy, hepatitis, rash, and a lupus-like syndrome. Pyrazinamide can cause hepatitis, rash, gastrointestinal upset, and hyperuricemia. Rifampin can cause hepatitis, gastrointestinal upset, rash, and orange coloring of body fluids. All patients should be evaluated at least monthly for adherence to these medications as well as possible adverse reactions.

Baseline audiogram and vestibular testing (including Romberg testing) is recommended for patients receiving streptomycin, an aminoglycoside with adverse effects, including ototoxicity (hearing and vestibular disturbances), neurotoxicity, and nephrotoxicity. Monthly questioning regarding vestibular/auditory symptoms and monthly assessments of kidney function are recommended.

Patients with HIV who become infected with tuberculosis should have a CD4 cell count performed as part of baseline monitoring.

### KEY POINT

- Before starting ethambutol, patients should be evaluated for color discrimination and visual acuity because an adverse effect of the drug is a retrobulbar neuritis manifesting as decreased green-red color discrimination or decreased visual acuity.

### Bibliography

American Thoracic Society; CDC; Infectious Diseases Society of America. Treatment of tuberculosis [erratum in MMWR Recomm Rep. 2005 Jan 7;53(51):1203]. MMWR Recomm Rep. 2003 Jun 20;52(RR-11):1–77 [PMID: 12836625]

## Item 6    Answer:    D

**Educational Objective: Diagnose Rocky Mountain spotted fever.**

The most likely diagnosis for this patient, who presents with fever, lymphocytic meningitis, and petechial rash following tick exposure, is Rocky Mountain spotted fever (RMSF).

Headache is common in RMSF, and meningoencephalitis is seen in as many as 20% of cases. A rash is present in 85% to 90% of cases of RMSF, although the onset of skin findings may be delayed several days after the initial fever. Early on, the rash is often macular and localized to the wrists and ankles. Over time, this evolves to a diffuse petechial eruption, usually sparing the face. Involvement of palms and soles is characteristic of RMSF, although it is not universal. The low platelet counts and elevated liver enzyme levels also suggest RMSF. Finally, the rapid clinical response to doxycycline is characteristic of RMSF and would make viral entities less likely. The negativity for RMSF antibodies should not discount this diagnosis. During the acute presentation, antibodies to *Rickettsia rickettsii* are often undetectable because of insufficient time to mount a serologic response to the infection. Testing a convalescent serum specimen obtained more than 14 days after symptom onset allows for retrospective confirmation of RMSF infection. Skin biopsy frequently reveals evidence of vasculitis, and the diagnosis may be confirmed by immunohistochemistry; however, this test is not widely available. A clinically compelling presentation for RMSF should prompt initiation of doxycycline treatment, and this should be continued despite the absence of detectable antibodies.

Rash caused by enterovirus is distinguishable from RMSF because it appears morbilliform rather than petechial. Hematologic abnormalities are uncommon with enterovirus infection.

Heartland virus is a newly identified phlebovirus transmitted by the same tick that causes ehrlichiosis. Although this infection is associated with thrombocytopenia and elevated liver enzyme levels, it can be distinguished from RMSF by lack of a rash or response to doxycycline treatment.

Lyme disease can cause neurologic manifestations, including meningitis, but is associated with erythema migrans rather than a petechial rash.

West Nile virus causes neuroinvasive disease in less than 1% of infected patients. It may be associated with a nonspecific rash; however, symptoms would not improve with doxycycline.

### KEY POINT

- Following a tick bite, symptoms of fever, petechial rash, and lymphocytic meningitis suggest Rocky Mountain spotted fever and should be treated with doxycycline.

### Bibliography

Lin L, Decker CF. Rocky Mountain spotted fever. Dis Mon. 2012 Jun;58(6):361–9. [PMID: 22608123]

## Item 7    Answer:    B

**Educational Objective: Treat hospital-acquired diarrhea with an antimotility medication.**

This patient, whose diarrhea began more than 3 days after hospitalization, tested negative for *Clostridium difficile*

Answers and Critiques

infection (CDI), so she should be prescribed an antimotility agent for symptomatic relief. CDI is the most common infectious cause of diarrhea in hospitalized patients. Antibiotic administration is a major risk factor; however, infection can also be acquired through person-to-person spread or environmental contamination. Diagnostic evaluation for CDI is appropriate for all patients with hospital-acquired diarrhea, regardless of antibiotic history. Nucleic acid amplification tests, such as polymerase chain reaction (PCR) for *C. difficile* toxin genes, are highly sensitive and specific and offer the advantage of rapid results. Antiperistaltic agents should be avoided in CDI treatment because they may obscure symptoms and increase risk for toxic megacolon. In this patient, however, the negative PCR test result essentially excludes this diagnosis. For noninfectious diarrhea, antimotility agents may relieve symptoms.

Hospital-acquired bacterial gastroenteritis, other than CDI, is exceedingly rare, with one study identifying an alternative bacterial enteropathogen in less than 1% of stool cultures submitted at 3 days of hospitalization or longer. Because of the low yield, many laboratories reflexively reject stool cultures submitted on patients who develop diarrhea more than 72 hours after admission.

Patients with confirmed CDI require antimicrobial treatment. Oral metronidazole, as well as vancomycin, is effective in the treatment of mild to moderate CDI. However, it is not indicated in the setting of a negative PCR test result.

Repeat PCR testing after a negative result is rarely indicated and only increases the probability of a false-positive result. Stool enzyme immunoassay, which detects glutamate dehydrogenase, an enzyme ubiquitous in *C. difficile*, is an accepted alternative to PCR in diagnosing CDI. When the result of stool enzyme immunoassay is negative, no further testing is necessary; however, when it is positive, a second, more specific test, such as PCR, is required for diagnosis.

### KEY POINT

- Patients with hospital-acquired diarrhea who test negative for *Clostridium difficile* infection should be treated with antimotility agents to suppress symptoms and not undergo additional testing or treatment for *C. difficile*.

### Bibliography

Slimings C, Riley TV. Antibiotics and hospital-acquired Clostridium difficile infection: update of systematic review and meta-analysis. J Antimicrob Chemother.2014 Apr;69(4):881-91. [PMID: 24324224]

### Item 8    Answer:    C

**Educational Objective: Diagnose immune reconstitution inflammatory syndrome caused by disseminated *Mycobacterium avium* complex infection.**

This patient has immune reconstitution inflammatory syndrome (IRIS) caused by disseminated *Mycobacterium avium* complex (DMAC) infection. She developed symptoms typical for DMAC (fever, chills, sweats, fatigue, weight loss)

approximately 1 month after starting antiretroviral therapy (ART). The infection was likely present before therapy initiation, but her improved immune response, made possible by treating her HIV infection, resulted in development of symptoms (the so-called "unmasking" of a preexisting infection). Her lymphadenopathy, hepatosplenomegaly, anemia, leukopenia, and elevated alkaline phosphatase level are typical signs. DMAC is usually seen in patients whose CD4 cell count is, or recently was, less than 50/μL. The diagnosis can be confirmed by culture of the blood or other normally sterile site, such as bone marrow, lymph node, or liver. A macrolide-based multidrug regimen, usually clarithromycin and ethambutol, and continued ART are the recommended treatment. IRIS is most common with mycobacterial or fungal infections but also has been reported with various opportunistic infections and with non-Hodgkin lymphoma.

Cytomegalovirus occurs in patients with AIDS with low CD4 cell counts and can present with nonspecific systemic symptoms, cytopenias, and hepatitis. However, it usually presents with focal organ involvement, most often in the gastrointestinal tract as esophagitis or colitis or in the eye as retinitis.

Candidal infection usually does not disseminate in HIV infection (compared with the risk in neutropenia) but rather causes mucocutaneous disease (such as esophagitis), which is not clinically present in this patient. Candidal infection also should not cause systemic symptoms or this patient's CT findings.

Gastrointestinal adverse effects are common with ART and often improve with time. Elevated liver enzymes may occur but often involve aminotransferases, not only alkaline phosphatase. Abacavir is associated with an uncommon hypersensitivity reaction consisting of fever, rash, gastrointestinal symptoms, hepatitis, and malaise, although abacavir toxicity would not explain this patient's lymphadenopathy or cytopenias and usually occurs shortly after therapy initiation.

### KEY POINT

- Treatment of HIV infection improves immune response, which can result in immune reconstitution inflammatory syndrome and symptomatic infection that may have been present at the time of antiretroviral therapy initiation.

### Bibliography

Panel on Opportunistic Infections in HIV-Infected Adults and Adolescents. Guidelines for the prevention and treatment of opportunistic infections in HIV-infected adults and adolescents: recommendations from the Centers for Disease Control and Prevention, the National Institutes of Health, and the HIV Medicine Association of the Infectious Diseases Society of America. http://aidsinfo.nih.gov/contentfiles/lvguidelines/adult_oi.pdf. Updated April 16, 2015. Accessed July 21, 2015.

### Item 9    Answer:    B

**Educational Objective: Treat a patient with *Coccidioides immitis* meningitis.**

This patient should be treated with fluconazole. She has coccidioidal meningitis caused by *Coccidioides immitis*.

*Coccidioides* species are endemic in desert regions of the southwestern United States and Central and South America. Primary infection is subclinical or manifests as self-limited chest pain, cough, and fever in most patients. However, disseminated coccidioidal infection may occur, and meningeal disease is the most serious form of disseminated infection, with significant associated morbidity and mortality. Patients at highest risk for coccidioidal meningitis are those with immunodeficiency (such as HIV/AIDS infection), diabetes mellitus, alcohol abuse, and pregnancy. Headache, vomiting, and change in mental status are the most common presenting findings. Cerebrospinal fluid (CSF) demonstrates a lymphocytic pleocytosis with elevated protein and low glucose. Eosinophils in the CSF are seen in up to 70% of patients with coccidioidal meningitis. Detection of complement-fixing antibodies in the CSF is more sensitive than is culture in diagnosing coccidioidal meningitis. Complement-fixing IgG is present in up to 90% of patients. Fluconazole is the treatment of choice. It offers a good response rate and a favorable safety profile; therefore, it has replaced intrathecal amphotericin B as the therapy of choice. Intrathecal amphotericin B is now used only in those who have not responded to fluconazole.

Caspofungin does not have activity against *C. immitis* and does not penetrate into CSF. Therefore, it would not be the best choice of therapy in this patient with coccidioidal meningitis.

Experience with the use of itraconazole for coccidioidal meningitis has been less than that with fluconazole; therefore, it is considered second line-therapy and should not be chosen before first-line therapy with fluconazole is provided.

> **KEY POINT**
>
> - Fluconazole is the treatment of choice for coccidioidal meningitis, because it offers a good response rate and a favorable safety profile.

**Bibliography**

Mathisen G, Shelub A, Truong J, Wigen C. Coccidioidal meningitis: clinical presentation and management in the fluconazole era. Medicine (Baltimore). 2010 Sep;89(5):251-84. [PMID: 20827104]

## Item 10    Answer:    A

**Educational Objective: Evaluate for neurosyphilis with cerebrospinal fluid analysis.**

This patient, who has serologic results consistent with syphilis of unknown duration, should undergo cerebrospinal fluid (CSF) analysis to exclude the possibility of neurosyphilis as a contributing factor to her cognitive decline. CSF should be sent for protein, glucose, cell count with differential, and VDRL testing. Neurosyphilis must be confirmed or excluded in this patient because this will determine the appropriate therapeutic approach.

A positive CSF VDRL result in the absence of visible blood contamination or any other unexplained abnormality of the spinal fluid (elevated protein, elevated leukocyte count) should prompt treatment of neurosyphilis with intravenous penicillin. If the CSF analysis yields normal results, treatment for late-latent syphilis with intramuscular benzathine penicillin is appropriate.

Both rapid plasma reagin and VDRL are nonspecific tests. The positive serum rapid plasma reagin result in this case was confirmed by a positive specific test (the fluorescent treponemal antibody absorption test). Therefore, syphilis is confirmed by serologic testing, and it would not be necessary to perform an additional nonspecific test for syphilis. Neurosyphilis must be diagnosed by CSF analysis.

> **KEY POINT**
>
> - Patients who have syphilis of unknown duration and an abnormal neurologic examination should undergo cerebrospinal fluid analysis to confirm or exclude the diagnosis of neurosyphilis before treatment is started.

**Bibliography**

Workowski KA, Berman S; Centers for Disease Control and Prevention (CDC). Sexually transmitted diseases treatment guidelines, 2010 [erratum in MMWR Recomm Rep. 2011 Jan 14;60(1):18]. MMWR Recomm Rep. 2010 Dec 17;59(RR-12):1-110. [PMID: 21160459]

## Item 11    Answer:    B

**Educational Objective: Determine treatment duration for a patient with active pulmonary tuberculosis.**

This patient has pulmonary tuberculosis and is completing a 2-month initial phase of treatment with the three-drug regimen of rifampin, isoniazid, and ethambutol and will require a 7-month continuation phase consisting of isoniazid and rifampin. Although most patients with active tuberculosis are treated with a four-drug regimen, usually consisting of rifampin, isoniazid, ethambutol, and pyrazinamide, pyrazinamide is contraindicated for use in patients with active gout and should be used with caution in chronic gout because it inhibits renal tubular excretion of uric acid. In most patients, a continuation phase of 4 months of isoniazid and rifampin is recommended for treatment of drug-susceptible tuberculosis. However, a 7-month continuation phase of isoniazid and rifampin is recommended in patients who do not receive pyrazinamide during the initial phase, in patients receiving once-weekly isoniazid and rifapentine whose sputum cultures are still positive at the end of the initial treatment phase, and in patients with cavitary pulmonary tuberculosis whose sputum cultures are positive at end of the initial phase of treatment. Because this patient did not receive pyrazinamide as part of his initial drug regimen, he should be treated with a 7-month continuation phase.

In the absence of drug resistance, 6 to 9 months of total treatment is sufficient. Longer courses extending beyond 9 months are reserved for multidrug-resistant tuberculosis.

- A 7-month therapy continuation phase is recommended in patients with active tuberculosis who have certain comorbidities or positive sputum cultures after completing initial therapy.

**Bibliography**

Centers for Disease Control and Prevention. Treatment for TB Disease. www.cdc.gov/tb/topic/treatment/tbdisease.htm. Updated December 9, 2011. Accessed July 21, 2015.

## Item 12          Answer:    C

**Educational Objective: Manage immunizations in a patient after transplantation.**

This patient should receive a booster immunization with the tetanus-diphtheria-acellular pertussis (Tdap) vaccine because he has not received it as an adult. The childhood version of this vaccine, DTaP, is highly effective, but immunity against pertussis may wane into the adult years, increasing the risk for infection in this population. Because of this, the Advisory Committee on Immunization Practices recommends that all adults receive a single booster administration with Tdap, regardless of the timing of a previous diphtheria-tetanus booster. This recommendation does not differ for patients who have undergone transplantation; because the Tdap is not a live vaccine, administration to immunocompromised patients carries no contraindication.

This patient was immunized for *Streptococcus pneumoniae*, including receiving the pneumococcal conjugate and polysaccharide vaccines, before transplantation as appropriate for immunocompromised patients. Therefore, he does not require a booster of the pneumococcal conjugate vaccine and should receive instead a one-time booster of the pneumococcal polysaccharide vaccine, but not until 5 years after the first administration.

The varicella vaccine is a live-attenuated vaccine. As such, its administration is contraindicated after transplantation. Ideally, it should be given before transplantation, if needed. The zoster vaccine, indicated later in life, is also a live-attenuated vaccine and is contraindicated in immunosuppressed patients.

**KEY POINT**

- All adults, including immunocompromised patients, should receive a one-time booster immunization with the tetanus-diphtheria-acellular pertussis vaccine.

**Bibliography**

Rubin LG, Levin MJ, Ljungman P, et al; Infectious Diseases Society of America. 2013 IDSA clinical practice guideline for vaccination of the immunocompromised host [erratum in Clin Infect Dis. 2014 Jul 1;59(1):144]. Clin Infect Dis. 2014 Feb;58(3):309-18. [PMID: 24421306]

## Item 13          Answer:    B

**Educational Objective: Interpret tuberculin skin test results in a person with recent exposure to tuberculosis.**

This patient should start receiving isoniazid therapy for latent tuberculosis infection (LTBI). He is asymptomatic and has a normal chest radiograph; however, a tuberculin skin test (TST) reaction of 5-mm or larger induration is interpreted as positive in patients who have recently been in contact with a person with active tuberculosis. A TST reaction of 10-mm or larger induration is interpreted as positive in patients who use injection drugs, are recent arrivals from countries with a high prevalence of tuberculosis, or reside in homeless shelters. Treatment for LTBI with isoniazid for 9 months is recommended. Other possible treatment regimens for LTBI include a 12-week regimen of directly observed once-weekly isoniazid and rifapentine. This regimen is not recommended for patients suspected of having infection with isoniazid- or rifampin-resistant tuberculosis strains. Four months of daily rifampin therapy is acceptable for patients with LTBI that is suspected to be resistant to isoniazid or who cannot take isoniazid.

This asymptomatic patient with a normal chest radiograph has LTBI. CT may be helpful in detecting abnormalities in the lung not seen with plain radiographs. However, this patient has no indications of active disease, so CT is not indicated.

Four-drug therapy with isoniazid, rifampin, pyrazinamide, and ethambutol would be recommended as initial therapy for a patient with active tuberculosis. This patient, who has no symptoms or evidence of active infection and a normal chest radiograph, has LTBI. Therefore, four-drug therapy would not be appropriate.

Pursuing no additional evaluation or therapy would not be appropriate for this patient. Treatment of LTBI significantly reduces the risk of progression to active disease.

**KEY POINT**

- Tuberculin skin test results must be accurately interpreted in patients who are asymptomatic and were recently exposed to active tuberculosis so that treatment for latent tuberculosis infection can be initiated.

**Bibliography**

Targeted tuberculin testing and treatment of latent tuberculosis infection. American Thoracic Society. MMWR Recomm Rep. 2000 Jun 9;49(RR-6): 1-51. [PMID: 10881762]

## Item 14          Answer:    D

**Educational Objective: Treat a patient with necrotizing fasciitis with empiric antimicrobial therapy.**

This patient has necrotizing fasciitis and should receive empiric treatment with vancomycin plus piperacillin-tazobactam. Clues to a potential necrotizing skin infection include systemic toxicity (abnormal liver and kidney function, metabolic acidosis) with fever, chills, and hypotension. The patient's pain may be disproportionate to the physical examination findings. Skin changes can evolve rapidly and become ecchymotic, vesiculobullous, and gangrenous in appearance. "Woody" induration is also characteristic. Prompt surgical intervention is indicated as the primary treatment, with concurrent antibiotic therapy. The

CONT.

microbiologic cause can be monomicrobial or polymicrobial. Until the microbiology is determined, empiric therapy should be broad and consist of coverage against mixed aerobic and anaerobic gram-positive and gram-negative organisms, including methicillin-resistant *Staphylococcus aureus* (MRSA). Recommended regimens include vancomycin, linezolid, or daptomycin plus one of the following: piperacillin-tazobactam, a carbapenem (such as imipenem or meropenem), or metronidazole with either ceftriaxone or a fluoroquinolone. Polymicrobial infections are generally seen in patients with gastrointestinal and genitourinary infections, pressure ulcers, or at injection sites in patients using illicit drugs.

Ceftriaxone plus metronidazole alone provides broad-spectrum coverage against many organisms, but lacks MRSA activity. The addition of vancomycin or linezolid to this regimen would be needed until the microbiologic causes of necrotizing fasciitis are determined.

Doxycycline plus ciprofloxacin or ceftriaxone is the recommended regimen for patients with monomicrobial *Aeromonas hydrophila*–associated necrotizing skin infection. Patients who are immunocompromised, including those with liver disease and cancer, are at increased risk for serious skin infections and bacteremia/sepsis with this gram-negative bacillus. Wound infection usually occurs by inoculation through the skin. *A. hydrophila* is found in freshwater environments, but may also be present in brackish water. This regimen would not provide reliable empiric coverage against anaerobic bacteria or MRSA.

If *Streptococcus pyogenes* is confirmed by Gram stain and culture as the cause of necrotizing fasciitis, then penicillin plus clindamycin are recommended, particularly with associated toxic shock syndrome. Clindamycin is included because it inhibits toxin production and remains effective even in the presence of a high inoculum of bacteria. This regimen also would not provide adequate empiric coverage against gram-negative aerobic bacteria.

**KEY POINT**

- Patients with necrotizing fasciitis should receive empiric treatment with broad-spectrum antimicrobials that include coverage of aerobic and anaerobic gram-positive and gram-negative organisms, including methicillin-resistant *Staphylococcus aureus*, until microbiology is determined.

### Bibliography
Stevens DL, Bisno AL, Chambers HF, et al. Practice guidelines for the diagnosis and management of skin and soft tissue infections: 2014 update by the Infectious Diseases Society of America. Clin Infect Dis. 2014 Jul 15; 59(2):147-59. [PMID: 24947530]

 **Item 15      Answer:   A**

**Educational Objective: Evaluate pyelonephritis not responding to appropriate therapy.**

This patient has had a persistent, high fever after 72 hours of appropriate antibiotic therapy; therefore, ultrasonography or contrast-enhanced CT should be performed to exclude an intrarenal or perinephric abscess. Both are acceptable imaging modalities, but CT is considered the gold standard because it offers better anatomic detail. MRI could also be performed to investigate for these complications. Abscess formation is an uncommon complication of urinary tract infection (UTI). The most common predisposing factors for perinephric abscess are diabetes mellitus and the presence of urinary tract calculi. Abscess formation within the kidney usually occurs from infective disruption of the kidney parenchyma secondary to obstruction, frequently by a stone. Perinephric abscesses may result from rupture of an abscess in the corticomedullary region of the kidney through the fascia surrounding the kidney and into the perinephric space. A smaller number of abscesses associated with UTI result from hematogenous spread of bacteria from the highly vascular kidney. Most intrarenal or perinephric abscesses are caused by gram-negative enteric bacilli, whereas gram-positive cocci are generally seen when the abscess occurs secondary to bacteremia. Infection may also be polymicrobial, and fungal organisms such as *Candida* may be causative in some abscesses. Abscess drainage is usually required except for very small collections or those for which the causative factor (such as a kidney stone) may be removed to allow drainage.

This patient is receiving appropriate therapy for pyelonephritis caused by *Escherichia coli*, and the isolate is known to be susceptible to ceftriaxone. Therefore, a change in antibiotic to gentamicin, which has significant toxicity, is not indicated, and changing the antibiotic therapy might delay diagnosis of a complication from her UTI.

Repeating the urine culture is not indicated. A culture was performed on admission and has already revealed the causative organism with susceptibility testing. It is highly unlikely that another pathogen would be identified or a resistant *E. coli* strain would emerge during appropriate and adequate therapy.

Because most patients respond to antibiotic therapy with defervescence within 72 hours, continued observation without any further diagnostic interventions would be inappropriate.

**KEY POINT**

- Patients with pyelonephritis who remain febrile after 72 hours of appropriate antibiotic therapy should undergo kidney ultrasonography, CT, or MRI to investigate for complications, such as perinephric or intrarenal abscess.

### Bibliography
Gardiner RA, Gwynne RA, Roberts SA. Perinephric abscess. BJU Int. 2011 Apr;107(Suppl 3):20-3. [PMID: 21492371]

**Item 16      Answer:   C**

**Educational Objective: Treat nonoccupational exposure to HIV.**

The patient should be treated with postexposure prophylaxis with tenofovir-emtricitabine and raltegravir while awaiting the results of HIV testing. This management of significant HIV exposure is the same whether the exposure was occupational or nonoccupational. Baseline HIV testing is performed as soon as possible after exposure to ensure the exposed person is not already infected. Postexposure prophylaxis must begin immediately, however, without waiting for results. The preferred regimen for postexposure prophylaxis is a three-drug regimen of combination tenofovir-emtricitabine and raltegravir, which has been shown to be effective in reducing acquisition of HIV when used prophylactically.

Although higher levels of viral load are associated with an increased risk for transmission, knowing the partner's recent viral load level would not alter appropriate prophylactic treatment because even an undetectable viral load does not indicate no risk is present. Beginning prophylactic therapy should not be delayed while this information is obtained.

Combination tenofovir-emtricitabine is FDA approved for preexposure prophylaxis in those at significant risk for exposure. However, postexposure prophylaxis should involve a three-drug regimen of these two nucleoside analogues and a third agent, with raltegravir being the preferred agent.

Receptive anal intercourse qualifies as a potential significant HIV exposure and puts the exposed person at risk for infection. Although the likelihood of transmission may be reduced if the person who is the source of the exposure is receiving antiretroviral therapy, as in this patient, it is not lowered to zero. Therefore, awaiting the results of HIV testing without postexposure prophylaxis would be inappropriate.

**KEY POINT**

- Patients who have experienced a significant HIV exposure should immediately begin postexposure prophylaxis with a three-drug regimen of tenofovir-emtricitabine and raltegravir.

**Bibliography**

Kuhar DT, Henderson DK, Struble KA, et al; US Public Health Service Working Group. Updated US Public Health Service guidelines for the management of occupational exposures to human immunodeficiency virus and recommendations for postexposure prophylaxis [erratum in Infect Control Hosp Epidemiol. 2013 Nov;34(11):1238]. Infect Control Hosp Epidemiol. 2013 Sep;34(9):875-92. [PMID: 23917901]

**Item 17        Answer:   C**

**Educational Objective: Manage encephalitis.**

This patient has symptoms consistent with encephalitis (obtundation, fever, elevated cerebrospinal fluid [CSF] leukocyte count) and should undergo electroencephalography (EEG). Recent consensus guidelines promote standardized evaluation for encephalitis, which includes lumbar puncture, brain MRI, and EEG. EEG is indicated to confirm the diagnosis of encephalitis, provide information that may help identify a causative organism, and assess the need for antiepileptic therapy. Nonconvulsive seizures, defined as the pres-

ence of seizure activity on EEG in the absence of myoclonic movements or other clinical evidence of seizures, could contribute to alterations in consciousness. Nonconvulsive status epilepticus may be focal or generalized and has been reported with viral and autoimmune encephalitides. Nonconvulsive status epilepticus in patients with encephalitis is associated with a delay in initiating antiepileptic therapy and an increased risk for death.

Cerebral edema is a poor prognostic factor in encephalitis, and patients with evidence of increased intracranial pressure based on neuroimaging or increased opening pressure are best managed in an intensive care setting. The opening CSF pressure for this patient is within normal limits, indicating the absence of cerebral edema or increased intracranial swelling. Therefore, intracranial pressure monitoring or initiating mannitol, which is used to decrease intracranial edema, is not necessary.

Transcranial Doppler ultrasonography is useful for monitoring patients at risk for vasospasm after subarachnoid hemorrhage. It has not been found to be beneficial in the management of patients with encephalitis and would not be indicated in this patient.

**KEY POINT**

- Standardized evaluation for encephalitis includes lumbar puncture, brain MRI, and electroencephalography.

**Bibliography**

Venkatesan A, Tunkel AR, Bloch KC, et al; International Encephalitis Consortium. Case definitions, diagnostic algorithms, and priorities in encephalitis: consensus statement of the international encephalitis consortium. Clin Infect Dis. 2013 Oct;57(8):1114-28. [PMID: 23861361]

**Item 18        Answer:   C**

**Educational Objective: Diagnose late complement component deficiency.**

This patient most likely has a late complement component deficiency. He has a history of meningococcal meningitis, and the current episode suggests recurrent meningococcal meningitis with bacteremia. Patients with late (terminal) complement component deficiencies (C5, C6, C7, C8, C9) may present with recurrent, invasive meningococcal or gonococcal infections. Complement deficiency can be acquired or inherited. The likelihood of complement deficiency is increased to greater than 30% among persons who have had more than one episode of meningococcal infection or who have a family history of meningococcal infection; for those with inherited late complement component deficiencies, the mode of inheritance is autosomal codominant. C5 deficiency confers impaired chemotaxis and absent serum bactericidal activity. C6, C7, and C8 deficiencies result in absent serum bactericidal activity, and C9 deficiency results in impaired serum bactericidal activity. The susceptibility to systemic neisserial infections, especially meningococcal disease, is greatest for those deficient in C5,

C6, C7, or C8 compared with those deficient of C9. Meningococcal disease is the most common infection in those with complement deficiency. Up to 60% of those with a deficiency of a late complement component or of the circulating complement-potentiating protein properdin will experience at least one episode of infection during their lifetime. Meningococcal disease in patients with complement deficiencies also tends to be caused by uncommon serogroups, especially groups Y, W-135, and X relative to nondeficient patients with meningococcal meningitis. Recurrent meningococcal disease occurs in approximately 45% of those deficient in C5, C6, C7, or C8.

Common variable immunodeficiency (CVID) involves B- and T-cell abnormalities, and the usual manifestation is hypogammaglobulinemia. Bacterial infections, often of the sinus tract and lungs, are common, and the immune dysregulation seen in CVID is associated with autoimmunity and malignant disease. However, CVID is not associated with recurrent meningococcal infection.

Selective IgA deficiency is a common B-cell immunodeficiency. Most patients are asymptomatic or have sinopulmonary infections or gastrointestinal involvement with inflammatory bowel disease, sprue-like illness, or celiac disease. Giardiasis may also be seen. It is not associated with recurrent meningococcal infection.

Classical complement pathway (C1, C4, C2) deficiencies are often associated with a rheumatologic disorder, such as systemic lupus erythematosus, vasculitis, dermatomyositis, or scleroderma. Frequency of infection is relatively low in those with C1, C4, or C2 deficiency compared with deficiencies of other complement components. When they do occur, common infections are caused by encapsulated bacteria, especially *Streptococcus pneumoniae*.

**KEY POINT**

- Patients with late complement component deficiencies may present with recurrent, invasive meningococcal or gonococcal infections.

**Bibliography**
Tichaczek-Goska D. Deficiencies and excessive human complement system activation in disorders of multifarious etiology. Adv Clin Exp Med. 2012 Jan-Feb;21(1):105-14. [PMID: 23214307]

**Item 19**     **Answer:**   **B**

**Educational Objective: Treat a patient with a brain abscess resulting from dental sepsis with intravenous penicillin and metronidazole.**

This patient should begin empiric antibiotic treatment with intravenous penicillin and metronidazole. She has severe, unremitting headache and focal neurologic findings, both indicating a presumed brain abscess with an odontogenic source. Abscesses resulting from dental sepsis are usually caused by mixed *Fusobacterium*, *Prevotella*, and *Bacteroides* species and by streptococci. Penicillin covers most mouth flora, including both aerobic and anaerobic streptococci, and metronidazole provides additional anaerobic coverage with excellent tissue penetration.

Meropenem would be an appropriate antibiotic choice if there was concern about *Pseudomonas aeruginosa* infection, which would be more common in a brain abscess involving neurosurgical procedures. However, *P. aeruginosa* is not a typical source of brain abscess resulting from an odontogenic focus.

Trimethoprim-sulfamethoxazole and vancomycin would provide inadequate coverage against the pathogens typically found in brain abscesses with an odontogenic source. Intravenous vancomycin and a third-generation cephalosporin would be most appropriate for management of brain abscess related to neurosurgery or trauma. This patient's brain abscess is from an odontogenic source, so treatment with penicillin and metronidazole is most appropriate.

**KEY POINT**

- Patients suspected of having brain abscess from a likely odontogenic source should begin empiric antibiotic therapy with intravenous penicillin and metronidazole.

**Bibliography**
Helweg-Larsen J, Astradsson A, Richhall H, Erdal J, Laursen A, Brennum J. Pyogenic brain abscess, a 15 year survey. BMC Infect Dis. 2012 Nov 30;12:332. [PMID: 23193986]

**Item 20**     **Answer:**   **B**

**Educational Objective: Manage potential bioterrorism-related anthrax exposure.**

This patient likely has been exposed to anthrax and should be treated with ciprofloxacin. Although this woman's cutaneous lesion may be a methicillin-resistant *Staphylococcus aureus* furuncle resulting from contact with her infected husband, the distinctive "coal-like" black eschar, together with similar lesions on two coworkers, requires that anthrax be considered in the differential diagnosis. Oral monotherapy with ciprofloxacin, levofloxacin, moxifloxacin, or doxycycline is recommended as treatment of uncomplicated cutaneous anthrax. Uncomplicated cutaneous anthrax is defined as the absence of systemic symptoms and involvement of the head or neck in the absence of extensive swelling. Moreover, suspicion of any bioterrorism event must immediately be reported to local health authorities.

The addition of one or two preferably bactericidal antibiotic agents is indicated for treating anthrax when systemic disease is clinically suspected or confirmed. Because this patient does not have systemic disease, doxycycline, imipenem, and rifampin are not necessary.

Trimethoprim-sulfamethoxazole (TMP-SMX) is an appropriate antibiotic for treating most methicillin-resistant *S. aureus* soft tissue infections, but TMP-SMX is not adequate treatment for anthrax because it has unreliable activity.

In cases of suspected bioterrorism, deferring treatment until culture and biopsy results are available could have serious adverse consequences. Untreated cutaneous anthrax is associated with an estimated mortality rate of 10% to 20% because of secondary bacteremic spread. Treatment should be initiated as soon as the diagnosis is suspected.

---

**KEY POINT**

- Uncomplicated cutaneous anthrax should be treated with ciprofloxacin, levofloxacin, moxifloxacin, or doxycycline and should be reported to local health authorities.

---

**Bibliography**

Hendricks KA, Wright ME, Shadomy SV, et al; Workgroup on Anthrax Clinical Guidelines. Centers for disease control and prevention expert panel meetings on prevention and treatment of anthrax in adults. Emerg Infec Dis. 2014 Feb;20(2). [PMID: 24447897]

## Item 21    Answer:    A

**Educational Objective: Treat asymptomatic bacteriuria in a pregnant woman.**

This patient is pregnant and has asymptomatic bacteriuria caused by *Escherichia coli* susceptible to multiple antibiotics, so she should begin a course of amoxicillin. Asymptomatic bacteriuria during pregnancy increases the risk of pyelonephritis and has been associated with preterm birth and low-birthweight infants. Therefore, pregnancy is one of the few indications for screening for bacteriuria in asymptomatic patients and should occur in the first and third trimesters. Bacteriuria is defined as bacterial counts of $10^5$ or greater colony-forming units/mL on urine culture; the prevalence of asymptomatic bacteriuria in pregnancy is approximately 4% to 7%. Risk factors for bacteriuria during pregnancy include lower socioeconomic status, increased parity, older age, increased sexual activity, diabetes mellitus, sickle cell trait, and history of urinary tract infection. In patients with untreated bacteriuria early in pregnancy, approximately 20% to 40% will develop acute symptomatic pyelonephritis later in pregnancy. Antibiotic therapy should be culture guided using an antibiotic with a known safety profile in pregnancy, such as amoxicillin. Amoxicillin-clavulanate and cephalexin are also effective and safe for many cases of asymptomatic bacteriuria. Urine cultures should be obtained 1 to 2 weeks after completing therapy and monthly for the remainder of the pregnancy.

Nitrofurantoin is an effective agent for uncomplicated cystitis but is contraindicated in the third trimester of pregnancy.

Trimethoprim-sulfamethoxazole is also an effective agent for uncomplicated cystitis when the rate of resistance of *E. coli* in the community is less than 20%. However, trimethoprim-sulfamethoxazole should not be used in pregnant patients near term because it may cause hyperbilirubinemia and kernicterus in the newborn.

No treatment is necessary for asymptomatic bacteriuria except during pregnancy or if a patient is scheduled to undergo an invasive urologic procedure, which is the only other indication for screening asymptomatic persons. Because this patient is pregnant, treatment for identified bacteruria is indicated.

---

**KEY POINT**

- Asymptomatic bacteriuria should be treated in patients who are pregnant, and amoxicillin is safe to use in the third trimester of pregnancy.

---

**Bibliography**

Nicolle LE. Asymptomatic bacteriuria. Curr Opin Infect Dis. 2014 Feb;27(1). [PMID: 24275697]

## Item 22    Answer:    D

**Educational Objective: Manage a false-positive HIV test result.**

No further testing is needed for this patient, who does not have HIV infection. The fourth-generation antigen/antibody combination assay, which evaluates for the presence of HIV antibodies and the p24 viral nucleic acid protein, is recommended for initial HIV testing. This patient's initial testing was reactive, so further testing was indicated. The preferred follow-up testing for a positive result on an antigen/antibody combination assay includes an HIV-1/HIV-2 antibody differentiation assay and HIV nucleic acid amplification testing (NAAT) if the antibody differentiation assay finding is indeterminate or negative. HIV-1/HIV-2 antibody differentiation assay can identify the presence of HIV-1 or HIV-2 antibodies in the serum; HIV NAAT can detect viral RNA and is used to rule out the antibody-negative "window period" of acute HIV infection. Despite her initial positive test results, both follow-up test results were negative, and the appropriate interpretation is that her initial positive result on the screening test was a false positive. Although the recommended initial screening test has a reported specificity of 99.6%, in persons at low risk with very low pretest probability, the rate of false-positive results may still be significant. If the patient is at low risk and has no symptoms to suggest acute HIV infection, she should be reassured that the initial test result was a false positive (on the basis of her negative follow-up testing) and she does not have HIV.

T-cell subsets should never be used in diagnostic testing for HIV infection because a reduced CD4 cell count is neither sensitive nor specific for HIV infection.

Western blot testing for HIV antibody is no longer recommended for confirmatory testing of immunoassay results because of a higher risk for false-negative or indeterminate results early in the course of HIV infection.

Repeating HIV screening testing is unnecessary because the antibody differentiation immunoassay and NAAT have already clarified that the result of the initial combination assay was falsely positive. Repeating this study is therefore not indicated.

**KEY POINT**

- A reactive HIV-1/2 antigen/antibody combination immunoassay followed by negative result on confirmatory testing indicates that the initial combination assay result was a false positive.

**Bibliography**

Branson BM, Owen SM, Wesolowski LG, et al; Centers for Disease Control and Prevention; Association of Public Health Laboratories. Laboratory testing for the diagnosis of HIV infection: updated recommendations. http://stacks.cdc.gov/view/cdc/23447. Published June 27, 2014. Accessed July 21, 2015.

## Item 23     Answer:    C

**Educational Objective: Treat a nonimmune immunocompromised adult exposed to varicella infection.**

This patient should be given varicella-zoster immune globulin. Varicella-zoster is transmitted through infected respiratory secretions and, much less frequently, after direct contact with virus-containing cutaneous vesicular fluids. Persons with active varicella infection can shed virus beginning a few days before developing the typical rash. Susceptible household contacts are at greatest risk for contracting disease, which is estimated to occur at a rate of 90%. Historically, varicella is a childhood exanthem illness with limited morbidity and mortality providing life-long immunity thereafter, but infection in adults, pregnant women, and immunocompromised persons can result in more severe disease, at times resulting in death.

Following a known exposure to a person with varicella, the recommended postexposure prophylaxis to prevent varicella infection in nonimmune patients should be based on the type of exposure, susceptibility assessment, and risk factors for development of serious disease. When clinically warranted, postexposure preventive measures include active immunization or passive immunoprophylaxis. When administered within 3 to 5 days of exposure, the varicella vaccine has proved beneficial in preventing infection and diminishing disease severity in susceptible persons when infection occurs. However, this is a live-attenuated vaccine and is contraindicated in patients who are immunocompromised or taking immunosuppressive therapies, as well as in pregnant women. Under such circumstances, passive immunoprophylaxis using a purified human varicella-zoster immune globulin containing high levels of varicella-specific IgG antibodies is recommended and has been found to be most effective when administered within 4 days of exposure.

The efficacy of antiviral agents, such as acyclovir, to prevent postexposure development of varicella has not been proved and is not recommended.

Observation without providing postexposure prophylaxis may result in serious consequences in specific patient populations, including this patient, who is taking an immunosuppressive medication.

**KEY POINT**

- In patients with contraindication to vaccination, passive immunoprophylaxis with varicella-zoster immune globulin is the postexposure prevention of choice for varicella infection.

**Bibliography**

Gershon AA, Gershon MD. Pathogenesis and current approaches to control of varicella-zoster virus infections. Clin Microbiol Rev. 2013;26(4):728-43. [PMID: 24092852]

## Item 24     Answer:    B

**Educational Objective: Diagnose a superficial incisional surgical site infection.**

This patient should undergo Gram stain and culture of the fluid drainage from the incision site. Most surgical site infections (SSIs) occur within 30 days of the surgical procedure, except in procedures involving an implant, which may present up to a year after the operation. SSIs are categorized as superficial incisional, deep incisional, and organ/deep space infections. They are differentiated on the basis of presenting clinical signs and symptoms as well as the implicated organism (for example, some organisms cause minimal to no drainage). A superficial incisional infection involves only the skin and subcutaneous tissues, whereas a deep incisional infection involves the underlying soft tissue. Signs and symptoms of a superficial incisional infection include inflammatory changes at the incision site, with or without purulent drainage, and generally without systemic signs of infection such as fever, as seen in this patient. In such situations, the infection is usually managed with antibiotics alone and does not require debridement. Although the organisms obtained from a drainage culture may only reflect skin flora, the culture and Gram stain are helpful for identifying possible antibiotic-resistant organisms not covered by empiric therapy. Deep incisional SSIs generally present with more systemic signs of infection (fever, leukocytosis), and management requires debridement and antibiotic therapy guided by results of deep tissue cultures.

A patient with a superficial incisional SSI would not be expected to be bacteremic, so a blood culture would not be helpful in guiding management. Obtaining blood cultures should be guided by the clinical presentation and may be useful in some patients with organ/deep space SSIs.

Surgical site imaging with ultrasonography or CT may be helpful in patients with suspected organ/deep space SSIs to localize the site of infection, identify any fluid collections, and help to plan a drainage procedure. However, imaging would not be helpful in this patient who has a superficial SSI.

- Patients with superficial incisional surgical site infection typically have inflammatory changes at the incision site, with or without purulent drainage, and generally without systemic signs of infection such as fever.

**Bibliography**

Stevens DL, Bisno AL, Chambers HF, et al. Practice guidelines for the diagnosis and management of skin and soft tissue infections: 2014 update by the Infectious Diseases Society of America [erratum in Clin Infect Dis 2014; 59:147-59]. Clin Infect Dis. 2014;59:e10-52. [PMID: 24973422]

## Item 25     Answer:     A

**Educational Objective: Treat a patient with bacterial meningitis with the appropriate empiric antimicrobial regimen.**

This patient should begin treatment with intravenous ampicillin, ceftriaxone, and vancomycin. She has bacterial meningitis, and although the definitive cause has not been determined, empiric treatment should be initiated to cover the most likely infecting organisms. The most common causes of bacterial meningitis are *Streptococcus pneumoniae* and *Neisseria meningitides*, which account for more than 80% of cases. Therefore, primary empiric antibiotic therapy must adequately cover these two organisms. Common empiric regimens include the third-generation cephalosporins ceftriaxone or cefotaxime, which are bactericidal β-lactams that penetrate the central nervous system (CNS) well with excellent coverage of these organisms. One of these agents is combined with vancomycin, which also penetrates the CNS adequately when it is inflamed and provides coverage of possible penicillin-resistant organisms until specific identification and sensitivities are known. Additional antibiotic coverage is needed in patients with risk factors for specific infections. Although *Listeria monocytogenes* makes up only a small percentage (<5%) of meningitis cases in immunocompetent persons, the incidence increases significantly with age. Therefore, in patients older than 50 years, such as this patient, or persons with impaired cell-mediated immunity, ampicillin is added to empiric therapy because *Listeria* is not adequately covered by the usual components of empiric antibiotic regimens. Therefore, in this patient, the combination of ampicillin, ceftriaxone, and vancomycin provides the most appropriate empiric coverage of the suspected pathogens while culture results are pending.

Ceftazidime and vancomycin without ampicillin would be inadequate for this patient because it lacks coverage for *Listeria*.

Meropenem is used primarily in patients with impaired cell-mediated immunity or nosocomial or neurosurgery-related meningitis in which more extensive coverage of gram-negative organisms, including *Pseudomonas aeruginosa*, is indicated.

Fluoroquinolones, such as moxifloxacin, have not been well studied for treatment of bacterial meningitis, and their use is typically limited to patients who cannot tolerate typical empiric therapies, such as those with a severe allergic response to β-lactam antibiotics.

- Empiric antibiotic therapy for bacterial meningitis in the older adult should include ampicillin, ceftriaxone, and vancomycin.

**Bibliography**

van de Beek D, Brouwer MC, Thwaites GE, Tunkel AR. Advances in treatment of bacterial meningitis. Lancet. 2012 Nov 10;380(9854):1693-702. [PMID: 23141618]

## Item 26     Answer:     B

**Educational Objective: Treat cervicitis with ceftriaxone and azithromycin.**

This patient most likely has cervicitis and should be treated with ceftriaxone and azithromycin. It is important to differentiate cervicitis from vaginitis because the treatments differ. Cervicitis, characterized by an inflamed and friable cervix, is typically caused by gonorrhea and chlamydia. Vaginitis refers to inflammation of the vagina and is caused by infections such as candidiasis and trichomoniasis or by noninfectious conditions such as atrophic vaginitis or vaginal irritation. Bacterial vaginosis is a syndrome that appears noninflammatory, is characterized by alterations in the microbial composition of the vaginal flora, and may cause vaginal discharge and odor. In this patient with cervicitis, it is appropriate to give empiric therapy to cover *Neisseria gonorrhoeae* and *Chlamydia trachomatis*. The regimen of choice is a single intramuscular dose of ceftriaxone, 250 mg, and a single oral dose of azithromycin, 250 mg. Oral cefixime can be used but only if ceftriaxone is unavailable; cefixime is associated with increasing minimum inhibitory concentrations of *N. gonorrhoeae*.

Cefotetan plus doxycycline is preferred for the treatment of patients with pelvic inflammatory disease who require hospitalization. The absence of cervical motion, uterine, or adnexal tenderness makes ascending genital tract infection unlikely in this patient.

Fluconazole is used to treat *Candida* vaginitis, a disease that would not result in clinical findings of cervicitis. Additionally, fungal organism would be visualized on the potassium hydroxide preparation.

Metronidazole is used to treat bacterial vaginosis and trichomonas. The pH of vaginal secretions would be elevated, clue cells would be visible on the wet mount (rather than numerous leukocytes), and the whiff test would have a positive result in bacterial vaginosis. Trichomonas would result in numerous leukocytes on the wet mount, but motile organisms would also be visible; the clinical findings should include vulvar and vaginal mucosal erythema.

- Cervicitis is characterized by an inflamed, friable cervix and should be treated with ceftriaxone and azithromycin.

**Bibliography**

Wilson JF. In the clinic. Vaginitis and cervicitis. Ann Intern Med. 2009 Sep 1;151(5):ITC3-1–ITC3-15. [PMID: 19721016]

## Item 27          Answer:     D

### Educational Objective: Diagnose West Nile neuroinvasive disease.

This patient, who has a fever and acute flaccid paralysis of a lower extremity after outdoor activity, should be screened for the West Nile virus (WNV) antibody. Transmission is most often from an infected mosquito, and infections often occur during the summer and fall when mosquito populations are largest. Focal motor weakness is a common finding in West Nile neuroinvasive disease (WNND), either combined with meningoencephalitis or as an isolated myelitis. In its most severe form, infection of the anterior horn cells can cause a symmetric or asymmetric flaccid paralysis, analogous to that seen with polio in the prevaccination era. Respiratory failure may occur when diaphragmatic nerves are involved. The diagnosis of WNND can be confirmed through identification of the IgM antibody in the cerebrospinal fluid (CSF). Positivity for serum antibodies suggests infection but is less specific because WNV IgM remains detectable more than 1 year after acute infection. Furthermore, cross-reactivity occurs with other flaviviruses (such as Saint Louis encephalitis virus or Japanese encephalitis virus), which may produce a false-positive antibody result after natural infection or vaccination. WNV polymerase chain reaction of the CSF is of limited diagnostic utility in most patients because when symptoms become apparent, the virus has cleared the bloodstream and spinal fluid.

Eastern equine encephalitis virus infection is also caused by transmission from an infected mosquito. However, it predominantly occurs along the Atlantic and Gulf states, and encephalitic illness is characterized by fever, headache, vomiting, diarrhea, and convulsions.

La Crosse encephalitis virus infection is also transmitted by mosquito but typically occurs in the Eastern and central United States. Motor weakness is not associated with this infection, and symptoms are generally mild.

Powassan virus is spread by ticks rather than mosquitos, and infections are limited to the northeastern and north central United States. Symptoms include fever, headache, weakness, and other neurologic complications.

- Fever, headache, and focal limb weakness following outdoor activities suggest West Nile neuroinvasive disease, and the most appropriate diagnostic test is for West Nile virus antibodies within cerebrospinal fluid.

**Bibliography**

Hart J Jr, Tillman G, Kraut MA, et al; NIAID Collaborative Antiviral Study Group West Nile Virus 210 Protocol Team. West Nile virus neuroinvasive disease: neurological manifestations and prospective longitudinal outcomes. BMC Infect Dis. 2014 May 9;14:248. [PMID: 24884681]

## Item 28          Answer:     C

### Educational Objective: Prevent catheter-associated urinary tract infection.

This patient's indwelling urinary catheter should be removed now. The prevention of catheter-associated urinary tract infection (CAUTI) relies on using urinary catheters only if they are essential to the patient's care and only for as brief a period of time as possible. The risk for a CAUTI increases by 3% to 7% each day a urinary catheter is in place. This translates to a risk for CAUTI of up to 70% when a urinary catheter has been in place for 10 days. Although urinary catheters are useful in select patients when fluid balance must be managed carefully, they should not be used routinely in hospitalized patients, in patients not requiring detailed information about urine output, or for convenience of the patient or staff. Appropriate indications for a urinary catheter include perioperative use for selected surgeries (should be removed before the end of the second postoperative day), need for accurate measurement of urine output in critically ill patients in the ICU, management of acute urinary retention or bladder outlet obstruction, assistance in open sacral or perineal wound healing for patients who are incontinent, and, as an exception, end-of-life patient comfort if needed. Urinary catheters should be inserted by trained personnel following aseptic technique and maintained in a manner that minimizes the chance of contamination or introduction of organisms into the bladder (that is, using a closed drainage system, gravity drainage, and keeping the drainage bag off the floor).

Changing a urinary catheter, whether at the time of hospital admission from the emergency department or routinely (such as every 3 or 5 days), does not decrease the risk for a CAUTI and should not be done for that purpose.

In this patient with chronic kidney disease and decompensated heart failure, monitoring diuretic effect with standard urine collection procedures should be adequate to guide therapeutic decision making. Kidney function remaining above baseline is not an indication for continuing the indwelling urinary catheter. Therefore, continued use of an indwelling catheter has no clear indication.

- Preventing catheter-associated urinary tract infection relies on using urinary catheters only if they are essential to the patient's care and only for as short a period of time as possible.

**Bibliography**

Lo E, Nicolle LE, Coffin SE, et al; Society for Healthcare Epidemiology of America (SHEA). Strategies to Prevent Catheter-Associated Urinary Tract Infections in Acute Care Hospitals: 2014 Update. Infect Control Hosp Epidemiol. 2014;35:32–47. [PMID: 25026611]

**Answers and Critiques**

H **Item 29**     **Answer:**   **D**

**Educational Objective: Manage a central line-associated fungal bloodstream infection.**

Removal of the peripherally inserted central venous catheter and initiation of antifungal therapy is the most appropriate management in this patient. When candidemia is likely to be the result of an intravenous catheter, the catheter must be removed promptly because it serves as a nidus for ongoing candidemia. The duration is shorter and mortality rate is lower for candidemia related to intravenous catheters when the catheter is removed than when it remains in place. Additionally, catheter salvage is extremely difficult with fungal colonization, almost always requiring removal of the catheter. Although removal of long-term catheters may be a management challenge in patients being treated with a prolonged course of antibiotics, such as this patient, alternative short-term access is indicated to continue treatment and allow antifungal therapy to be given.

Empiric antifungal therapy should be based on the most likely organism (such as *Candida albicans*) because candidemia can be prolonged and may lead to metastatic complications (endophthalmitis, endocarditis, osteomyelitis) if not already present at the time of diagnosis. Other considerations in choosing empiric therapy include a history of recent azole exposure, prevalence of different species and susceptibility data in a particular institution, the severity of illness, comorbidities (such as neutropenia), and evidence of disseminated involvement (such as the central nervous system or eyes). Some experts recommend an echinocandin as the preferred agent for all patients with candidemia and not just for those who may have recently received an azole or are moderately to severely ill. Blood cultures should always be repeated until candidemia clearance is documented. Treatment should be given for 2 weeks after symptoms resolve and blood cultures are negative for candidemia or longer if metastatic complications are present.

**KEY POINT**

- In patients with candidemia associated with an intravenous catheter, the catheter should be removed and empiric antifungal therapy initiated.

**Bibliography**
Pappas PG, Kauffman CA, Andes D, et al; Infectious Diseases Society of America. Clinical Practice Guidelines for the Management of Candidiasis: 2009 Update by the Infectious Diseases Society of America. Clin Infect Dis. 2009;48:503-535. [PMID: 19191635]

**Item 30**     **Answer:**   **B**

**Educational Objective: Treat secondary syphilis with benzathine penicillin.**

This man presents with a rash consistent with secondary syphilis and should be treated with benzathine penicillin. The most common clinical manifestation of secondary syphilis is a generalized rash that is typically nonpruritic and often involves the palms and soles. Lesions may be macular, papular, or pustular. Silvery gray erosions with an erythematous border may be visualized on mucosal surfaces (mucus patches). Patients with secondary syphilis frequently have generalized lymphadenopathy and systemic symptoms. A single dose of 2.4 million units given intramuscularly is the treatment of choice, preferably at the time of presentation if follow-up cannot be guaranteed. Syphilis among men who have sex with men, particularly in urban areas, has increased significantly in the past several years, so recognition of the characteristic clinical presentation is essential. Diagnostic testing with syphilis serologic assessment should still be obtained to confirm the diagnosis and provide a baseline titer that can be followed to assess the adequacy of therapy. In addition, the patient should be screened for other sexually transmitted infections including HIV, *Neisseria gonorrhoeae*, and *Chlamydia trachomatis* infections; specimens for *N. gonorrhoeae* and *C. trachomatis* should be obtained from all potentially exposed anatomic sites (throat, urethra, and anus) on the basis of the sexual history obtained.

A single 2-g dose of azithromycin is effective for the management of early syphilis; however, resistance associated with treatment failure has been reported recently. Azithromycin should be used only when treatment with penicillin or doxycycline (the recommended alternative in the setting of penicillin allergy) is not possible.

Ceftriaxone may be used to treat neurosyphilis as an alternative in a patient allergic to penicillin whose reaction is not life threatening, but it is not recommended in any other setting.

Although an allergic reaction may be in the differential diagnosis of a rash, involvement of the palms and soles is uncommon. Empiric treatment with methylprednisolone in a person with a high-risk sexual history is inappropriate.

**KEY POINT**

- A high-risk sexual history and erythematous macules and papules on the palms and soles indicate secondary syphilis, which should be treated with benzathine penicillin.

**Bibliography**
Workowski KA, Berman S; Centers for Disease Control and Prevention (CDC). Sexually transmitted diseases treatment guidelines, 2010 [erratum in MMWR Recomm Rep. 2011 Jan 14;60(1):18]. MMWR Recomm Rep. 2010 Dec 17;59(RR-12):1-110. [PMID: 21160459]

**Item 31**     **Answer:**   **C**   H

**Educational Objective: Diagnose cytomegalovirus infection after transplantation.**

This patient likely has colitis resulting from cytomegalovirus (CMV) infection. CMV infection is a common complication of transplantation, especially in the first few months after transplantation when immunosuppression is typically highest. Unless donor and recipient are CMV seronegative and the risk is low, prophylaxis with valganciclovir is often used during this time period. This patient recently finished the

**CONT.** prophylaxis period and is at risk for CMV reactivation. She has symptoms typical for colitis; the colon and esophagus are common sites for CMV disease after transplantation. Hepatitis, gastritis, and small bowel enteritis may also occur, although less often. Quantitative polymerase chain reaction testing in serum for CMV can be suggestive, but colonoscopy with biopsy for characteristic histopathology and viral tissue culture provide a definitive diagnosis.

Candidal infection does not cause colitis, even in immunocompromised patients. *Candida* species are part of the normal bowel flora, with positive stool cultures commonly occurring in the absence of systemic disease. This patient has no evidence of invasive candidal infection, which makes this an unlikely cause of her presenting symptoms.

Although she is at risk for *Clostridium difficile* colitis, her negative results on nucleic acid testing makes this a less likely cause of her clinical findings than CMV disease.

Although mycophenolate can cause diarrhea as an adverse effect, this patient is at significant risk for opportunistic infections, which must be considered more likely, especially in the presence of fever.

Polyoma BK virus is a DNA virus present in approximately 5% of kidney transplant recipients. Its activity is usually related to the degree of immunosuppression and can occur at this stage or later after transplantation. However, it primarily causes tubulointerstitial nephropathy, not colitis.

**KEY POINT**

- Cytomegalovirus is a common complication of transplantation, especially in the first few months after transplantation when immunosuppression is typically highest, and patients who have just finished prophylaxis against cytomegalovirus are at risk for reactivation.

**Bibliography**
Lemonovich TL, Watkins RR. Update on cytomegalovirus infections of the gastrointestinal system in solid organ transplant recipients. Curr Infect Dis Rep. 2012 Feb;14(1):33-40. [PMID: 22125047]

**Item 32      Answer:   C**
**Educational Objective: Manage osteomyelitis of the foot in a patient with type 2 diabetes mellitus.**

This patient with type 2 diabetes mellitus most likely has osteomyelitis of the foot and should be treated with vancomycin and piperacillin-tazobactam. Surgical debridement is also important to ensure removal of all nonviable and purulent tissue and allows for collecting more representative tissue specimens for microbiologic studies. Infections in the feet of patients with diabetes may come on suddenly, present with sepsis, and rapidly become limb-threatening. Most often these infections result from ulcerations created by prior surgical procedures, trauma, or local pressure. Diminished sensation, decreased blood flow, and poor glycemic control are frequent contributing factors. Empiric broad-spectrum antimicrobial therapy aimed at gram-positive cocci (β-hemolytic streptococci and staphylococci)

along with aerobic and anaerobic gram-negative bacilli should be initiated as soon as possible in patients with suspected osteomyelitis and systemic findings. Methicillin-resistant strains of *Staphylococcus aureus* should be considered potential pathogens in these clinical situations and included in the antimicrobial coverage until proven absent. Vancomycin and a broad-spectrum β-lactam/β-lactamase inhibitor, such as piperacillin-tazobactam, would be an appropriate empiric regimen; it is appropriate to narrow the antibiotic spectrum once bone culture results are known. Surgical debridement is essential in the treatment of this patient's obviously gangrenous foot.

Antimicrobial therapy with the combination of cefazolin and metronidazole has too narrow a spectrum under these clinical circumstances. Coverage against a greater variety of aerobic, gram-negative bacilli is required.

Clindamycin has activity against most of the gram-positive cocci and anaerobic gram-negative bacilli associated with diabetic foot infections. However, gentamicin to provide coverage against aerobic gram-negative bacilli in complex diabetic foot infections is not recommended because of its narrow toxicity-to-benefit ratio.

Grossly visible bone or the ability to probe to bone is highly predictive of osteomyelitis, making the need for a bone biopsy and delay in treatment inadvisable.

**KEY POINT**

- Osteomyelitis of the foot in a patient with a diabetic foot infection with sepsis should be immediately treated with broad-spectrum antibiotics and surgical debridement.

**Bibliography**
Game FL. Osteomyelitis in the diabetic foot: diagnosis and management. Med Clin North Am. 2013 Sep;97(5):947-56. [PMID: 23992902]

**Item 33      Answer:   C**
**Educational Objective: Diagnose dengue fever.**

This patient, who recently travelled to the Caribbean, has symptoms characteristic of dengue fever (DF), a flavivirus transmitted by the *Aedes* mosquito. DF is the most common arthropod-borne viral infection in humans. Endemic areas include Southeast Asia, the South Pacific, South and Central America, and the Caribbean. Most infections encountered in the United States are diagnosed in persons visiting or returning from endemic geographic areas. Recently, the incidence of infection from the Caribbean islands has increased. The hallmarks of DF are sudden high fever, frontal headache and retro-orbital pain, myalgia and arthralgia, severe lower back pain ("break-bone fever"), and a maculopapular rash that often appears as the fever abates. Mild hemorrhagic symptoms and the development of petechiae, elicited by a tourniquet test, can occur. A more severe and rare form of infection (dengue hemorrhagic fever) can be seen in patients previously infected by one of the four dengue virus serotypes who subsequently become infected with another serotype.

**CONT.**

Typical laboratory findings in DF include leukopenia with relative lymphocytosis, hemoconcentration, thrombocytopenia, and elevation of hepatocellular enzymes. Diagnosis confirmation generally relies on specific serologic assays.

Human granulocytic anaplasmosis is one of the forms of ehrlichiosis transmitted by ticks. This febrile illness is accompanied by laboratory abnormalities similar to those seen with DF; however, rash with human granulocytic anaplasmosis is rare. This obligate, intracellular, gram-negative organism can be seen in the cytoplasm of neutrophils in 20% to 80% of infected patients. Although ehrlichiosis can occur worldwide, the *Ixodes* tick vector is infrequently found in the Caribbean. The diagnosis usually is made using serologic assays.

Chikungunya virus is also transmitted by the bite of an *Aedes* mosquito and recently has become an epidemic in several Caribbean islands. Although it shares many clinical features with DF, an important distinction is its severe joint pain and stiffness. Other distinguishing features include high fever, which often recurs after a brief afebrile period ("saddle-back fever"); more significant polyarticular and migratory joint pains involving the small joints of the hands, wrists, and ankles; and much less thrombocytopenia.

Leptospirosis may be confused with DF but typically involves more organ systems, including the pulmonary, renal, hepatic, and central nervous systems. Characteristically, conjunctival suffusion occurs but a generalized rash is rare. Aseptic meningitis is a common feature of the immune or delayed phase of this spirochetal infection. A more severe form of infection, known as icteric leptospirosis (Weil syndrome), presents with profound jaundice, hepatic necrosis, kidney disease, and pulmonary manifestations.

### KEY POINT

- Dengue fever is characterized by sudden high fever, frontal headache and retro-orbital pain, myalgias and arthralgias, severe lower back pain, and rash that appears as the fever abates.

**Bibliography**
Ratnam I, Leder K, Black J, Torresi J. Dengue fever and international travel. J Travel Med. 2013 Nov-Dec:20(6):384–93. [PMID: 24165383]

### Item 34    Answer:    B

**Educational Objective: Evaluate a patient with nonresponsive community-acquired pneumonia using chest CT.**

A chest CT should be obtained in this patient with nonresponsive pneumonia. He presents with severe community-acquired pneumonia (CAP) and has been treated with appropriate empiric antibiotics. Most patients with uncomplicated CAP will show improvement in clinical symptoms (fever, cough, dyspnea) within 2 to 3 days; nonresponsive pneumonia is defined as a lack of significant clinical response within 72 hours of initiating therapy. Chest CT or, possibly, high-resolution chest CT is the usual initial radiographic

study used to evaluate patients with nonresponsive pneumonia. Compared with plain chest radiography, chest CT provides improved detection of parenchymal abnormalities, including foci of infection such as a lung abscess or cavitary lesions and occult empyema. These findings may help guide additional therapy, or CT may identify other causes of failure to improve that were not previously considered, particularly in a patient whose baseline plain radiograph may be difficult to interpret.

Fiberoptic bronchoscopy with bronchoalveolar lavage and transbronchial biopsy may be helpful in the diagnosis of nonresponsive pneumonia but is typically performed after chest CT, particularly if there are findings (focal areas of fluid collection or consolidation or lymphadenopathy) that help guide bronchoscopic evaluation or be amenable to bronchoscopic biopsy.

Chest ultrasonography is used primarily to diagnose pleural effusions and guide therapeutic thoracentesis and may be helpful in diagnosing pleural abnormalities such as thickening or nodules. It is less helpful for evaluating the lung parenchyma. This patient has not had evidence of pleural effusions on chest radiography, so the diagnostic yield of chest ultrasonography would be low, particularly compared with chest CT.

More invasive biopsy procedures such as thoracoscopic or open lung biopsy are typically reserved for instances when a specific disorder requiring direct tissue evaluation is needed or if other diagnostic interventions are unrevealing in a patient requiring a diagnosis. Therefore, lung biopsy would not be an appropriate next step before additional imaging.

### KEY POINT

- Chest CT, which provides improved detection of parenchymal abnormalities, is the usual initial radiographic study used to evaluate patients with nonresponsive pneumonia.

**Bibliography**
Mandell LA, Wunderink RG, Anzueto A, et al; Infectious Diseases Society of America, American Thoracic Society. Infectious Diseases Society of America/American Thoracic Society consensus guidelines on the management of community-acquired pneumonia in adults. Clin Infect Dis. 2007 Mar 1;44(Suppl 2):S27-72. [PMID: 17278083]

### Item 35    Answer:    B

**Educational Objective: Manage vertebral osteomyelitis by determining microbiologic cause for appropriate treatment.**

This patient has vertebral osteomyelitis and should undergo CT-guided needle biopsy and aspirate to determine a microbiologic diagnosis and the most adequate antimicrobial therapy. Single isolates of *Corynebacterium* species are generally regarded as blood culture contaminants and would be uncommon pathogens in this scenario. Furthermore, although the patient was recently treated for a central line–associated bloodstream infection caused by

CONT.

*Staphylococcus aureus*, it cannot be assumed the same organism is infecting the lumbar spine. Treatment of this patient should not be initiated until the infecting microbial agent has been identified. Neck or back pain that persists or increases in severity over weeks to months is the most common symptom associated with infection of the vertebral column or disc space. Bacteremia may result from infective endocarditis, intravenous drug use, intravenous catheters, or foci of infection at distant sites. The lumbar vertebrae are most frequently involved and, if left undiagnosed and untreated, may progress to an epidural abscess with subsequent neurologic deficits.

Spread of infection from the urinary tract through vertebral veins (Batson plexus) is considered unlikely; therefore, empiric antimicrobial treatment with ciprofloxacin aimed at the previous *Proteus* infection is not warranted. Likewise, initiating antimicrobial therapy with vancomycin before attempting to make a microbiologic diagnosis may adversely alter the culture result. However, it would be an appropriate choice if *S. aureus* was determined to be the causative pathogen considering the patient's allergy to penicillin. Empiric therapy is indicated in patients who are unable or unwilling to undergo an invasive diagnostic procedure.

The blood culture did not demonstrate persistent bacteremia, and no signs or symptoms were consistent with infective endocarditis. Therefore, performing echocardiography is unnecessary.

Three-phase nuclear bone scanning has a high sensitivity for diagnosing osteomyelitis but lacks the specificity provided by MRI, which this patient has already undergone. Additional imaging would add no relevant information in this patient.

**KEY POINT**

- When blood cultures are negative, the microbiologic cause of vertebral osteomyelitis should be determined by CT-guided needle aspiration biopsy to determine the most appropriate antimicrobial therapy.

**Bibliography**
Weissman S, Parker RD, Siddiqui W, Dykema S, Horvath J. Vertebral osteomyelitis: retrospective review of 11 years of experience. Scand J Infect Dis. 2014 Mar;46(3):193-9. [PMID: 24450841]

**Item 36          Answer:     D**

**Educational Objective: Manage immunizations in a patient with HIV infection.**

This patient should receive the 13-valent pneumococcal conjugate vaccine (PCV13) now. Vaccination against *Streptococcus pneumoniae* is indicated in all persons with HIV infection because of the increased risk of invasive pneumococcal disease. Immunocompromised persons, including those with HIV, should receive PCV13 first, followed by the 23-valent pneumococcal polysaccharide vaccine (PPSV23) at least 8 weeks later, in a "prime-boost" strategy that is used to improve the antibody response to immunization. This recommendation applies regardless of the patient's CD4 cell count.

HIV infection alone is not an indication to receive hepatitis A vaccination. Hepatitis A vaccination would be indicated if the patient had another risk factor, such as men who have sex with men or other liver disease, including chronic hepatitis B or C virus infection. She does not have hepatitis B or C virus infection, as shown by negative results on laboratory testing, so hepatitis A vaccination is unnecessary at this time.

All patients with HIV should be vaccinated for hepatitis B if not already immune or infected. However, this patient has positivity for hepatitis B surface antibody, demonstrating existing immunity. Therefore, she does not require hepatitis B immunization.

This patient is beyond the recommended age (approximately 11-26 years) for females in the general population to receive human papillomavirus vaccination. This recommendation does not change for patients with HIV infection.

This patient should receive PPSV23, but not until at least 8 weeks after PCV13, so giving it now would be inappropriate. Patients with HIV infection who have received PPSV23 in the past should receive PCV13 followed by another PPSV23 dose at least 8 weeks later.

**KEY POINT**

- Immunocompromised persons, including those with HIV, should receive the 13-valent pneumococcal conjugate vaccine first, followed 8 weeks later by the 23-valent pneumococcal polysaccharide vaccine.

**Bibliography**
Bridges CB, Coyne-Beasley T, Advisory Committee on Immunization Practices. Advisory Committee on Immunization Practices (ACIP) recommended immunization schedules for adults aged 19 years or older: United States, 2014. Ann Intern Med. 2014;160:190. [PMID: 24658695]

**Item 37          Answer:     B**

**Educational Objective: Prevent spread of infection of disseminated varicella-zoster virus.**

This patient should be placed on airborne and contact precautions. Varicella-zoster virus can be transmitted from persons with zoster to susceptible hosts (that is, those who have never had chickenpox and are not vaccinated against it) who may develop chickenpox as a result of the exposure. The virus can spread through direct contact with active lesions, which is most common with localized zoster. Localized zoster is defined as rash in one or two dermatomes, most commonly along a thoracic dermatome, that does not cross the midline. Patients with localized zoster who are not immunocompromised can be managed with contact precautions alone; a person is no longer infectious after all the lesions have crusted over. Disseminated zoster is defined as a more widespread rash involving three or more dermatomes. Disseminated zoster can appear similar to varicella (chickenpox). Vesicles usually appear in various stages of development and generally form over 3 to 5 days before they start to dry and crust over. Immunocompromised persons

**CONT.**

(such as this patient) are at increased risk for disseminated zoster, which may involve the respiratory tract. In patients with disseminated zoster or those who are immunocompromised, the virus may be transmitted via the airborne route from infected small (≤5 μm) respiratory droplet nuclei that can remain suspended for extended periods or travel long distances on air currents. Airborne (negative-pressure room) and contact precautions are appropriate management for patients who have disseminated zoster or localized zoster and are immunocompromised. Other organisms transmitted via the airborne route include those causing tuberculosis, measles, and chickenpox.

Droplet precautions are applied for organisms that are transmitted via large (>5 μm) droplets that travel less than 3 feet on air currents (such as respiratory, pertussis, and mumps viruses).

**KEY POINT**

- Airborne and contact precautions are indicated to prevent spread of infection in patients with disseminated zoster infection or those who are immunocompromised with localized zoster infection.

**Bibliography**

Siegel JD, Rhinehart E, Jackson M, Chiarello L, Healthcare Infection Control Practices Advisory Committee. 2007 Guideline for Isolation Precautions: Preventing Transmission of Infectious Agents in Healthcare Settings. www.cdc.gov/hicpac/2007IP/2007isolationPrecautions.html. Updated December 9, 2010. Accessed July 20, 2015.

## Item 38    Answer:    D

**Educational Objective: Manage mild travelers' diarrhea.**

Fluid replacement with aggressive oral hydration without further treatment is the most appropriate treatment recommendation for this patient with mild travelers' diarrhea. Travelers' diarrhea is defined as the occurrence of three or more unformed stools per day with abdominal pain or cramps, nausea or vomiting, bloody stools, or fever and is the most common travel-related infection. Depending on the geographic region, the incidence of gastrointestinal infection may occur in greater than 30% of travelers. Africa, Asia, South and Central America, and Mexico are considered the regions with the greatest risk. The diarrhea is usually self-limited, lasting 1 to 4 days. Enterotoxigenic and enteroaggregative *Escherichia coli* are the most common bacterial pathogens. Less often, *Salmonella, Shigella, Campylobacter, Aeromonas, Plesiomonas,* and noncholera *Vibrio* species are involved. With the exception of rotavirus and norovirus, travelers' diarrhea caused by viral infections is uncommon; norovirus has been associated with diarrheal disease outbreaks aboard cruise ships. Protozoan pathogens are isolated in less than 10% of cases. However, no definitive microbiologic agent is identified in approximately one third of patients. The use of prophylactic antibiotics is effective in reducing the risk for travelers' diarrhea, but, to avoid potential adverse effects, is generally reserved for patients with a

history of inflammatory bowel disease, immunosuppressive illnesses, or chronic diseases that could become more severe or be exacerbated by dehydration brought on with significant diarrhea.

Antibiotics lessen the duration of diarrhea by a few days, but their use is generally limited to patients with more severe disease, usually defined as more than four unformed stools per day with fever and blood, pus, or mucus in the stool. Antibiotic treatment may also be a reasonable option in patients with milder illness if it is markedly disruptive to travel plans.

Antimotility agents, such as loperamide, may relieve symptoms in patients with travelers' diarrhea. However, they do not treat the underlying infection. Concern exists that using antimotility agents alone may prolong dysenteric illnesses without treatment of the underlying infection. For this reason, antimotility agents are generally not recommended without concurrent use of antibiotics for treatment of travelers' diarrhea.

**KEY POINT**

- Fluid replacement with aggressive oral hydration without further treatment is the most appropriate treatment recommendation for otherwise healthy persons with mild travelers' diarrhea.

**Bibliography**

Steffen R, Hill DR, DuPont HL. Traveler's diarrhea: a clinical review. JAMA. 2015;313:71-80. [PMID: 25562268]

## Item 39    Answer:    B

**Educational Objective: Identify criteria for establishing that a patient with tuberculosis is noncontagious.**

The Centers for Disease Control and Prevention has established three criteria that must be met to establish that a patient with tuberculosis is noncontagious: adequate treatment for tuberculosis for at least 2 weeks, improvement of symptoms, and three consecutive negative sputum smears (collected at 8- to 24-hour intervals, including one early morning collection). This patient has met two of these criteria but must complete at least 2 weeks of treatment with rifampin, isoniazid, pyrazinamide, and ethambutol before he is considered noncontagious.

Factors associated with the contagiousness of a patient infected with tuberculosis include presence of a lung cavity, cough, or acid-fast bacilli on sputum smear; receiving inadequate treatment; pulmonary or laryngeal tuberculosis; coughing without covering the mouth; and sputum culture positivity. The absence of a cavity does decrease the contagiousness of a patient but is not a criterion for establishing that a patient is noncontagious.

A positive result on a tuberculin skin test (TST) indicates that a patient has been infected with *Mycobacterium tuberculosis*. A negative TST result makes it unlikely that the patient has been infected. However, false-negative results

**CONT.**

do occur. Physiologic causes of false-negative TST results include active tuberculosis infection, HIV infection, use of immunosuppressive agents (such as glucocorticoids), kidney injury, lymphoproliferative disorders, and recent vaccination with live virus. Therefore, the lack of a positive result does not correlate with contagiousness.

The leukocyte count may be normal, decreased, or increased in patients with active tuberculosis. It is not used as a criterion for determining whether a patient is contagious.

**KEY POINT**

- A patient with active tuberculosis must undergo adequate tuberculosis treatment for at least 2 weeks, demonstrate improvement of symptoms, and have three consecutive negative sputum smears to be considered noncontagious.

**Bibliography**

Centers for Disease Control and Prevention (CDC), National Center for HIV/AIDS, Viral Hepatitis, STD, and TB Prevention. Prevention and control of tuberculosis in correctional and detention facilities: recommendations from CDC. Endorsed by the Advisory Council for the Elimination of Tuberculosis, the National Commission on Correctional Health Care, and the American Correctional Association. MMWR Recomm Rep. 2006 Jul 7;55 (RR-9):1-44. [PMID: 16826161]

**Item 40      Answer:    D**

**Educational Objective: Treat candidemia in a postsurgical patient.**

This patient should be treated with micafungin. He most likely has candidemia. His risk factors include recent major abdominal surgery, the presence of an intravascular catheter, and exposure to antibiotics. Echinocandins (caspofungin, anidulafungin, and micafungin) are considered the therapy of choice for candidemia and most other forms of invasive candidiasis. All three agents are considered to be equally effective, are well tolerated, and have good safety profiles. Kidney disease does not necessitate dose adjustment, and the potential for drug interactions is low. Transition to fluconazole can occur after 5 to 7 days of therapy with an echinocandin if the patient is clinically stable, the isolate is susceptible to fluconazole, and repeat blood cultures are negative.

Amphotericin B deoxycholate would be an effective therapy but has an adverse effect profile that includes kidney injury and other systemic reactions that preclude it as a good treatment option, especially considering the availability of therapies that are equally effective and have better adverse effect profiles.

Although for many years fluconazole was considered the drug of choice for treating candidemia, recent studies show lesser efficacy compared with the echinocandins, even in treating *Candida albicans*. Additionally, the spectrum of fluconazole is limited compared with the echinocandins or amphotericin B–based compounds because it is inactive against *Candida krusei*, and resistance has been reported for *Candida glabrata*.

Liposomal amphotericin B has similar efficacy to the echinocandins but has a higher rate of nephrotoxicity. Because this patient already has kidney disease, liposomal amphotericin B would not be recommended.

**KEY POINT**

- In a patient with candidemia, echinocandins such as caspofungin, anidulafungin, and micafungin are the empiric therapy of choice.

**Bibliography**

Cornely OA, Bassetti M, Calandra T, et al; ESCMID Fungal Infection Study Group. ESCMID guideline for the diagnosis and management of Candida diseases 2012: non-neutropenic adult patients. Clin Microbiol Infect. 2012 Dec;18(Suppl 7):19-37. [PMID: 23137135]

**Item 41      Answer:    D**

**Educational Objective: Diagnose acute progressive disseminated histoplasmosis.**

This patient's clinical illness and laboratory findings are most consistent with acute progressive disseminated histoplasmosis. *Histoplasma* is the most common endemic mycosis in the United States (primarily in the Ohio and Mississippi river valleys) and is also prevalent in Central America. The causative agent, *Histoplasma capsulatum*, is typically found in soil contaminated with bird or bat droppings, which encourage spore formation. Infection is usually through inhalation of spores and, in immunocompetent patients, may be asymptomatic or cause mild, self-limited pulmonary symptoms. However, in patients who are severely immunosuppressed, especially those with AIDS or hematologic malignancies, disseminated histoplasmosis may occur. In persons with HIV infection, the risk factors for histoplasmosis are a CD4 cell count less 200/µL and a history of exposure. Clinical manifestations are nonspecific. Fever and weight loss are common. The most common findings on physical examination include hepatosplenomegaly and lymphadenopathy. Common laboratory abnormalities include anemia, thrombocytopenia and leukopenia, and elevated serum aminotransferases and alkaline phosphatase. Chest radiographs may be normal or show scattered nodular densities or a diffuse reticular pattern. Diagnosis is by detection of histoplasma antigen in body fluids, which is present in up to 90% of patients with acute progressive disseminated histoplasmosis, or by isolation of *H. capsulatum* from bodily fluids or tissues. Bone marrow and blood cultures may also be useful in establishing the diagnosis (blood smear shown top of next page). Therapy is typically with liposomal amphotericin B with long-term suppressive therapy following short-term treatment.

Disseminated blastomycosis most commonly manifests as skin lesions, which this patient does not have. Other sites of disseminated disease include bones, joints, and the male genitourinary tract. Blastomycosis has been reported as a late complication in patients with AIDS, in whom central nervous system complications of blastomycosis are common

Answers and Critiques

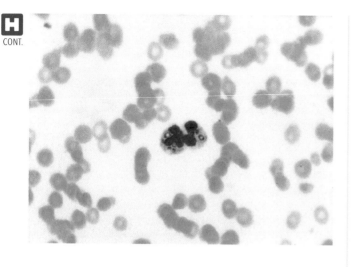

CONT.

and manifest as abscess or meningitis. The yeast forms of *Blastomyces dermatitidis* have a distinct appearance with broad-based budding.

Although mucosal candidiasis is common in advanced HIV infection, candidemia and disseminated candidiasis are rare.

Disseminated coccidioidomycosis most commonly presents with skin lesions, which this patient does not have. Other common sites of dissemination include bones, joints, and the meninges. Spherules (large, round, thick-walled structures containing endospores), noted by cytologic or histopathologic evaluation, are the classic finding.

### KEY POINT

- Acute progressive disseminated histoplasmosis is most often seen in patients who are severely immunosuppressed, especially those with AIDS or hematologic malignancies, and common signs and symptoms include fever, weight loss, and hepatosplenomegaly.

### Bibliography

Knox KS, Hage CA. Histoplasmosis. Proc Am Thorac Soc. 2010 May;7(3): 169-72. [PMID: 20463244]

## Item 42      Answer:    C

**Educational Objective: Manage conversion from an intravenous to an oral antimicrobial agent.**

Sequential antimicrobial therapy, also known as intravenous to oral antimicrobial switching, should be considered in patients who have an intact and functioning gastrointestinal tract and whose clinical status is improving. This patient meets criteria for changing from intravenous ceftriaxone to an oral antimicrobial agent to complete the course of treatment for *Escherichia coli* pyelonephritis. When making a parenteral-to-oral antimicrobial switch, the bioavailability of the oral antimicrobial option is important and depends on the infection being treated. In patients with bacteremia, an agent with excellent bioavailability should be used (quino-

lones, trimethoprim-sulfamethoxazole, metronidazole, clindamycin, linezolid). Trimethoprim-sulfamethoxazole has excellent bioavailability, so it is the oral antimicrobial agent of choice.

Oral ciprofloxacin would be an option for this patient rather than intravenous. However, ciprofloxacin has a broader spectrum of activity than trimethoprim-sulfamethoxazole, so it would not be preferred. The most focused, narrowest-spectrum agent possible is preferred when an antimicrobial agent is prescribed.

Nitrofurantoin is used for acute, uncomplicated urinary tract infections. It is not adequate treatment for pyelonephritis, with or without bacteremia, because active levels are achieved only in the urine and not in the kidney parenchyma.

### KEY POINT

- In patients taking intravenous antimicrobial therapy, a switch to oral therapy should be considered in all patients with an intact and functioning gastrointestinal tract and whose clinical status is improving.

### Bibliography

Masterton RG. Antibiotic de-escalation. Crit Care Clin. 2011;27(1):149-162. [PMID 21144991]

## Item 43      Answer:    A

**Educational Objective: Manage a reactive tuberculin skin test in an immunosuppressed patient.**

This patient should undergo chest radiography to exclude active tuberculosis infection. The patient is asymptomatic and is taking infliximab, a tumor necrosis factor α inhibitor, for management of her psoriasis. A tuberculin skin test (TST) reaction of 5-mm or larger induration is interpreted as positive in patients who are immunosuppressed, including those who are taking tumor necrosis factor α inhibitors or the equivalent of at least 15 mg/d of prednisone for 1 month or longer. Other patients for whom 5-mm or larger induration is considered positive include patients with HIV infection, organ transplants, and fibrotic changes on chest radiograph consistent with old tuberculosis, and recent contacts of a person with active tuberculosis. If the chest radiograph is negative, treatment for latent tuberculosis infection, usually consisting of daily isoniazid with pyridoxine (vitamin B$_6$) for 9 months, is recommended to decrease the risk for progression to active disease.

Testing with both the TST and interferon-γ release assay is not routinely recommended. According to the Centers for Disease Control and Prevention, using both tests may be helpful when the result of the initial test is positive and additional validation of infection is required before recommended treatment is initiated, such as in health care professionals who previously received the bacillus Calmette-Guérin vaccine or patients at low risk for infection and progression to active disease. Conversely, both tests may be helpful when the result of the initial test is negative and the risk for infection, active disease, and a poor outcome is increased, such as in patients infected with HIV or children younger than 5 years who have been exposed to a patient with active tuberculosis. Using both tests also may be helpful when the result of the initial test is negative but symptoms, signs, or imaging results are suspicious for TB and evidence of infection with *M. tuberculosis* is being sought. Because this patient does not fit into one of these categories, interferon-γ release assay would not be indicated.

Rifampin, isoniazid, pyrazinamide, and ethambutol would be recommended as initial therapy for a patient with active tuberculosis. This patient has no symptoms of active infection. Unless the chest radiograph suggests active tuberculosis, beginning four-drug antituberculous therapy is not indicated and would not be appropriate before further evaluation.

No additional intervention, including evaluation or therapy, would be inappropriate for this patient. Although she is asymptomatic, she is at risk for active tuberculosis if untreated for latent tuberculosis infection.

**KEY POINT**

- Patients who have a positive reaction to tuberculin skin testing should be further evaluated by chest radiography to rule out active tuberculosis infection.

**Bibliography**

Centers for Disease Control and Prevention. Latent Tuberculosis Infection: A Guide for Primary Health Care Providers. www.cdc.gov/tb/publications/LTBI/diagnosis.htm. Updated November 26, 2014. Accessed July 21, 2015.

## Item 44    Answer:    B

**Educational Objective: Diagnose a primary genital herpes simplex virus infection.**

A polymerase chain reaction (PCR) test of a lesion specimen should be performed for genital herpes simplex virus (HSV) infection. The patient has genital lesions characteristic of HSV infection (shallow ulcers on an erythematous base), and primary infection is likely because of the presence of multiple lesions, regional lymphadenopathy, and systemic symptoms. It is important that all first presentations of genital HSV infection be microbiologically confirmed. PCR is the most sensitive of the available testing modalities and can also distinguish between HSV-1 and HSV-2, which can help inform discussions with the patient regarding risk of recurrent genital ulcer disease. HSV-1 is the most common and is less likely to cause recurrent infection or asymptomatic shedding. If the diagnosis is confirmed, the patient should be offered screening for other sexually transmitted infections and counseled regarding the need to inform prospective sexual partners and her obstetrician should she become pregnant.

Direct florescent antibody testing of a genital lesion is a specific study for HSV infection and is also able to identify the type of virus present. However, it is less sensitive than

PCR testing and is no longer recommended for the diagnosis of genital HSV.

Type-specific serum antibodies to HSV develop within weeks of primary infection and persist indefinitely. However, their presence does not confirm that the genital ulcers are caused by HSV; therefore, this study would not be appropriate for this patient.

Tzanck smear is an older test that assesses the presence of multinucleate giant cells in a lesion specimen that demonstrates the cytopathic effects of the virus. However, the sensitivity and specificity of this test are low, and the test does not differentiate among serotypes of HSV; it is therefore no longer used frequently.

**KEY POINT**

- Polymerase chain reaction testing of genital lesions is the most sensitive diagnostic modality available for herpes simplex virus infection.

**Bibliography**

Workowski KA, Berman S; Centers for Disease Control and Prevention (CDC). Sexually transmitted diseases treatment guidelines, 2010 [erratum in MMWR Recomm Rep. 2011 Jan 14;60(1):18]. MMWR Recomm Rep. 2010 Dec 17;59(RR-12):1-110. [PMID: 21160459]

## Item 45    Answer:    B

**Educational Objective: Diagnose giardiasis.**

The most appropriate diagnostic test for this patient with subacute diarrheal illness is the stool *Giardia* antigen test. The constellation of steatorrhea, abdominal distention, and weight loss in the absence of fever suggests a parasitic gastrointestinal illness, most likely *Giardia* infection. *Giardia* is ubiquitous in the environment and can cause human infection through ingestion of contaminated food or water. Less commonly, transmission can occur through fecal-oral routes. Giardiasis is a common gastrointestinal infection in outdoor enthusiasts and international travelers, who may become infected after drinking contaminated water. Boiling or filtering water is protective, but chlorination does not prevent infection.

Amebiasis is an uncommon cause of dysentery in developed countries and would be unlikely in the absence of a history of travel, as is the case in this patient. Therefore, a stool *Entamoeba* antigen test would be inappropriate.

Stool microscopy is no longer the preferred diagnostic test for giardiasis, as *Giardia* antigen testing has a sensitivity greater than 80%. Identification of cysts or trophozoites by microscopy in stool samples is hindered by intermittent shedding of the parasite, and multiple stool samples are therefore required to exclude the diagnosis.

Several enteric parasites are not well visualized using traditional microscopy and require modified acid-fast stains for optimal diagnosis. These include *Cyclospora* and *Cystoisospora* species, both of which are uncommon causes of diarrhea in the absence of travel or HIV/AIDS. *Cyclospora* infections in the United States have been associated with outbreaks traced to imported fruits and vegetables, but this patient's history of backcountry camping makes giardiasis a much more likely diagnosis.

**KEY POINT**

- Steatorrhea, abdominal distention, and weight loss suggest giardiasis, most common in travelers and outdoor enthusiasts, who may become infected from drinking contaminated water.

**Bibliography**

Wright SG. Protozoan infections of the gastrointestinal tract. Infect Dis Clin North Am. 2012 Jun;26(2):323-39. [PMID: 22632642]

## Item 46　　Answer:　C

**Educational Objective: Identify preferred screening for *Mycobacterium tuberculosis* infection in a patient who is unlikely to return for follow-up.**

This patient uses injection drugs, so she is at higher risk for exposure to or infection with *Mycobacterium tuberculosis* and should be screened for the pathogen, preferably with an interferon-γ release assay (IGRA). An IGRA or a tuberculin skin test (TST) can be used to diagnose tuberculosis, although neither differentiates between active disease and latent tuberculosis infection (LTBI). An IGRA can be used instead of a TST in all cases in which TST is recommended; however, an IGRA is preferred for persons from groups who are at high risk for not returning for interpretation of their TST result (such as injection drug users or homeless persons) and those who have received bacillus Calmette-Guérin as a vaccine or for cancer treatment. Although IGRA tends to be more expensive than TST, the resultant increase in rates of test completion are likely more cost-effective in persons at high risk for noncompletion of TST testing and also allows for improved public health efforts in the management of infected persons at significant risk for infection.

If the IGRA result is positive, then an evaluation for active disease includes review of symptoms (fever, night sweats, weight loss, cough, fatigue, chest pain), chest radiography, and possibly microbiologic assessment of sputum (or other involved fluid). LTBI can be diagnosed when active disease is ruled out. However, chest radiography or induced sputum examination is not used for screening for LTBI.

**KEY POINT**

- Interferon-γ release assay is preferred for tuberculosis screening in groups at high risk for not returning for interpretation of skin test results and those who have received bacillus Calmette-Guérin as a vaccine or for cancer treatment.

**Bibliography**

Mazurek GH, Jereb J, Vernon A, LoBue P, Goldberg S, Castro K; IGRA Expert Committee; Centers for Disease Control and Prevention (CDC). Updated guidelines for using Interferon Gamma Release Assays to detect Mycobacterium tuberculosis infection - United States, 2010. MMWR Recomm Rep. 2010 Jun 25;59(RR-5):1-25. [PMID: 20577159]

## Item 47　　Answer:　A

**Educational Objective: Treat a patient with HIV infection with opportunistic infection prophylaxis.**

This patient should begin azithromycin. Because his CD4 cell count is less than 50/μL, he is at significant risk for disseminated *Mycobacterium avium* complex infection and should begin prophylaxis immediately with azithromycin. He has HIV infection and meets the definition for AIDS based on a CD4 cell count less than 200/μL. Although he has not yet had an opportunistic infection, he should also receive prophylaxis against *Pneumocystis jirovecii*, for which daily trimethoprim-sulfamethoxazole is the drug of choice.

Although this patient is at risk for candidal infections, such as oroesophageal disease, or infection by other fungi, including *Cryptococcus neoformans*, primary antifungal prophylaxis is not recommended in HIV infection. Therefore, fluconazole is not indicated in this patient.

The risk for tuberculosis (TB) infection increases in patients following HIV seroconversion and increases as loss of CD4 cells and immunosuppression progress. Therefore, all patients with HIV infection should be screened for latent TB, and close follow-up for primary TB infection should be maintained. However, this patient has no evidence of latent or active TB infection. The interferon-γ release assay result is indeterminate because of his very low CD4 count and consequent inability to react to the positive control used in the testing. He has no clinical symptoms or signs of TB and has not had any exposure. Therefore, treatment with isoniazid and vitamin B$_6$ is not indicated.

Pyrimethamine is an agent with activity against *Toxoplasma gondii*, which this patient is at risk for based on his positive serologic results and CD4 cell count less than 100/μL. Leucovorin is given concomitantly to lessen the risk for cytopenias, which are a common adverse effect associated with pyrimethamine therapy. However, the trimethoprim-sulfamethoxazole already being used for *Pneumocystis* prophylaxis will also protect against toxoplasmosis, so additional medication is unnecessary.

Although the patient is at risk for reactivation disease due to cytomegalovirus, primary prophylaxis is not recommended because of the hematologic toxicity of valganciclovir.

**KEY POINT**

- Patients with HIV/AIDS with CD4 cell counts less than 50/μL and less than 200/μL should undergo prophylaxis against *Mycobacterium avium* complex and *Pneumocystis jirovecii*, respectively.

**Bibliography**

Panel on Opportunistic Infections in HIV-Infected Adults and Adolescents. Guidelines for the prevention and treatment of opportunistic infections in HIV-infected adults and adolescents: recommendations from the Centers for Disease Control and Prevention, the National Institutes of Health, and the HIV Medicine Association of the Infectious Diseases Society of America. http://aidsinfo.nih.gov/contentfiles/lvguidelines/adult_oi.pdf. Updated April 16, 2015. Accessed July 21, 2015.

**Item 48**     **Answer:**   **C**

**Educational Objective: Manage opportunistic infection prophylaxis in a patient who has undergone solid organ transplantation.**

This patient's level of immunosuppression must be increased for this episode of acute rejection, and therefore prophylaxis for *Pneumocystis jirovecii* infection should be reinitiated. Because of defects in cell-mediated immunity resulting from antirejection drugs, patients who have undergone transplantation are at high risk for *P. jirovecii* infection and are usually treated with prophylaxis for *Pneumocystis* infection, especially for the first 6 to 12 months when immunosuppression is given at higher levels. Long-term prophylaxis is not typically required when immunosuppression for the transplant can be minimized. However, these patients are also at increased risk beyond the first year if episodes of rejection require increases in immunosuppression, such as in this patient. It is thus important to reinstitute prophylaxis for *Pneumocystis* infection under these circumstances, even if increased immunosuppression is temporary. Trimethoprim-sulfamethoxazole is the preferred prophylactic agent in most patients without a contraindication.

Pulmonary aspergillosis is more likely to occur in the neutropenic period after hematopoietic stem cell transplantation or after lung transplantation; it would be uncommon in a patient after other solid organ transplantation, and prophylaxis is not indicated.

Both recipient and donor in this case were seronegative for cytomegalovirus before transplantation and thus cytomegalovirus disease is unlikely, even with increased immunosuppression, and prophylaxis is not necessary.

In contrast to the high risk in patients with advanced AIDS, *Mycobacterium avium* complex infection is unusual after transplantation, and prophylaxis against this is not indicated.

> **KEY POINT**
>
> - Patients who have undergone transplantation are at high risk for *Pneumocystis jirovecii* infection, especially during the first 6 to 12 months and after episodes of rejection requiring increased immunosuppression.

**Bibliography**

Carmona EM, Limper AH. Update on the diagnosis and treatment of *Pneumocystis* pneumonia. Ther Adv Respir Dis. 2011 Feb;5(1):41-59. [PMID: 20736243]

**Item 49**     **Answer:**   **B**

**Educational Objective: Prevent hepatitis A in a traveler to South Asia.**

This patient should receive hepatitis A virus (HAV) vaccine and a dose of intramuscular immune globulin now. Travel-related risk for acquiring HAV depends on the person's immune status to HAV and level of endemicity of this hepatotropic pathogen in the geographic area being visited. The adoption of routine childhood HAV vaccination programs in recent years has greatly decreased the incidence of infection. However, only approximately 40% of adults are immune to HAV and, therefore, are at risk for infection, particularly when traveling to developing parts of South Asia, Africa, and South and Central America. Transmission occurs by the fecal-oral route from close contact with an infected person or ingestion of contaminated water or food. Therefore, active immunization using either of the two available inactivated vaccines is effective for preventing infection and is strongly recommended when traveling to areas of high disease prevalence, such as Cambodia.

One dose of vaccine administered any time before departure generally provides protection to most persons 40 years or younger, although a second dose given 6 to 12 months after the initial dose is required for long-term protection. However, persons older than 40 years, those with chronic medical conditions, immunocompromised persons, or those with chronic liver disease who plan to depart within 2 weeks to an endemic area should be treated with hepatitis A vaccination and intramuscular immune globulin given at a distant injection site to provide optimal protection. The use of immunosuppressive medications (as in this patient), including tumor necrosis factor $\alpha$ inhibitors, is not a contraindication to immunization with killed or inactivated vaccines.

Hepatitis A vaccine is the primary method for triggering immunity to the virus, with immune globulin providing additional protection in patients at high risk. The use of immune globulin alone without hepatitis A vaccination is not indicated or recommended.

Administering hepatitis A vaccine or immune globulin following exposure to hepatitis A in nonimmunized patients (postexposure prophylaxis) is effective in reducing attack rates of infection. However, preexposure prophylaxis is not contraindicated in this patient, and postexposure prophylaxis should not be necessary.

> **KEY POINT**
>
> - Hepatitis A virus vaccine, with a dose of intramuscular immune globulin to provide optimal protection to persons traveling within 2 weeks, should be given to any person planning travel to developing parts of South Asia, Africa, and South and Central America.

**Bibliography**

Centers for Disease Control and Prevention. Infectious Diseases Related to Travel, Hepatitis A. In: CDC Health Information for International Travel 2014. http://wwwnc.cdc.gov/travel/yellowbook/2014/chapter-3-infectious-diseases-related-to-travel/hepatitis-a. Updated July 10, 2015. Accessed July 20, 2015.

**Item 50**     **Answer:**   **E**

**Educational Objective: Treat a patient with a second recurrence of *Clostridium difficile* infection.**

This patient with a second recurrence of mild to moderate *Clostridium difficile* infection (CDI) should be treated with oral vancomycin for 6 weeks. Approximately 20% of patients with CDI will experience a relapse. In 2010, an expert panel outlined evidence-based recommendations for treatment of CDI. A recent study found that adherence to these guidelines resulted in significantly improved outcomes and fewer recurrences of CDI.

The initial treatment regimen is based on the severity of illness, with a 10- to 14-day course of oral metronidazole recommended for mild to moderate illness and a 10- to 14-day course of oral vancomycin for severe illness. For the first recurrence, guidelines specify that treatment decisions should be based on the severity of illness, similar to the determination of appropriate treatment with the initial presentation. However, for subsequent relapses, the probability of sustained response is significantly decreased, and it is therefore recommend that all patients receive a prolonged course of vancomycin, typically given at tapered doses over 6 to 8 weeks.

Metronidazole is not recommended for use in multiple recurrences of CDI because prolonged administration is associated with a risk for neurotoxicity, and luminal concentrations of the antibiotic decrease to subtherapeutic levels after resolution of colitis.

Small studies have suggested that rifaximin may be useful in multiple recurrences of CDI when given at the end of the vancomycin taper, but this agent is not recommended as a stand-alone therapy.

---

**KEY POINT**

- Patients who have more than one recurrence of *Clostridium difficile* infection should be treated with oral vancomycin given at tapered doses over 6 to 8 weeks.

---

**Bibliography**

Leffler DA, Lamont JT. Clostridium difficile infection. N Engl J Med. 2015 Apr; 16;372(16):1539-48. [PMID: 25875259]

## Item 51     Answer:   B

**Educational Objective: Treat a patient with community-acquired pneumonia who has reached clinical stability by switching to oral antibiotic therapy.**

This patient should be switched to an oral antibiotic agent, and he should be discharged when otherwise clinically ready. Empiric intravenous antibiotic therapy is usually started in patients requiring hospital admission for community-acquired pneumonia (CAP), as was done with this patient, to cover the most likely infecting organisms. He has had an appropriate response to therapy as indicated by improvement in his clinical symptoms (fever, cough, dyspnea) within the 3 days of treatment. Patients treated with intravenous antibiotics for CAP with an appropriate clinical response can be switched to an oral agent, generally of the same antimicrobial class and with similar spectrum of activity, when clinical stability has been attained. Parameters suggesting

clinical stability include 1) temperature of 37.8 °C (100.0 °F) or less, 2) heart rate of 100/min or less, 3) respiration rate of 24/min or less, 4) systolic blood pressure of 90 mm Hg or greater, 5) arterial oxygen saturation of 90% or more or $P_{O_2}$ of 60 mm Hg (8.0 kPa) or greater breathing ambient air (or requiring a similar amount of supplemental oxygen as before admission if the patient receives chronic oxygen therapy), 6) ability to maintain oral intake, and 7) normal mental status.

Extended intravenous antibiotic therapy in stable patients without another indication for prolonging this treatment has not been shown to be more beneficial than oral therapy. Similarly, overlapping intravenous and oral antibiotic therapy, or hospital monitoring of stable patients following the transition from parenteral to oral therapy, has not been shown to improve outcomes.

---

**KEY POINT**

- Patients treated with intravenous antibiotics for community-acquired pneumonia with an appropriate clinical response can be switched to an oral agent, generally of the same antimicrobial class and with similar spectrum of activity, when clinical stability has been attained.

---

**Bibliography**

Aliberti S, Zanaboni AM, Wiemken T, et al. Criteria for clinical stability in hospitalised patients with community-acquired pneumonia. Eur Respir J. 2013 Sep;42(3):742-9. [PMID: 23143544]

## Item 52     Answer:   B

**Educational Objective: Diagnose a traveler with coccidioidomycosis.**

The patient has coccidioidomycosis, most likely acquired during her recent trip to Arizona. *Coccidioides immitis*, a dimorphic fungus, is regularly found in the soil in the southwestern United States, along with parts of Mexico and Central and South America. Even limited exposure in endemic areas can result in inhalation of airborne spores of this pathogen. In most patients, the primary lung infection of coccidiomycosis is asymptomatic; patients who develop clinical disease often report influenza-like illness. Chest imaging studies are nonspecific; findings may be normal in asymptomatic patients or include diffuse infiltrates, nodules, and cavities, sometimes in combination. The endospore-containing spherule detected in the bronchoalveolar lavage specimen shown is characteristic of *C. immitis*.

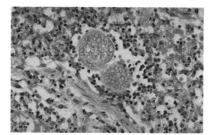

Unilateral hilar lymphadenopathy and pleural effusions are observed in approximately one fifth of symptomatic patients. Constitutional and pulmonary symptoms predominate, often beginning weeks after returning from travel. The presence of erythema nodosum lesions on the anterior lower extremities is also fairly common. Severe pulmonary disease and hematogenous dissemination of the organism to skin, bone, joints, peritoneum, and central nervous system occur infrequently, but patients with impaired T-cell–mediated immunity, such as this patient, are at significantly higher risk for more severe disease. Confirmation relies on isolation of the organism from clinical specimens, histologic identification, serologic assays, and DNA probes. *Coccidioides* infections generally resolve without antifungal therapy, but immunocompromised patients with severe or disseminated infection warrant antifungal therapy. An amphotericin B deoxycholate formulation is recommended in severely ill patients. In all others, fluconazole or itraconazole can be used.

Blastomycosis and histoplasmosis are dimorphic fungi that share clinical features with coccidioidomycosis but are mostly concentrated in the central river valleys and south-central and southeastern United States. Morphologically, the organisms are easily distinguishable from *Coccidioides* species on clinical specimens.

*Mycoplasma pneumoniae* is less common in adults and rarely presents as severe pneumonia. A single reactive IgM antibody assay may not be reliable in confirming the diagnosis because both the sensitivity and specificity of this test are suboptimal. Diagnosis is best confirmed by showing a four-fold increase or decrease in paired sera titers or by detecting *M. pneumoniae*–specific antigens in respiratory secretions using newer immunoassays.

**KEY POINT**

- Coccidioidomycosis should be considered in any patient with a respiratory illness who lives or has spent time in an endemic area, which includes the southwestern United States, Mexico, and South and Central America.

**Bibliography**
Galgiani JN, Ampel NM, Blair JE, et al; Infectious Diseases Society of America. Coccidioidomycosis. Clin Infect Dis. 2005;41(9):1217-23. [PMID: 16206093]

**Item 53      Answer:   A**
**Educational Objective: Manage *Enterococcus faecalis* bacteremia.**

This patient should receive ampicillin in place of meropenem. Distinguishing between bacteremia caused by *E. faecalis* versus *Enterococcus faecium* is necessary because *E. faecium* is relatively more resistant than *E. faecalis* and more likely to be vancomycin resistant, depending on local epidemiology. Intravenous ampicillin is the most appropriate treatment option for sensitive *E. faecalis* because it is the

most narrow-spectrum agent and antibiotic of choice for this organism. Antibiotic stewardship requires that empiric antimicrobial therapy be modified or de-escalated as soon as culture results are available, even when a patient is improving with the empiric antimicrobial regimen. Doing so helps preserve the effectiveness of broad-spectrum agents used to initially treat patients requiring aggressive therapy. Meropenem is highly effective against a wide range of organisms, and this breadth of coverage is unnecessary after the primary infecting organism has been identified. Additionally, it is less active against *E. faecalis* than ampicillin or vancomycin and should therefore be discontinued.

Adding gentamicin to ampicillin or vancomycin is not necessary in nonendocarditis *E. faecalis* infections, including bacteremia. In this patient, *E. faecalis* bacteremia occurred secondary to urinary tract infection; he has no evidence of endocarditis by history, examination, or clinical course. In patients with enterococcal endocarditis, adding gentamicin (if high-level aminoglycoside resistance is not present) to ampicillin or vancomycin for a limited period early in the treatment course improves clinical outcomes.

Vancomycin is used in patients who are allergic to penicillin or in ampicillin-resistant *E. faecalis* but is not the initial agent of choice for use against *E. faecalis*.

**KEY POINT**

- Empiric antimicrobial therapy should be modified or de-escalated as soon as culture results become available to provide the narrowest-spectrum agent available.

**Bibliography**
Masterton RG. Antibiotic de-escalation. Crit Care Clin. 2011;27(1):149-162. [PMID 21144991]

**Item 54      Answer:   A**
**Educational Objective: Diagnose invasive *Aspergillus* infection.**

This patient most likely has acute *Aspergillus* rhinosinusitis. Invasive fungal infections, such as sinusitis, are uncommon except in immunocompromised persons with prolonged neutropenia, such as this patient who has an underlying hematologic malignancy and is undergoing chemotherapy. His clinical symptoms (sinus pain), examination and radiographic findings (sinusitis and exophthalmos), and laboratory studies (positive result on galactomannan antigen immunoassay and characteristic histopathologic findings) support the diagnosis of *Aspergillus* rhinosinusitis. Direct invasion into the palate can occur from infection of the maxillary sinus. Infection of the ethmoid sinus may extend into the cavernous sinuses and cause cranial nerve deficits and internal carotid artery thrombosis. Central nervous system (CNS) involvement may also occur as a complication. Additionally, periorbital infection with subsequent loss of vision may occur. The mortality rate of *Aspergillus* rhinosinusitis is high. Definitive diagnosis requires a tissue biopsy demonstrating hyphae and a positive culture for *Aspergillus*.

**Answers and Critiques**

H
CONT.

The appearance of septate hyphae with acute angle branching on histopathologic testing can be diagnostic. The galactomannan assay is an important non-culture-based tool for the diagnosis of invasive aspergillosis. Detection of galactomannan in serum has a high sensitivity and specificity in patients at high risk; galactomannan can also be detected in cerebrospinal fluid specimens from patients with CNS aspergillosis and in bronchoalveolar lavage fluid from those with invasive pulmonary aspergillosis. It is useful in early detection and in therapeutic monitoring. Voriconazole is the therapy of choice for most patients with invasive aspergillosis because of its potent fungicidal activity against *Aspergillus* species. Culture confirmation is important to distinguish *Aspergillus* from other filamentous fungal infections.

*Candida* and *Cryptococcus* are yeasts that are unlikely causes of rhinosinusitis and do not result in a positive finding on galactomannan assay or have the characteristic morphologic features of *Aspergillus*.

Although rare in otherwise healthy patients, *Pseudomonas* rhinosinusitis is encountered most frequently in immunocompromised or severely traumatized patients. *Pseudomonas* is a gram-negative, bacillary bacterium that also does not cause a positive galactomannan test result.

**KEY POINT**

- Definitive diagnosis of *Aspergillus* sinusitis requires a tissue biopsy demonstrating hyphae and a positive culture for *Aspergillus*, and use of the galactomannan antigen immunoassay to detect galactomannan in serum has a high sensitivity and specificity in patients at high risk.

**Bibliography**

Karthaus M, Buchheidt. Invasive aspergillosis: new insights into disease, diagnostic and treatment. Curr Pharm Des. 2013;19(20):3569-94. [PMID: 23278538]

## Item 55      Answer:      C

**Educational Objective: Diagnose posttransplant lymphoproliferative disease.**

This patient most likely has posttransplant lymphoproliferative disease (PTLD). She is at increased risk for PTLD because she was seronegative for Epstein-Barr virus (EBV) and the organ donor was seropositive. PTLD is related to B-cell proliferation induced by infection with EBV in the setting of chronic immunosuppression and resulting decreased T-cell immune surveillance. She presents within a typical timeframe (first few months to 1 year after transplantation) with lymphadenopathy found on CT scan and systemic symptoms consistent with PTLD. In addition to PTLD, EBV after transplantation can cause a mononucleosis syndrome, leukopenia and thrombocytopenia, and hepatitis or pneumonitis. Quantitative serum polymerase chain reaction for EBV can suggest a diagnosis of PTLD, which is confirmed by biopsy and histopathologic evaluation of the swollen lymph nodes or extranodal mass. Management consists of reduction in

immunosuppression, if possible, and may require chemotherapy, which often includes rituximab.

Cytomegalovirus infection is common after transplantation, especially in seronegative recipients with seropositive donors, and can manifest as a nonspecific febrile syndrome. However, cytomegalovirus would be unlikely to cause a single, significantly enlarged lymph node; this presentation makes PTLD more likely.

Although this patient has whitish plaques in her oropharynx consistent with oral thrush, and disseminated fungal infections may cause systemic symptoms such as this patient is experiencing, an invasive *Candida* infection would not cause her isolated lymphadenopathy and is not supported by her negative fungal blood cultures.

Tuberculosis reactivation increases in incidence after solid organ transplantation and is more likely to have extrapulmonary findings. It could present with lymphadenopathy and fever but clear lungs, as in this patient. However, she had a negative result on a test for latent tuberculosis before transplantation, which makes reactivation of tuberculosis unlikely.

**KEY POINT**

- Patients are at high risk for posttransplant lymphoproliferative disease if they received an organ from a donor seropositive for Epstein-Barr virus when they are seronegative.

**Bibliography**

Kamdar KY, Rooney CM, Heslop HE. Posttransplant lymphoproliferative disease following liver transplantation. Curr Opin Organ Transplant. 2011 Jun;16(3):274-80. [PMID: 21467936]

## Item 56      Answer:      A

**Educational Objective: Treat a patient with a dog bite.**

This patient has experienced a dog bite and should receive treatment with amoxicillin-clavulanate. A 3- to 5-day course of prophylaxis (early preemptive therapy) with amoxicillin-clavulanate is recommended for patients who are immunosuppressed (including those with asplenia or significant liver disease); have moderate to severe wounds (particularly on the face or hand); have wounds near a joint or bone; or have wounds associated with significant crush injury or edema. Amoxicillin-clavulanate, an oral β-lactam/β-lactamase inhibitor, is a good choice because it has a broad spectrum of activity against the aerobic and anaerobic bacteria that constitute a dog's oral flora. Prompt wound irrigation and debridement, if appropriate, are also indicated. Each patient should also be evaluated for the need for tetanus and rabies prophylaxis.

Metronidazole provides anaerobic bacterial coverage but lacks coverage against aerobic bacteria in dogs' mouth flora. If used, it should be combined with a fluoroquinolone (such as ciprofloxacin or levofloxacin) or trimethoprim-sulfamethoxazole.

Patients with bite wounds should be vaccinated with tetanus toxoid if they have not received a tetanus immunization within the past 5 years because this type of wound is considered a "dirty" wound. Other wounds that are considered "dirty" include those contaminated with soil, saliva, dirt, or feces; avulsions; puncture wounds; and wounds resulting from burns, frostbite, crushing, or missiles. This patient has been immunized within this time period, so she does not require tetanus immunization. For a clean and minor wound, a booster dose of tetanus toxoid would be given to prevent tetanus if more than 10 years have elapsed since immunization.

Pursuing no additional therapy or evaluation would not be appropriate for this patient, who is receiving a tumor necrosis factor α inhibitor, which is an immunosuppressant. Although the patient has no signs or symptoms of infection, antibiotic prophylaxis is recommended as soon as possible after a bite to decrease the risk for infection.

**KEY POINT**

- A 3- to 5-day course of antibiotic prophylaxis with a broad-spectrum agent, such as amoxicillin-clavulanate, is recommended for patients who have received an animal bite and are immunosuppressed.

**Bibliography**

Stevens DL, Bisno AL, Chambers HF, et al. Practice guidelines for the diagnosis and management of skin and soft tissue infections: 2014 update by the Infectious Diseases Society of America. Clin Infect Dis. 2014 Jul 15;59(2):147-59. [PMID: 24947530]

**Item 57          Answer:    C**

**Educational Objective: Diagnose recurrent herpes simplex virus type 2 genital infection.**

Recurrent herpes simplex virus 2 (HSV-2) infection is the most likely cause of this patient's rash. HSV-2 is the leading cause of genital ulcerative disease in the world. Although herpes simplex virus 1 (HSV-1) is rapidly gaining prevalence as a cause of this form of herpetic infection in younger white populations, it tends to be milder, with significantly fewer recurrences; however, it is clinically indistinguishable from HSV-2. Therefore, the diagnosis of suspected HSV infection should be confirmed with viral culture, polymerase chain reaction assay, or type-specific serologic tests.

Primary infection follows introduction of the virus onto a mucosal surface or through damaged skin. The findings with primary infection are highly variable, ranging from no symptoms to severe, painful genital ulcers; fever; tender inguinal lymphadenopathy; and headache. However, this patient has had several episodes of a similar rash over the past year, suggesting recurrent disease from a primary infection that may have occurred in the distant past. Although HSV-2 lesions characteristically appear in the genital region, they may also present at locations not classically thought of as the genitalia, such as the gluteal and presacral surfaces. Sacral HSV infection may be accompanied by episodes of

aseptic meningitis. The pattern of recurrence may be influenced by diverse factors, including systemic infection, hormonal fluctuations associated with menstrual cycles, stress, and immune dysfunction. Long-term valacyclovir treatment taken on a daily basis decreases the frequency of recurrences and significantly diminishes asymptomatic viral shedding (which may occur without active skin lesions), which helps decrease transmission.

Dermatitis herpetiformis is an autoimmune disease associated with a gluten-sensitive enteropathy leading to skin deposition of IgA antibodies to gluten-tissue transglutaminase found in the gut. The lesions take the form of erythematous papules or plaques with clustered herpetiform vesicles and are usually located on the extensor surfaces of knees and elbows, but they may also be present on the shoulders and buttocks. Once present, the disease is chronic with periods of exacerbation and remission.

Fixed drug eruptions are cutaneous disorders associated with systemic exposure to various medications. The mechanism of disease is postulated to be a cell-mediated response to the offending drug acting as a hapten when it binds to specific cells in the skin. Outbreaks may occur on any cutaneous surface but seem to be more common on the lip and genitalia, where they appear as erythematous patches (often with blisters), postinflammatory necrosis, and hyperpigmentation. NSAIDs are included among the dozens of medications associated with this condition.

Sacral dermatomal distribution of HSV lesions is often confused with herpes zoster. However, multiple recurrences of zoster in a relatively young, immunocompetent woman would be very unusual.

**KEY POINT**

- Herpes simplex virus 2 is the most common cause of genital ulcer disease worldwide, although herpes simplex virus 1 as a cause of genital ulcer disease is increasing.

**Bibliography**

Hofstetter AM, Rosenthal SL, Stanberry LR. Current thinking on genital herpes. Curr Opin Infec Dis. 2014;27(1):75-83. [PMID: 24335720]

**Item 58          Answer:    E**

**Educational Objective: Treat mild nontyphoidal *Salmonella* gastroenteritis.**

This patient has acute diarrhea consistent with mild *Salmonella* gastroenteritis, which requires no therapy at this time. Nontyphoidal *Salmonella* infections typically cause an inflammatory diarrhea, sometimes associated with fever and abdominal pain. In young, healthy persons, such as this patient, the illness is usually self-limited and resolves without antibiotic therapy. In this population, antibiotic therapy is associated with prolonged asymptomatic fecal shedding with no decrease in duration of diarrhea. In contrast, *Salmonella* gastrointestinal infection in older patients, immunocompromised patients, or patients with sickle cell disease is associated with an increased risk for bacteremia and endovascular infection. In these populations, as well as in patients with severe salmonellosis or those requiring hospitalization, antibiotic therapy is warranted.

Azithromycin is the preferred empiric treatment option for *Campylobacter* gastroenteritis, considering increasing rates of quinolone resistance for this bacterium.

Ciprofloxacin is effective for most bacterial agents causing gastroenteritis but should be reserved for febrile patients with moderate to severe inflammatory diarrhea when the suspicion for *Salmonella* or Shiga toxin–producing *Escherichia coli* is low.

Loperamide and other antimotility agents are not recommended for inflammatory diarrhea because of the potential for delaying bacterial clearance and prolonging the illness.

Most studies of probiotics for infectious diarrhea have been performed in children. In that population, probiotics have been associated with an average decrease in the duration of symptoms by 1 day; however, the benefit for adults is less certain.

### KEY POINT

- Therapy for mild nontyphoidal *Salmonella* gastroenteritis should be withheld in otherwise healthy patients because treatment may increase duration of bacterial shedding.

### Bibliography

Onwuezobe IA, Oshun PO, Odigwe CC. Antimicrobials for treating symptomatic non-typhoidal Salmonella infection. Cochrane Database Syst Rev. 2012 Nov 14;11:CD001167. [PMID: 23152205]

## Item 59     Answer:    C

### Educational Objective: Treat a patient with acute, uncomplicated prostatitis.

This patient with likely acute bacterial prostatitis should begin empiric treatment with a fluoroquinolone, such as ciprofloxacin. Acute prostatitis most commonly results from an ascending urethral infection, although bacterial cystitis or epididymo-orchitis may be an underlying source of infection. Patients most often present with fever, chills, malaise, nausea and vomiting, dysuria, urgency, frequency, and pain in the lower abdomen, perineum, and rectum. The onset of symptoms is typically rapid. On physical examination, the prostate is tender and tense or boggy. Excessive palpation of the prostate should be avoided because it may contribute to bacteremia. As was done with this patient, blood and urine cultures should be obtained, and empiric broad-spectrum antibiotics should be started. Gram-negative bacillary organisms, including *Escherichia coli*, *Serratia* species, and *Klebsiella* species, are the most common causative agents in patients with uncomplicated acute bacterial prostatitis who are at low risk for sexually transmitted infections (STIs). The course of therapy with a fluoroquinolone is at least 14 days and up to 4 weeks. Trimethoprim-sulfamethoxazole is also

an appropriate first-line choice if the isolate is known to be susceptible or if the rate of *E. coli* resistance in the community is less than 20%.

Ampicillin, which had been an alternative therapeutic option for prostatitis, can no longer be recommended as empiric therapy because of the high rate of resistance among community-acquired microorganisms.

A single dose of ceftriaxone, 250 mg intramuscularly, is indicated for uncomplicated acute bacterial prostatitis in patients at risk for STIs with *Neisseria gonorrhoeae* or *Chlamydia trachomatis*. Generally, men younger than 35 years are at risk for infection with these organisms. Doxycycline, 100 mg twice daily for 10 days, is also indicated in these patients. This patient is not sexually active and therefore does not require coverage for possible STIs.

Treatment with a carbapenem, such as meropenem, should be reserved for systemically ill patients who require hospitalization or when a fluoroquinolone-resistant organism is a concern. The incidence of fluoroquinolone-resistant *E. coli* is very high (up to 90%) following prostate biopsy.

### KEY POINT

- Patients with uncomplicated acute bacterial prostatitis, most commonly caused by *Escherichia coli*, *Serratia* species, and *Klebsiella* species, who are at low risk for sexually transmitted infections should be treated empirically with ciprofloxacin.

### Bibliography

Wagenlehner FM, Weidner W, Pilatz A, Naber KG. Urinary tract infections and bacterial prostatitis in men. Curr Opin Infect Dis. 2014 Feb;27(1):97-101. [PMID: 24253463]

## Item 60     Answer:    C

### Educational Objective: Manage potential influenza exposure in a person who has not had an annual influenza vaccination.

This patient should be given postexposure prophylaxis with the inactivated influenza vaccine and oseltamivir chemoprophylaxis. Outbreaks of seasonal influenza virus infection generally occur during autumn and winter but may last into the spring. Most severe outbreaks are related to influenza A viruses, but they may also occur with type B influenza virus. Yearly preexposure immunization is recommended for all persons age 6 months or older, assuming no contraindications. In patients who have not been immunized, chemoprophylaxis with the neuraminidase inhibitors oseltamivir or zanamivir is recommended for persons who have been exposed to someone known or suspected of having active influenza, but only if the antivirals can be started within 48 hours of the most recent exposure. Both medications have activity against influenza A and B viruses, with resistance occurring in less than 1% of strains. However, zanamivir, which is administered by oral inhalation, is contraindicated in persons with chronic respiratory conditions, including those with asthma, such as this patient. Because chemoprophylaxis lowers but does not eliminate the risk for influenza, immunization with an influenza vaccine preparation should also be provided. Despite this patient's concern, the relative and attributable risks of neurologic sequelae such as Guillain-Barré syndrome after seasonal influenza vaccination are lower than those that occur in association with influenza infection.

The adamantine medication amantadine does not have activity against influenza B, and increasing drug resistance among influenza A strains make it an inappropriate medication for chemoprophylaxis.

The live-attenuated influenza vaccine given by nasal mist is approved only for persons age 2 to 49 years and would therefore not be appropriate in this patient.

**KEY POINT**

- Chemoprophylaxis with oseltamivir or zanamivir lowers but does not eliminate the risk for influenza, so immunization with an influenza vaccine preparation should also be provided to persons who may have been exposed to active influenza virus infection.

**Bibliography**

Fiore AE, Fry A, Shay D, et al; Centers for Disease Control and Prevention (CDC). Antiviral agents for the treatment and chemoprophylaxis of influenza – recommendations of the Advisory Committee on Immunization Practices (ACIP). MMWR Recomm Rep. 2011;60(1):1-24. [PMID: 21248682]

## Item 61    Answer:    B

**Educational Objective: Diagnose herpes simplex encephalitis.**

Despite the negative result on a herpes simplex virus (HSV) polymerase chain reaction (PCR) test, herpes simplex encephalitis remains the most likely cause of this patient's illness. HSV type 1 infection of the central nervous system causes a necrotizing infection of the temporal lobes, although atypical presentations may occur. Localization of inflammation to one or both temporal lobes on neuroimaging strongly suggests herpes simplex encephalitis and should prompt diagnostic testing and empiric therapy for this life-threatening infection. The sensitivity and specificity of cerebrospinal fluid (CSF) PCR for the diagnosis of herpes simplex encephalitis are greater than 95%, and PCR has replaced brain biopsy as the gold standard for laboratory confirmation of that condition. However, early in the course of infection, the PCR result may be falsely negative. Therefore, when clinical suspicion for herpes simplex encephalitis is high on the basis of the clinical presentation, acyclovir should be continued with repeat CSF PCR 3 to 7 days later. Delay in initiation of acyclovir therapy or premature cessation of treatment for herpes simplex encephalitis is associated with a significantly worse prognosis.

Enteroviruses are a common cause of lymphocytic meningitis but rarely cause meningoencephalitis in adults. In the case of enterovirus, no anatomic localization would be seen on imaging.

Pneumococcal meningitis is a life-threatening infection most commonly affecting the very old or very young; however, the absence of a neutrophilic pleocytosis (typically a CSF leukocyte count >1000/µL [1000 × 10$^6$/L]) and the focal involvement of brain parenchyma would essentially exclude this diagnosis.

West Nile virus may cause meningoencephalitis that is more common and severe in older adults, but neuroimaging findings are typically normal or show abnormalities of the thalami, basal ganglia, or spinal cord.

**KEY POINT**

- Initial cerebrospinal fluid polymerase chain reaction assay may be falsely negative early in herpes simplex encephalitis and should be repeated 3 to 7 days later (in addition to empiric acyclovir) in patients with high clinical suspicion for herpes simplex encephalitis.

**Bibliography**

Adler AC, Kadimi S, Apaloo C, Marcu C. Herpes simplex encephalitis with two false-negative cerebrospinal fluid PCR tests and review of negative PCR results in the clinical setting. Case Rep Neurol. 2011 May;3(2):172-8. [PMID: 21941494]

## Item 62    Answer:    A

**Educational Objective: Treat a patient with bacterial meningitis caused by *Streptococcus pneumoniae*.**

Treatment with adjunctive dexamethasone is the most likely intervention to improve neurologic outcomes in this patient with a presumptive diagnosis of bacterial meningitis due to *Streptococcus pneumoniae*. Meningitis leads to severe central nervous system (CNS) inflammatory changes that may cause acute neurologic changes and result in permanent, long-term neurologic damage. Neurologic sequelae associated with pneumococcal meningitis include seizures, hearing loss, cranial nerve deficits, and paralysis. The glucocorticoid dexamethasone decreases inflammation in the CNS and leads to lower mortality, fewer short-term neurologic sequelae, and decreased hearing loss in pneumococcal meningitis when used as adjunctive therapy in developed countries. Because of these potential benefits, guidelines recommend early dexamethasone treatment of possible or suspected pneumococcal meningitis; it should be given approximately 15 minutes before administration of antimicrobial agents and should be continued for the duration of antibiotic therapy.

Of interest, several recent studies have investigated therapeutic hyperthermia as a possible treatment of severe bacterial meningitis, but results have been conflicting and data not definitive enough to recommend this therapy.

Although excess intravascular volume has been associated with poorer outcomes in patients with severe bacterial meningitis, no evidence supports the benefit of fluid restriction or diuresis in euvolemic patients early in the management of bacterial meningitis compared with maintaining normal intravascular volume.

CONT.

Patients with meningitis frequently have increased intracranial pressure (ICP), and several interventions may lower the ICP, including maintaining the head of the bed at greater than 30 degrees, administering a hyperosmolar agent (such as glycerol), and placing a ventricular drain. However, monitoring and treating increased ICP are beneficial primarily in patients with bacterial meningitis who are stuporous or comatose, unlike this patient. The effect of interventions to lower ICP in patients without significant neurologic findings associated with meningitis is unclear.

Experimental animal models of pneumococcal meningitis have shown that infusions of mannitol modulate and reduce ICP. The mechanism for this effect on ICP may be related to reduction of hydroxyl radicals, which are implicated in CNS injury from ischemia and neuronal damage. The use of mannitol in this patient who has no clinical evidence of ICP is not appropriate.

### KEY POINT

- Adjunctive dexamethasone will improve outcomes in patients with a presumptive diagnosis of bacterial meningitis due to *Streptococcus pneumoniae*.

### Bibliography

Brouwer MC, McIntyre P, Prasad K, van de Beek D. Corticosteroids for acute bacterial meningitis. Cochrane Database Syst Rev. 2013;6:CD004405. [PMID: 23733364]

### Item 63      Answer:      C

**Educational Objective: Treat a patient with multidrug-resistant ventilator-associated pneumonia with empiric antibiotic therapy.**

This patient should be treated empirically with a carbapenem, such as meropenem, for a possible infection with a multidrug-resistant organism (MDRO). She is at high risk for ventilator-associated pneumonia (VAP) with multidrug-resistant *Klebsiella pneumoniae* as suggested by gram-negative rods on sputum Gram stain and the presence of other patients in the same ward with extended-spectrum β-lactamase (ESBL)–producing *K. pneumoniae* infection. ESBLs are enzymes that confer resistance to most β-lactam antibiotics, including penicillins, cephalosporins, and the monobactam aztreonam; they occur only in gram-negative organisms, primarily *K. pneumoniae*, *Klebsiella oxytoca*, and *Escherichia coli*. Carbapenems are less susceptible to ESBLs and provide adequate empiric coverage against this organism, as well as coverage for other possible gram-negative organisms such as *Pseudomonas* species, which is the second most common cause of VAP following *Staphylococcus aureus*. With any empiric regimen, antibiotic de-escalation should occur when culture results are available. Meropenem should be changed to ertapenem, a carbapenem without antipseudomonal activity, if an ESBL-producing organism is isolated without *Pseudomonas*. MDROs are more commonly associated with late-onset (>4 days) VAP. ESBL-producing *K. pneumoniae* are transmitted by health care personnel using improper hand hygiene or not following contact precautions. Contaminated shared patient care equipment that is not appropriately disinfected between patient uses is another possible route of transmission.

Because extended-spectrum penicillins and cephalosporins share susceptibility to ESBL, cefepime, ceftazidime, and piperacillin-tazobactam would not be optimal empiric therapy in this patient.

### KEY POINT

- Carbapenems, such as meropenem, are the appropriate choice for empiric therapy in patients with ventilator-associated pneumonia likely caused by extended-spectrum β-lactamase–producing *Enterobacteriaceae* species.

### Bibliography

Kalanuria AA, Zai W, Mirski M. Ventilator-associated pneumonia in the ICU. Crit Care. 2014;18:208-215. [PMID: 25029020]

### Item 64      Answer:      D

**Educational Objective: Manage HIV infection accompanied by serum creatinine elevation.**

This patient should continue his current antiretroviral regimen. Antiretroviral therapy for HIV usually comprises a "backbone" of two nucleoside/nucleotide reverse transcriptase inhibitors (NRTIs) plus a third agent, which may be a boosted protease inhibitor, a nonnucleoside reverse transcriptase inhibitor, or an integrase inhibitor. This patient's initial regimen contains the backbone of tenofovir and emtricitabine, primarily because these agents also have activity against hepatitis B. The third agent is elvitegravir, which is an integrase inhibitor; cobicistat is a cytochrome P-450 inhibitor used to boost the level of elvitegravir, which is metabolized through this pathway. This particular combination is available as a once-daily formulation, which is convenient for patients and encourages medication adherence. However, cobicistat also inhibits tubular secretion of creatinine, leading to increased levels of serum creatinine that do not reflect an actual change in the glomerular filtration rate (GFR). The creatinine level increases by an average of 0.14 mg/dL (12.4 µmol/L) with cobicistat. Because this does not actually affect the GFR, it is an expected occurrence and is not a reason to change the antiretroviral regimen, which is successful in this patient as demonstrated by the reduction in his viral load to undetectable levels. Investigation for true kidney dysfunction is recommended if the increase in creatinine level in patients taking cobicistat is 0.4 mg/dL (35.4 µmol/L) or more.

Changing the patient's antiretroviral regimen to an alternative NRTI backbone, such as abacavir-lamivudine or zidovudine-lamivudine, plus a third agent would be reasonable if a change in medications from his currently effective regimen were indicated, but this is not the case. Additionally, changing regimens from tenofovir and emtricitabine would lose the dual treatment effect of these agents for the patient's hepatitis B.

Even a brief discontinuation of antiretroviral therapy would be inappropriate because the patient is tolerating therapy well and it has been effective. Moreover, in this patient with chronic active hepatitis B, discontinuing agents with hepatitis B activity (tenofovir and emtricitabine) can lead to an acute flare in activity of the hepatitis, which can be severe.

Although this patient is at risk for several potential kidney diseases, including HIV-associated nephropathy, hepatitis B–associated kidney disease, and tenofovir renal toxicity, the likely artifactual increase in his serum creatinine level in combination with his negative urinalysis result and bland urine sediment does not suggest active kidney disease requiring further evaluation, such as by kidney biopsy.

### KEY POINT

- Cobicistat can inhibit tubular secretion of creatinine but does not actually affect glomerular filtration rate, so an increase in the creatinine level is expected when this agent is used.

### Bibliography

Panel on Antiretroviral Guidelines for Adults and Adolescents. Guidelines for the use of antiretroviral agents in HIV-1-infected adults and adolescents. Department of Health and Human Services. https://aidsinfo.nih.gov/contentfiles/lvguidelines/adultandadolescentgl.pdf. Accessed July 21, 2015.

## Item 65        Answer:     B

### Educational Objective: Treat a severe case of *Clostridium difficile* infection.

This patient has severe *Clostridium difficile* infection (CDI) and should be treated with oral vancomycin. Consensus guidelines for the treatment of CDI indicate that the specific antibiotic and route of administration should be guided by the severity of disease. Severe CDI is defined by the Infectious Diseases Society of America as a leukocyte count of 15,000/µL ($15 \times 10^9$/L) or greater and a serum creatinine level greater than 1.5 times the baseline level. Although more recent guidelines (see citation) use slightly different measures for defining severity, infectious disease and gastroenterology specialties concur that the preferred treatment for severe CDI is oral vancomycin. This is based on lower cure rates with oral metronidazole compared with vancomycin for patients with severe disease.

Oral metronidazole is the recommended initial therapy for patients with mild to moderate CDI (leukocyte count <15,000/µL [$15 \times 10^9$/L] and serum creatinine level <1.5 times baseline) based on cure rates similar to those of vancomycin and lower cost. A newer antimicrobial agent, fidaxomicin, showed noninferiority to vancomycin in the treatment of patients with mild to moderate CDI and, in a subset of patients, was associated with fewer relapses. However, the cost difference is substantial. A 10-day course of fidaxomicin approaches $3000, whereas metronidazole costs less than $30 and oral vancomycin costs less than $700. The indications for fidaxomicin will likely evolve, but as of publication it is not recommended as initial therapy for mild to moderate CDI.

Complicated CDI is defined as severe disease with the additional findings of hypotension, ileus, or megacolon. Patients with ileus may have limited transit of oral antibiotics to distal sites of infection in the colon. Therefore, in this critically ill group, the recommendation is to give vancomycin orally or through a rectal tube in addition to intravenous metronidazole. Parenteral metronidazole has variable penetration but provides some delivery to the distal colon in the setting of ileus. In contrast, intravenous vancomycin does not achieve appreciable levels intraluminally, and this route of administration is not indicated for treatment of CDI.

No treatment benefit results from combination therapy with oral metronidazole and oral vancomycin for CDI regardless of severity of infection.

### KEY POINT

- Severe *Clostridium difficile* infection should be treated with oral vancomycin.

### Bibliography

Surawicz CM, Brandt LJ, Binion DG, et al. Guidelines for diagnosis, treatment, and prevention of Clostridium difficile infections. Am J Gastroenterol. 2013 Apr;108(4):478-98. [PMID: 23439232]

## Item 66        Answer:     D

### Educational Objective: Diagnose sporadic Creutzfeldt-Jakob disease.

This patient most likely has sporadic Creutzfeldt-Jakob disease (CJD). She has a compatible clinical presentation, with acute onset of rapidly progressive dementia, ataxic gait, and myoclonus. In addition, the cerebrospinal fluid (CSF) demonstrates elevated 14-3-3 protein. Brain biopsy would be required for definitive diagnosis. Sporadic CJD is the most common form of human prion disease, with onset usually in the seventh decade of life. Myoclonus is seen in 90% of patients. In the appropriate clinical setting, the CSF test for the 14-3-3 protein is relatively specific and sensitive for this diagnosis. Other disorders that increase CSF 14-3-3 protein, such as acute stroke or multiple sclerosis, are rarely confused with CJD clinically.

Patients with Alzheimer disease have a more insidious and chronic presentation of dementia and other neurologic findings than seen in this patient.

Kuru was the first prion disease recognized to be transmissible and was linked to cannibalism among tribes of Papua, New Guinea. Common initial manifestations of kuru include headaches and joint pain. Subsequent symptoms include ataxia, dysarthria, and tremors. Myoclonus and dementia are generally seen only late in the illness. The incidence of kuru has decreased with the cessation of the practice of cannibalism.

Neurosyphilis may be asymptomatic or may manifest as syphilitic meningitis, meningovascular syphilis, tabes dorsalis (demyelination of the posterior columns of the spinal cord), or general paresis. General paresis is a chronic meningoencephalitis that results in gradual, progressive loss of cortical function. The CSF is nearly always abnormal, with a lymphocytic pleocytosis and increased protein.

### KEY POINT

- Patients with sporadic Creutzfeldt-Jakob disease usually present in the seventh decade of life and have disordered cognition, ataxia or spasticity, myoclonus, and elevated 14-3-3 protein in the cerebrospinal fluid.

### Bibliography

Lee J, Hyeon JW, Kim SY, Hwang KJ, Ju YR, Ryou C. Review: Laboratory diagnosis and surveillance of Creutzfeldt-Jakob disease. J Med Virol. 2015 Jan;87(1):175-86. [PMID: 24978677]

## Item 67          Answer:   C

**Educational Objective: Diagnose a patient with smallpox.**

Smallpox (variola) infection is the most likely diagnosis in this patient. Smallpox was once a significant worldwide cause of morbidity and mortality but was declared eradicated by the World Health Organization in 1980. Routine active vaccination against this viral illness ended more than 35 years ago. However, owing to its highly contagious nature, ability to cause illness and death, and a population largely nonimmune to infection, smallpox has gained a position on the category A list of potential bioterrorism agents. Because natural infection no longer occurs and most physicians are unfamiliar with the clinical presentation of smallpox, a high level of suspicion must be maintained for the possibility of infection in persons at potential risk, such as this patient with recent travel to an area where bioterrorism agents might be used. An incubation period of 10 to 14 days precedes clinical infection; patients are not contagious during that time. Most infected persons present with a prodromal phase characterized by fever, back pain, headache, vomiting, and pharyngitis. The rash begins as small red dots on the pharyngeal and buccal mucosa, at which time patients become contagious. The lesions then spread in centrifugal fashion to the hands and face, followed by the arms, legs, and feet. Classically, the rash of smallpox progresses in synchronous fashion, from macules to papules to vesicles and pustules before crusting over. Patients remain contagious until all crusts are shed.

Measles, or rubeola, is characterized by fever, malaise, and prominent upper respiratory infection manifestations consisting of the classic triad of conjunctivitis, cough, and coryza. Generally, the exanthem begins 2 to 4 days later, often with small, whitish spots on the buccal mucosa (Koplik spots), followed by a morbilliform rash on the face and neck, which eventually spreads to the extremities. Unlike the rash of smallpox, these lesions typically blanch and do not become vesicular. Additionally, universal measles vaccination has resulted in almost complete elimination of this

childhood disease; therefore, if this patient had been immunized, it would make measles infection much less likely.

Rickettsial pox, caused by *Rickettsia akari*, occurs following the bite of a mite found on a reservoir mouse. A papular lesion initially forms at the site of inoculation, later becoming vesicular before eventually forming an eschar and then healing. Occasionally, the rash may become more generalized but can be differentiated from that seen with smallpox by its asynchronous mode of development. Fever and muscle aches accompany the skin lesion.

Chickenpox (varicella) is the viral infection most resembling smallpox, but clearly differs by fact that the rash is mostly localized to the trunk and spreads centripetally to the periphery of the body. Additionally, varicella lesions can be found in various stages on the same body area at any one time and rarely involve the palms and soles.

### KEY POINT

- The rash of smallpox begins as small red dots on the pharyngeal and buccal mucosa with centrifugal spreading to the hands and face, followed by the arms, legs, and feet; the rash progresses in synchronous fashion, from macules to papules to vesicles and pustules before crusting over.

### Bibliography

Christian MD. Biowarfare and bioterrorism. Crit Care Clin. 2013 Jul;29(3):717-56. [PMID: 23830660]

## Item 68          Answer:   B

**Educational Objective: Identify acute HIV infection as a cause of aseptic meningitis.**

An HIV antigen/antibody combination immunoassay would be most likely to confirm the diagnosis of meningitis due to acute HIV infection in this patient. Acute HIV infection, clinically known as acute retroviral syndrome, is frequently associated with the clinical findings seen in this patient, including fever, lymphadenopathy, pharyngitis, myalgias and arthralgias, and a generalized maculopapular rash. Neurologic findings are also common, with headache occurring in one third of patients and meningitis in a smaller percentage.

Polymerase chain reaction of the cerebrospinal fluid (CSF) is used to test for enterovirus infection. Although enterovirus infections can produce aseptic meningitis, the presence of other findings, such as rash and pharyngitis and the lack of gastrointestinal symptoms characteristic of enterovirus infections, makes this diagnosis less likely than acute HIV infection.

This patient does not have a clear exposure history suggesting Lyme disease, and his clinical presentation, including the lack of the characteristic erythema migrans rash associated with *Borrelia burgdorferi* infection, makes this a less likely diagnosis.

This patient does not have parotitis or orchitis or other findings consistent with acute mumps infection. Also, given

CONT.

his age and the likelihood that he received a primary immunization series against mumps infection as a child, it would be unlikely for him to develop acute mumps infection causing aseptic meningitis in adulthood. Aseptic meningitis can be seen with mumps infection, although the CSF profile typically has a low glucose level.

**KEY POINT**

- Because acute HIV infection can cause aseptic meningitis, patients with meningitis and clinical signs and symptoms of HIV infection–such as pharyngitis, rash, and lymphadenopathy–should undergo testing by nucleic acid amplification.

**Bibliography**

Hanson KE, Reckleff J, Hicks L, Castellano C, Hicks CB. Unsuspected HIV infection in patients presenting with acute meningitis. Clin Infect Dis. 2008 Aug 1;47(3):433–4. [PMID: 18605915]

## Item 69     Answer:    A

**Educational Objective: Diagnose acute osteomyelitis with imaging studies.**

This patient has focal signs and symptoms of an acute bacterial skin and skin-structure infection or osteomyelitis and should undergo contrast-enhanced CT. Physical findings and laboratory data often cannot distinguish soft tissue from bone infection in the acute setting; therefore, imaging studies are heavily relied on in making the diagnosis. Plain radiographs are often not sufficiently sensitive to detect any bony abnormality early on in cases of acute osteomyelitis. MRI would be the imaging modality of choice for evaluating acute or chronic osteomyelitis. However, this patient is unable to undergo MRI because of his metallic implant. CT is helpful in evaluating bone anatomy and delineating the adjacent soft tissues and is the next best choice when MRI with contrast is contraindicated.

Tagged leukocyte nuclear scanning has a relatively high sensitivity for detecting bone infection but is limited by diminished specificity in clinical situations when alternative reasons for accumulation of the radionuclide tracer at the suspected site exist, such as trauma, recent surgery, malignancy, and degenerative bone or joint disease. This is particularly true in assessment of small bones, such as in the feet.

Three-phase nuclear bone scanning carries similar specificity limitations as tagged leukocyte nuclear scanning. However, a negative test result is very good evidence of no bone infection.

**KEY POINT**

- Contrast-enhanced CT is the next best choice when MRI with contrast, the study of choice in evaluating for acute or chronic osteomyelitis, is contraindicated.

**Bibliography**

Lindbloom BJ, James ER, McGarvey WC. Osteomyelitis of the foot and ankle: diagnosis, epidemiology, and treatment. Foot Ankle Clin. 2014 Sep;19(3):569–88. [PMID: 25129362]

## Item 70     Answer:    A

**Educational Objective: Diagnose *Mycobacterium fortuitum* skin infection.**

This patient has *Mycobacterium fortuitum*–associated skin infection. Nontuberculous mycobacteria can colonize salon water, and *M. fortuitum* furunculosis has been well described in patients who obtain pedicures at nail salons that use contaminated whirlpool footbaths. Recent leg shaving with a razor increases the risk for these infections, likely owing to resultant skin nicking. The distal lower-extremity skin lesions, which usually arise 3 to 4 weeks after inoculation of the organism, appear in areas that have been exposed to spa water. Initially papular, these progress to a boil before ulcerating. The fast growth of the organism in culture (<7 days) is consistent with rapidly growing mycobacteria, such as *M. fortuitum*, *Mycobacterium chelonae*, or *Mycobacterium abscessus*.

*Mycobacterium gordonae*, *Mycobacterium kansasii*, and *Mycobacterium marinum* are slowly growing bacteria (that is, growth on solid media requires more than 7 days and usually 2 to 4 weeks). *M. gordonae* is a ubiquitous organism that rarely causes infection in immunocompetent hosts. Isolation of the organism in patients who are not immunosuppressed usually reflects colonization or contamination.

An environmental pathogen, *M. kansasii* typically causes a lung infection that mimics tuberculosis. Risk factors include COPD, HIV, alcohol abuse, exogenous immunosuppression, and cancer. Skin infection is uncommon and usually occurs in immunosuppressed patients with disseminated disease.

*M. marinum* can cause trauma-associated skin infection after exposure to fresh or salt water, including fish tanks and swimming pools. Initially papular before ulcerating, skin lesions are sometimes referred to as "fish tank granuloma." The rapid growth of the culture from this patient's lesions (<7 days) makes *M. marinum* unlikely.

**KEY POINT**

- *Mycobacterium fortuitum* furunculosis is a well-described skin infection in patients who obtain pedicures at nail salons that use contaminated whirlpool footbaths.

**Bibliography**

Winthrop KL, Abrams M, Yakrus M, et al. An outbreak of mycobacterial furunculosis associated with footbaths at a nail salon. N Engl J Med. 2002 May 2;346(18):1366–71. [PMID: 11986410]

## Item 71     Answer:    B

**Educational Objective: Provide empiric antimicrobial therapy with meropenem and vancomycin for a patient with nosocomial bacterial meningitis.**

This patient should begin empiric antimicrobial therapy with intravenous meropenem and vancomycin. He developed

**CONT.**

fever, nuchal rigidity, and altered mental status after a neurosurgical intervention, and analysis of the cerebrospinal fluid is consistent with bacterial meningitis following an invasive central nervous system (CNS) surgical procedure. In the setting of nosocomial meningitis, empiric antimicrobial therapy must cover a broad spectrum of pathogens, including gram-negative organisms (including *Pseudomonas aeruginosa*, *Acinetobacter* species, and Enterobacteriaceae) and *Staphylococcus aureus* (including methicillin-resistant *S. aureus* [MRSA]). Meropenem, a monobactam, is a broad-spectrum, bactericidal β-lactam with excellent coverage of gram-positive and gram-negative organisms that effectively penetrates the CNS, making it an excellent agent for empiric treatment of nosocomial meningitis. Vancomycin is necessary to provide coverage for possible β-lactam gram-positive organisms, including MRSA. Therefore, the combination of meropenem and vancomycin is the most appropriate antibiotic regimen to cover the potential causative pathogens in this patient.

Because the combination of vancomycin and ceftriaxone, with or without ampicillin, would not provide adequate coverage for *P. aeruginosa*, this regimen would not be the most appropriate treatment choice in this patient.

Moxifloxacin may cover appropriate gram-negative and gram-positive organisms; however, fluoroquinolones have not been well studied for use in bacterial meningitis and are generally reserved for patients with an allergy to β-lactam antibiotics. Fluoroquinolones also do not provide empiric coverage for MRSA.

**KEY POINT**

- Empiric antimicrobial therapy for nosocomial meningitis must cover a broad spectrum of pathogens, including gram-negative organisms and *Staphylococcus aureus*, particularly methicillin-resistant *S. aureus*.

**Bibliography**
van de Beek D, Drake JM, Tunkel AR. Nosocomial bacterial meningitis. N Engl J Med. 2010 Jan 14;362(2):146-54. [PMID: 20071704]

## Item 72    Answer:    C

**Educational Objective: Manage initiation of treatment for a patient with newly diagnosed HIV infection.**

The most appropriate next step in management is to defer initiation of antiretroviral therapy (ART) or other HIV-associated treatment pending further discussion of this patient's diagnosis and its management. Although ART initiation is recommended in all patients regardless of CD4 cell count and there are public health benefits to early treatment to reduce transmission of infection, this patient raises several concerns for possible poor adherence to therapy and the likelihood of suboptimal treatment. Adherence to HIV treatment may be influenced by numerous factors, including behavioral (denial, nondisclosure of HIV status, fear of

stigma), psychosocial (mental illness or low levels of social support), and structural (poverty, homelessness, inconsistent access to medications) barriers; low health literacy; active substance use; and age (young adults have increased difficulty with adherence). It is important for patients with any of these risk factors to discuss their disease and the goals of therapy to optimize the chance for adequate adherence to treatment. Therefore, the most prudent strategy is to take additional time for counseling and education to prepare this patient for success in adhering to ART and other HIV treatments. Because his CD4 cell count is still high and viral load is low, his risk for rapid progression of disease is low, allowing additional time to accomplish this.

The patient's CD4 cell count is not less than 200/μL and is unlikely to decrease that low in the near future considering his high CD4 cell count now and low level of viral activity. Therefore, providing *Pneumocystis jirovecii* prophylaxis with trimethoprim-sulfamethoxazole before initiating ART is unnecessary.

Because of the concerns for adherence with this patient, initiation of any ART is best delayed until the chances for medication adherence are improved. Once that is accomplished, however, it would be inappropriate to wait for an arbitrary CD4 count to begin therapy. There are benefits to initiating ART early, in terms of both improving the patient's health and reducing potential transmission to others.

**KEY POINT**

- For patients with high CD4 cell counts and low viral loads, it is safe to defer antiretroviral therapy until chances for medication adherence are improved.

**Bibliography**
Panel on Antiretroviral Guidelines for Adults and Adolescents. Guidelines for the use of antiretroviral agents in HIV-1-infected adults and adolescents. Department of Health and Human Services. https://aidsinfo.nih.gov/contentfiles/lvguidelines/adultandadolescentgl.pdf. Accessed July 21, 2015.

## Item 73    Answer:    E

**Educational Objective: Manage asymptomatic candiduria.**

This patient has asymptomatic candiduria, which requires no antifungal therapy. Candiduria is a common finding in patients in the ICU. *Candida albicans* is the most common colonizing and infecting species, and most strains are fluconazole susceptible. The presence of candiduria may represent a contaminated urine sample, colonization of the bladder or catheter, upper or lower urinary tract infection (UTI), or a manifestation of candidemia rather than true UTI. In patients who have candiduria and an indwelling urinary catheter, the catheter should be removed, if possible, and a urine sample obtained several days later to assess whether the candiduria has resolved. If the catheter cannot be removed, it should be replaced and a urine sample collected through the new catheter. Most patients with candiduria are asymptomatic, and asymptomatic candiduria rarely results

**CONT.**

in candidemia. Asymptomatic candiduria should not be treated with antifungal agents except in certain populations at risk for candidemia, including patients who are neutropenic or who are undergoing urinary tract procedures. Patients who have symptoms of UTI should be treated. If treatment becomes necessary, oral fluconazole is the drug of choice.

Amphotericin B and flucytosine are less desirable alternatives to fluconazole. Local instillation of amphotericin B into the bladder is effective in eliminating the organism, but the effect is short lived and guidelines on the management of urinary tract candidiasis do not recommend it except for a few situations, including as adjunctive treatment for *Candida glabrata* or *Candida krusei* cystitis.

The echinocandins (micafungin, anidulafungin, and caspofungin), voriconazole, and posaconazole are not recommended for treatment of *Candida* UTI because very little active drug is found in the urine.

**KEY POINT**

- Patients with asymptomatic candiduria require no antifungal therapy, except in certain populations at risk for candidemia; however, if an indwelling catheter is present, it should be removed if possible.

**Bibliography**

Revankar SG, Hasan MS, Revankar VS, Sobel JD. Long-term follow-up of patients with candiduria. Eur J Clin Microbiol Infect Dis. 2011 Feb;30(2):137-40. [PMID: 20857164]

## Item 74      Answer:   C

**Educational Objective: Monitor a patient receiving outpatient parenteral nafcillin therapy.**

Serum creatinine level, complete blood count, and liver enzyme tests should be monitored weekly in this patient. Outpatient parenteral antimicrobial therapy (OPAT) is becoming more common, with some patients receiving therapy for extended periods (≥6 weeks for osteomyelitis). Outpatient monitoring for adverse drug effects and other potential complications resulting from intravenous administration (such as intravenous catheter infection) are part of an OPAT management plan. The plan should be confirmed with all physicians involved in the care of the patient. The monitoring schedule for adverse drug effects depends on the agent being used; the most common antibiotics used for OPAT require weekly laboratory monitoring. For nafcillin, this includes monitoring for bone marrow suppression with a complete blood count (CBC) and liver enzyme tests. Kidney function testing with a serum creatinine level should also be performed weekly, because the dosage of nafcillin may require adjustment if significant deterioration of kidney function occurs or if the patient already has kidney injury and it improves while receiving therapy. Nafcillin does not affect potassium levels, so no monitoring is needed. Monitoring of oxacillin and carbapenems is similar to that of nafcillin, and monitoring of other β-lactam antibiotics is similar to that of nafcillin except that liver enzyme testing

is not necessary; antipseudomonal penicillins necessitate checking the serum potassium level weekly.

**KEY POINT**

- Patients undergoing outpatient parenteral antimicrobial therapy must undergo weekly monitoring for adverse drug effects.

**Bibliography**

Tice AD, Relm SJ, Dalovision JR, et al. Practice guidelines for outpatient parenteral antimicrobial therapy. Clin Infect Dis. 2004;38:1651-1672. [PMID: 15227610]

## Item 75      Answer:   D

**Educational Objective: Treat a patient with potential drug-resistant *Streptococcus pneumoniae* community-acquired pneumonia with appropriate antibiotic therapy.**

This patient should begin empiric antibiotic therapy with moxifloxacin. He has community-acquired pneumonia (CAP) confirmed by chest radiograph. Because he is lacking other risk factors or associated comorbid conditions that would make other pathogens more likely, his CAP infection is probably caused by *Streptococcus pneumoniae*. The possibility of drug-resistant *S. pneumoniae* (DRSP) should be assessed because it will determine which agents are appropriate for empiric treatment. Factors that increase the risk for DRSP include age greater than 65 years, alcoholism, immunosuppression, certain medical comorbidities (COPD, chronic liver or kidney disease, cancer, diabetes, functional or anatomic asplenia, chronic heart disease), and recent (within the past 3-6 months) antimicrobial therapy with a β-lactam, macrolide, or fluoroquinolone antibiotic. Recent β-lactam use is associated with an increased risk for β-lactam resistance, while recent use of macrolides or fluoroquinolones is associated with pneumococcal resistance to the same class of antibiotic. Because this patient received treatment with a β-lactam within the past 3 months, he is at increased risk for DRSP. Recommended empiric therapy for patients with possible DRSP includes a respiratory fluoroquinolone (such as moxifloxacin) or a β-lactam plus a macrolide or doxycycline; however, because he was recently treated with a β-lactam antibiotic, treatment with a respiratory fluoroquinolone would be preferable.

Combination therapy with a β-lactam plus a macrolide or doxycycline is recommended, rather than monotherapy with a β-lactam, to provide coverage for atypical pathogens (such as *Mycoplasma* species), which are common causes of CAP. However, this therapy is not optimal for this patient with recent β-lactam use.

Patients with CAP who are otherwise healthy and without risk factors for DRSP are eligible for monotherapy with a macrolide (such as azithromycin) or doxycycline. However, this patient's recent use of antibiotics and subsequent increased risk for DRSP make either of these agents an inappropriate therapeutic choice.

### KEY POINT

- Patients with uncomplicated community-acquired pneumonia who are suspected of having infection with drug-resistant *Streptococcus pneumoniae* should be treated empirically with a respiratory fluoroquinolone or a β-lactam plus a macrolide or doxycycline.

### Bibliography

Mandell LA, Wunderink RG, Anzueto A, et al; Infectious Diseases Society of America, American Thoracic Society. Infectious Diseases Society of America/American Thoracic Society consensus guidelines on the management of community-acquired pneumonia in adults. Clin Infect Dis. 2007 Mar 1;44(Suppl 2):S27-72. [PMID: 17278083]

## Item 76        Answer:    A

### Educational Objective: Diagnose a tick-borne coinfection.

This patient most likely has coinfection with *Anaplasma phagocytophilum,* a bacterium spread by the *Ixodes* tick (the same vector associated with Lyme disease). The constellation of fever, leukopenia, thrombocytopenia, and mild elevation in liver enzymes in a patient with recent Lyme disease is highly suggestive of anaplasmosis. Among patients with erythema migrans, up to 10% are coinfected with anaplasmosis. Although amoxicillin is active against Lyme disease, it is not effective therapy for *A. phagocytophila.* Doxycycline would have offered the advantage of treating the Lyme disease and an incubating asymptomatic infection with *Anaplasma.* Recrudescent symptoms of Lyme disease would not be expected in a patient receiving treatment, and patients with erythema migrans rarely develop later-stage disease after completing therapy.

*Babesia microti* is a parasite also transmitted by the *Ixodes* tick. Patients with symptomatic babesiosis often present with fever and signs of hemolysis, including jaundice, scleral icterus, and splenomegaly. This patient has leukopenia, thrombocytopenia, and a normal hematocrit and haptoglobin level, making babesiosis unlikely.

Powassan virus is also spread by *Ixodes* ticks but causes meningoencephalitis. No human coinfection has been documented with both Lyme disease and Powassan virus infection.

Serial episodes of erythema migrans can occur, and, until recently, it has been debated whether a second episode of erythema migrans represents relapse of inadequately treated disease. Genotyping of sequential erythema migrans lesions has shown that these cases are caused by a genetically distinct strain of *Borrelia* and represent reinfection rather than latent infection.

### KEY POINT

- Fever, leukopenia, and thrombocytopenia in a patient undergoing treatment for Lyme disease suggest coinfection with *Anaplasma phagocytophilum.*

### Bibliography

Horowitz HW, Aguero-Rosenfeld ME, Holmgren D, et al. Lyme disease and human granulocytic anaplasmosis coinfection: impact of case definition on coinfection rates and illness severity. Clin Infect Dis. 2013 Jan;56(1):93-9. [PMID: 23042964]

## Item 77        Answer:    B

### Educational Objective: Manage cystitis in an older woman.

This older adult patient most likely has cystitis and should begin nitrofurantoin therapy. Although the most common symptoms of cystitis in premenopausal women are dysuria, frequency, urgency, and suprapubic discomfort, postmenopausal women with cystitis may experience incontinence. Fever is unusual. The urine dipstick reveals pyuria and bacteriuria with positivity for leukocyte esterase and nitrites, respectively. With her symptoms and positive results on urine dipstick, cystitis is highly likely. Urinary tract infection (UTI) is one of the most commonly diagnosed infections in older adults, and *Escherichia coli* is the most frequently isolated organism. In one study, *E. coli* accounted for more than 80% of UTIs in this population. The treatment of cystitis in older adults who do not have significant concurrent medical illnesses is the same as that used in younger patients. This patient should begin nitrofurantoin, 100 mg twice daily for 5 days. Nitrofurantoin should not be used in patients whose creatinine clearance is less than 50 mL/min. Trimethoprim-sulfamethoxazole, one double-strength tablet twice daily for 3 days, is first-line therapy in the absence of a sulfa allergy and if local *E. coli* resistance to trimethoprim-sulfamethoxazole is less than 20%. Most women with lower UTI have only a superficial mucosal infection and can be cured with short courses of therapy. The advantages of short-course therapy include better adherence, lower cost, fewer adverse effects, and less selective pressure for the emergence of resistant organisms. Three days of therapy is considered superior to single-dose therapy. Nitrofurantoin for 5 days demonstrates better efficacy than a 3-day course of this medication. Treatment is indicated because this patient is symptomatic. If she were asymptomatic, treatment would not be indicated.

Fluoroquinolones, such as levofloxacin and ciprofloxacin, are considered second-line therapy because of their higher cost and the concern for emergence of resistance with widespread use.

A urine culture is indicated if pyelonephritis, complicated UTI, recurrent UTI, multiple antibiotic allergies, or a resistant organism is suspected; in pregnant women with asymptomatic bacteriuria; and for patients undergoing urologic procedures. Urine cultures are not generally indicated to diagnose cystitis.

### KEY POINT

- Treatment is indicated in all patients with symptomatic cystitis, and nitrofurantoin for 5 days is the regimen of choice in patients allergic to sulfa drugs.

**Bibliography**

Matthews SJ, Lancaster JW. Urinary tract infections in the elderly population. Am J Geriatr Pharmacother. 2011 Oct;9(5):286-309. [PMID: 21840265]

**Item 78      Answer:      B**

**Educational Objective: Treat suspected methicillin-resistant *Staphylococcus aureus* cellulitis and bacteremia in a patient who is intolerant of vancomycin.**

The most appropriate treatment for this patient is daptomycin. He has a history of methicillin-resistant *Staphylococcus aureus* (MRSA) skin infections and now presents with injection drug use–associated cellulitis and bacteremia with gram-positive cocci in clusters, presumably MRSA. Because of his history of vancomycin intolerance, daptomycin, an alternative to vancomycin for the empiric treatment of MRSA-associated bacteremia and infective endocarditis, should be given. Daptomycin is a lipopeptide-type antibiotic and is bactericidal against MRSA. He will require echocardiography and repeat blood cultures after intravenous antibiotics have been initiated. Additionally, patients receiving daptomycin should be assessed regularly for clinical or laboratory signs of muscle weakness or pain, particularly in those receiving statin-based lipid-lowering agents or with kidney disease. Intravenous antibiotics must be administered for at least 2 weeks for *S. aureus* bacteremia.

Ceftriaxone could be used to treat nonpurulent cellulitis because β-hemolytic streptococci are the likely cause. However, it does not provide effective coverage against MRSA.

Imipenem, a broad-spectrum β-lactam antibiotic with activity against many aerobic and anaerobic bacteria, does not provide effective coverage against MRSA.

Additionally, *S. aureus* that may be resistant to methicillin also may be resistant to oxacillin, nafcillin, and other β-lactam agents, including ceftriaxone and imipenem. Nafcillin or oxacillin would be appropriate choices if the infection were found to be caused by methicillin-susceptible *S. aureus*. Until that time, however, empiric therapy should reliably target MRSA. The only β-lactam with reliable activity against MRSA is ceftaroline, a fifth-generation cephalosporin approved by the FDA for treatment of skin infections and community-acquired bacterial pneumonia.

**KEY POINT**

- Daptomycin is an effective alternative to vancomycin for the treatment of methicillin-resistant *Staphylococcus aureus* cellulitis and bacteremia in patients unable to take vancomycin.

**Bibliography**

Liu C, Bayer A, Cosgrove SE, et al; Infectious Diseases Society of America. Clinical practice guidelines by the Infectious Diseases Society of America for the treatment of methicillin-resistant Staphylococcus aureus infections in adults and children [erratum in Clin Infect Dis. 2011 Aug 1;53(3):319]. Clin Infect Dis. 2011 Feb 1;52(3):e18-55. [PMID: 21208910]

**Item 79      Answer:      B**

**Educational Objective: Treat urethritis due to *Chlamydia trachomatis* with azithromycin.**

This patient has urethritis due to *Chlamydia trachomatis* and should be treated with azithromycin. Azithromycin, a macrolide antibiotic, is the preferred treatment of urethritis and cervicitis due to *C. trachomatis* because it can be given as single-dose therapy. The patient should be screened for other sexually transmitted infections and encouraged to refer his sexual partner for evaluation and treatment. Doxycycline is also effective against chlamydia; however, a 7-day regimen is required. The single-dose therapy of azithromycin is preferred to enhance adherence.

Penicillins have activity against *C. trachomatis* but have far lower cure rates than do azithromycin, doxycycline, or the fluoroquinolones ofloxacin or levofloxacin. Because of the lower cure rate, a test of cure is indicated when these agents are used.

Cefixime, an oral third-generation cephalosporin, has no activity against *C. trachomatis*, although it is an alternative for the treatment of *Neisseria gonorrhoeae* infections if ceftriaxone is unavailable. It would provide adequate antimicrobial coverage for treatment of urinary tract infection; however, this patient's colony count of *Escherichia coli* in the urine culture is insignificant and does not warrant therapy.

Dual treatment with ceftriaxone plus azithromycin for *N. gonorrhoeae* and *C. trachomatis* would be appropriate if empiric therapy were given before availability of the nucleic acid amplification test results. If only *N. gonorrhoeae* is diagnosed, dual therapy with ceftriaxone and azithromycin is recommended because of the high incidence of concomitant infection with *C. trachomatis*. Dual therapy also offers potential increased efficacy for treating gonorrhea in men, considering increasing minimum inhibitor concentrations for cephalosporins among gonorrhea isolates.

**KEY POINT**

- The preferred therapy for urethritis due to *Chlamydia trachomatis* is single-dose azithromycin for optimum adherence; alternative treatments include longer courses of doxycycline or the fluoroquinolones ofloxacin or levofloxacin.

**Bibliography**

Workowski K. In the clinic. Chlamydia and gonorrhea [erratum in Ann Intern Med. 2013 Mar 19;158(6):504]. Ann Intern Med. 2013 Feb 5;158(3): ITC2-1. [PMID: 23381058]

**Item 80      Answer:      B**

**Educational Objective: Treat a patient with acute, uncomplicated pyelonephritis.**

This patient should begin treatment with ciprofloxacin. She has signs and symptoms most consistent with acute pyelonephritis. Cystitis is infection of the bladder and lower urinary tract and commonly presents with dysuria, frequency, and urgency. However, the presence of fever or other systemic symptoms (chills, nausea, vomiting) and back or flank pain are more consistent with pyelonephritis, or kidney infection. Lower urinary tract symptoms may antedate fever and upper urinary tract symptoms by approximately 2 days. Most cases of pyelonephritis may be managed in the ambulatory setting; indications for hospitalization include hemodynamic instability, inability to tolerate oral medications, host factors such as pregnancy or presence of kidney stones or other obstructions, presence of comorbidities, and an unstable social situation that may compromise adherence or follow-up. A urine culture and susceptibility testing should always be performed in patients with suspected pyelonephritis to confirm the diagnosis and guide therapy. However, empiric treatment should be provided pending culture results, with initial therapy modified appropriately when the infecting organism is identified and susceptibilities are known. A fluoroquinolone is the preferred agent for empiric therapy when resistance in the community does not exceed 10%. If fluoroquinolone resistance exceeds 10%, an initial, one-time intravenous dose of a long-acting agent such as ceftriaxone or a 24-hour dose of an aminoglycoside should be administered. A 7-day course of a fluoroquinolone is as effective as a 14-day course in women. If high-dose levofloxacin (750 mg) is administered, the duration is 5 days. If once-daily oral ciprofloxacin (1000 mg extended release) is administered, it should be given for 7 days.

Ampicillin with gentamicin is an appropriate regimen for treating acute pyelonephritis in patients requiring hospitalization. Other choices for hospitalized patients include therapy with a fluoroquinolone, an extended-spectrum cephalosporin, an extended-spectrum penicillin, or a carbapenem such as ertapenem. However, despite this patient's systemic findings, she is clinically stable and can undergo outpatient therapy. Therefore, intravenous, broad-spectrum antibiotic therapy with either ampicillin with gentamicin or ertapenem is not indicated.

Nitrofurantoin or fosfomycin are indicated for treatment of uncomplicated cystitis and are not effective for pyelonephritis because they do not achieve adequate tissue levels in the kidney parenchyma. Therefore, they are not appropriate for patients with pyelonephritis.

### KEY POINT

- Patients with acute pyelonephritis who do not require hospitalization should begin empiric treatment with an oral fluoroquinolone, such as ciprofloxacin.

### Bibliography

Gupta K, Hooton TM, Naber KG, et al; Infectious Diseases Society of America; European Society for Microbiology and Infectious Diseases. International clinical practice guidelines for the treatment of acute uncomplicated cystitis and pyelonephritis in women: a 2010 update by the Infectious Diseases Society of America and the European Society for Microbiology and Infectious Diseases. Clin Infect Dis. 2011;52(5):3103-20. [PMID: 21292654]

## Item 81        Answer:    A

**Educational Objective: Diagnose chronic osteomyelitis with histopathologic and microbiologic studies.**

The most appropriate management for this patient is bone biopsy and culture. He has classic signs of long-bone osteomyelitis related to his previous fracture. The presence of chronic or intermittent drainage from a demonstrable sinus tract overlying an area of previous trauma, along with consistent clinical findings and radiographic evidence of a bone sequestra (dead bone) or involucrum (new bone formation), are hallmarks of chronic osteomyelitis. Other than local signs of ongoing infection, patients with chronic osteomyelitis rarely manifest systemic symptoms. Laboratory studies are generally not diagnostically helpful because leukocyte counts are almost always normal and inflammatory markers (erythrocyte sedimentation rate and C-reactive protein), although supportive of chronic infection when elevated, are very nonspecific for focal infection. Bone biopsy for histopathologic assessment and full microbiologic studies is important for diagnosing osteomyelitis, excluding other entities (such as neoplasm), and isolating the causative pathogen(s).

With the exception of *Staphylococcus aureus*, microorganisms from the surface of wounds or draining sinus tracts rarely correlate with cultures obtained from bone specimens and should not be acted upon. However, when *S. aureus* is isolated, it may be considered the causative pathogen, and therapy may be initiated without bone biopsy when the clinical picture is consistent with osteomyelitis. This patient's bone infection likely resulted from the introduction of bacteria at the time of his military injury. Although osteomyelitis resulting from hematogenous entrance of bacteria most often involves a single organism (such as *S. aureus*), infection that arises from a contiguous focus of infection or open trauma may comprise a multitude of potential pathogens alone or in combination.

Initiating empiric antimicrobial therapy without an attempt at confirming a histologic and microbiologic diagnosis is strongly discouraged and best delayed until more information is available to best select specific antimicrobial agent(s), route of administration, and duration of therapy.

MRI is the most sensitive and specific imaging modality for diagnosing osteomyelitis but is unnecessary in the presence of a chronic draining sinus. The demonstration of microorganisms coupled with characteristic features of osteomyelitis eliminates the need for MRI confirmation of the diagnosis.

### KEY POINT

- Histopathology and full microbiologic studies are important for diagnosing osteomyelitis and isolating the causative pathogen in order to direct appropriate treatment.

### Bibliography

Hatzenbuehler J, Pulling TJ. Diagnosis and management of osteomyelitis. Am Fam Physician. 2011 Nov 1;84(9):1027-33. [PMID: 22046943]

## Item 82    Answer:    D

**Educational Objective: Interpret results of serologic testing for Lyme disease.**

This patient has inflammatory arthritis and tests negative for *Borrelia burgdorferi*, so she requires no additional evaluation or treatment for Lyme disease. Arthritis is a late manifestation of Lyme disease, typically occurring months to years after infection. This typically presents as inflammatory arthritis, involving a single or limited number of large joints, with the knee most commonly affected. Even without treatment, symptoms wax and wane, with spontaneous remission of inflammation often followed several months later by involvement of the same or a different joint. Because the clinical presentation of Lyme arthritis is nonspecific, laboratory confirmation of infection is required using a two-tiered serologic testing strategy. The initial test, an enzyme immunoassay (EIA), is exquisitely sensitive but not specific. If the result of this test is negative, no further evaluation is necessary. When the EIA finding is positive or equivocal, a more specific Western blot test is recommended for confirmation. A negative Western blot result is interpreted as a negative serologic result. A positive result must be further interpreted with respect to acuity of symptoms. When symptoms are present for less than 1 month, an isolated positive IgM Western blot result may be diagnostic of acute infection. However, symptoms present for more than 1 month provide ample time for IgG seroconversion. Many laboratories perform the IgM and IgG Western blots reflexively on any sample with a positive EIA finding. When this is the case, a positive Western blot IgM result without associated positive IgG result in a patient with more than 30 days of symptoms should be interpreted as a false-positive result. Therefore, results of Lyme serologic testing for this patient would be interpreted as negative, and the diagnosis of Lyme arthritis excluded. Further evaluation or treatment for Lyme disease is not necessary at this time, and other causes for this patient's inflammatory arthritis should be evaluated.

Detection of *Borrelia* bacteria in synovial fluid or tissue is not necessary to diagnose Lyme arthritis and would be indicated only in selected scenarios, such as new-onset arthritis in a patient previously known to be seropositive for Lyme disease.

If the Western blot IgG had returned positive, the recommended treatment would be a 28-day course of doxycycline or amoxicillin. Parenteral therapy with ceftriaxone would be indicated for patients with Lyme arthritis who do not experience a clinical response to oral antibiotics.

### KEY POINT

- Lyme arthritis is excluded if symptoms have been present for longer than 1 month and Western blot IgG result is negative; there is no need for further evaluation or treatment for Lyme disease in these patients.

### Bibliography

DeBiasi RL. A concise critical analysis of serologic testing for the diagnosis of Lyme disease. Curr Infect Dis Rep. 2014 Dec;16(12):450. [PMID: 25351855]

## Item 83    Answer:    C

**Educational Objective: Diagnose *Vibrio* gastroenteritis.**

This patient's dysentery is most likely caused by *Vibrio parahaemolyticus* gastrointestinal infection. Bloody stools, fever, and vomiting commonly occur with *Vibrio* infection. The fact that other diners developed a gastrointestinal illness suggests a common source associated with the shared meal. *Vibrio* species are widespread in salt or brackish water, and human infections are associated with ingestion of contaminated seafood, particularly shellfish. In a large case series of *V. parahaemolyticus* infections reported to the U.S. Centers for Disease Control and Prevention, bloody diarrhea was noted in 29% of cases. Chronic liver disease is a risk factor for severe infection with this organism, and sepsis is a common and often fatal complication in this population. *Vibrio* species do not grow well on traditional stool culture media, so when this diagnosis is being considered, the laboratory should be notified to allow plating onto saline-enriched agar.

*Clostridium difficile* colitis has a similar presentation with diarrhea, fever, and abdominal pain and cramping, but gross blood in the stool is uncommon. *C. difficile* infection is not a foodborne illness, and therefore a clustering of cases following a shared meal would not be expected.

Norovirus is the leading cause of foodborne outbreaks in the United States, with spread through fecal-oral contamination. This virus causes a watery stool, often with associated vomiting; however, fever is uncommon and grossly bloody stools would exclude this diagnosis.

Yersiniosis typically occurs following ingestion of contaminated food or water. Outbreaks of *Yersinia enterocolitica* have been traced to consumption of chitterlings (pork intestines). *Yersinia* gastroenteritis is clinically indistinguishable from other forms of inflammatory diarrhea and is most commonly identified in young children. It does not cause grossly bloody stools. In some cases, diarrhea may be absent with bacteria localizing to lymphoid tissue in Peyer patches and associated mesenteric lymph nodes. This presentation may mimic appendicitis clinically.

### KEY POINT

- Gastrointestinal infections caused by *Vibrio* species are associated with ingestion of contaminated seafood, particularly shellfish, and can be severe in patients with liver dysfunction.

### Bibliography

Newton AE, Garrett N, Stroika SG, Halpin JL, Turnsek M, Mody RK; Centers for Disease Control and Prevention (CDC). Increase in Vibrio parahaemolyticus infections associated with consumption of Atlantic Coast shellfish–2013. MMWR Morb Mortal Wkly Rep. 2014 Apr 18;63(15):335-6. [PMID: 24739344]

## Item 84    Answer:    E

**Educational Objective: Manage selective IgA deficiency.**

Clinical follow-up without directed treatment is indicated for this patient. She has selective IgA deficiency, which has no specific therapy except for antibiotic treatment as needed for those with recurrent sinopulmonary infections. Selective IgA deficiency is the most common of the congenital immune defects, with an incidence of about 1:500. The disease is usually sporadic, but autosomal dominant and autosomal recessive inheritance is found. Most people with IgA deficiency are asymptomatic, although the most common clinical manifestation is sinopulmonary infection, which is often the reason quantitative serum immunoglobulin levels are obtained. IgA deficiency is defined as a serum IgA level less than 7 mg/dL (0.07 g/L). A less common but potentially severe finding in selective IgA deficiency is anaphylaxis with blood product transfusion. IgA deficiency is also frequently associated with autoimmune illnesses, including systemic lupus erythematosus, rheumatoid arthritis, hemolytic anemia, and immune thrombocytopenic purpura. Additional manifestations include atopic eczema, asthma, urticaria, and a variety of other allergic disorders. Gastrointestinal disorders, including infection with *Giardia lamblia*, may also occur. Despite these multiple potential clinical consequences associated with IgA deficiency, the indicated treatment approach is primarily preventive and supportive.

Patients with terminal complement deficiencies are at higher risk for meningococcal disease, but those with immunoglobulin deficiency are not. Therefore, the meningococcal conjugate vaccine is not indicated specifically for IgA deficiency.

Secreted IgA is produced and generally acts locally. Therefore, administration of intravenous concentrates of IgA would not achieve adequate levels in mucosal secretions, so it would not be helpful in this patient.

IgA deficiency is selective, occurring without deficits in other immunoglobulins in these patients. Therefore, administration of intravenous immune globulin would not be indicated in this patient. Intravenous immune globulin is used in patients with severe deficiencies in most immunoglobulins, as is seen in X-linked agammaglobulinemia and common variable immunodeficiency.

Stem cell or bone marrow transplantation is appropriate treatment for severe combined immune deficiency syndrome, but not selective IgA deficiency. Selective IgA deficiency is usually asymptomatic or has mild symptoms that are easily treated or managed; therefore, the potential risks and long-term immunosuppression associated with stem or bone marrow transplantation are greater than the potential benefits of this treatment for selective IgA deficiency.

### KEY POINT

• Patients with selective IgA deficiency require no specific therapy except for preventive measures against known potential complications and as-needed antibiotic therapy for those with recurrent sinopulmonary infections.

**Bibliography**
Singh K, Chang C, Gershwin ME. IgA deficiency and autoimmunity. Autoimmun Rev. 2014 Feb;13(2):163-77. [PMID: 24157629]

## Item 85    Answer:    A

**Educational Objective: Treat a patient with early localized Lyme disease.**

This patient has an enlarging erythematous skin lesion with central clearing suggestive of erythema migrans and should be prescribed doxycycline. Erythema migrans is the most common presentation of Lyme disease, seen in up to 80% of patients, although an initial heterogenous patch of erythroderma is more common than the classic target-like appearance. Erythema migrans is often the only manifestation of early localized Lyme disease because fevers or constitutional symptoms are uncommon at this stage. Treatment of early stage Lyme disease with doxycycline prevents progression to later-stage cardiac, neurologic, or rheumatologic complications in more than 90% of patients. Amoxicillin or cefuroxime axetil could be alternative options for the treatment of Lyme disease; however, these agents have not been evaluated for the treatment of southern tick–associated rash illness (STARI). STARI also presents as erythema migrans and can be identical to Lyme disease. Therefore, in a patient presenting with erythema migrans, treatment with an oral antibiotic active against localized Lyme disease and STARI, such as doxycycline, would be most appropriate.

Babesiosis is a parasitic disease that is spread by the same tick as Lyme disease but does not cause erythema migrans. Although coinfection with *Borrelia burgdorferi* can occur, serologic testing is not recommended in the absence of signs or symptoms, which include fever, jaundice, and scleral icterus. Lyme disease and human granulocytic anaplasmosis coinfection has also been reported; however, doxycycline is active against the bacterium causing this infection as well.

Laboratory testing for Lyme disease is insensitive at the early stage of infection, with less than 50% of patients having detectable titers to *B. burgdorferi*. In addition, laboratory confirmation is not necessary when erythema migrans is present.

### KEY POINT

• Early localized Lyme disease and southern tick–associated rash illness present with erythema migrans and are clinically indistinguishable; therefore, patients with erythema migrans should be treated with doxycycline, which is effective in both conditions.

## Bibliography

Shapiro ED. Clinical practice. Lyme disease. N Engl J Med. 2014 May 1;370(18):1724–31. [PMID: 24785207]

## Item 86        Answer:    C

**Educational Objective: Identify the most common complication of *Escherichia coli* O157:H7 dysentery.**

This patient with dysentery most likely has *Escherichia coli* infection and is at risk for hemolytic uremic syndrome (HUS). *E. coli* O157:H7, a Shiga toxin–producing *E. coli* (STEC) serotype, is the most common cause of acute bloody diarrhea in the United States. It differs from other causes of dysentery in that fever is distinctly uncommon. STEC organisms are widespread in the gastrointestinal tract of domesticated animals, particularly cattle, and cause disease through ingestion of contaminated food or, as in this case, unpasteurized milk. One of the most serious complications of STEC infection is the development of HUS, which occurs in 5% to 10% of cases, most frequently in children. HUS is a form of thrombotic microangiopathy characterized by fever, hemolytic anemia, consumptive thrombocytopenia, neurologic findings, and kidney failure. Antibiotic and antimotility therapies are both associated with increased risk for HUS and should not be prescribed when there is clinical concern for STEC gastrointestinal disease.

The other choices are complications associated with bacterial causes of dysentery, but unlike STEC infections, these are usually associated with fevers. Aortitis is an inflammation of the aortic wall and can potentially be caused by *Salmonella* infection, which has a propensity for causing endovascular infection, particularly when there is significant atherosclerosis or graft material. Guillain-Barré syndrome is a rare complication of *Campylobacter* infection, occurring in less than 1% of cases; however, up to 40% of cases of Guillain-Barré are triggered by an antecedent *Campylobacter* infection. Several strains of *Yersinia* cause infection of the mesenteric lymph nodes and can mimic acute appendicitis. Grossly bloody stools are uncommon with *Yersinia* infection. Reactive arthritis can occur following *Campylobacter*, *Shigella*, *Salmonella*, or *Yersinia* infections in patients who are positive for the HLA-B27 gene.

### KEY POINT

- One of the most serious complications of *Escherichia coli* O157:H7 infection is hemolytic uremic syndrome, with this risk increased if antibiotics or antimotility therapy is administered.

## Bibliography

Frank C, Werber D, Cramer JP, et al; HUS Investigation Team. Epidemic profile of Shiga-toxin-producing Escherichia coli O104:H4 outbreak in Germany. N Engl J Med. 2011 Nov 10;365(19):1771–80. [PMID: 21696328]

## Item 87        Answer:    B

**Educational Objective: Manage an asymptomatic patient who has babesiosis.**

This patient has asymptomatic babesiosis and should undergo repeat polymerase chain reaction (PCR) assay in 3 months. No treatment is indicated at this time, but the patient should be followed closely for clearance of the parasite. Babesiosis is a protozoal infection that is primarily spread through *Ixodes* ticks and is most commonly found among residents or travelers to the coastal northeastern United States. Following infection, the parasite lives inside erythrocytes. More than 150 cases of transmission have been documented through transfusion of blood products from asymptomatically infected donors. This probably significantly underestimates the true frequency of this route of transmission because up to 1% of donors from highly endemic regions are seropositive for *Babesia microti*. Microscopy using Giemsa or Wright staining on a thin blood smear will show trophozoites, appearing as ring forms inside erythrocytes. PCR is the most sensitive method for diagnosing infection, particularly when there is relatively low-level parasitemia, as is the case for asymptomatic infections. Although many *Babesia* infections resolve spontaneously, an asymptomatic infection that has persisted for more than 3 months after the initial diagnosis is an indication for treatment.

Patients with severe anemia and greater than 10% parasitemia may benefit from exchange transfusion, in which the patient's blood is removed by catheter and replaced with healthy donor blood, but would not be indicated in this patient with asymptomatic disease.

Symptomatic infection is an indication for treatment. Atovaquone combined with azithromycin is the recommended treatment for mild babesiosis. This regimen is equally effective as quinine plus clindamycin, with significantly fewer adverse effects. Severe disease is characterized by significant hemolysis and requires hospitalization for supportive care and monitoring. Quinine plus clindamycin is the preferred therapy for severe disease.

### KEY POINT

- Patients diagnosed with babesiosis who are asymptomatic should undergo a repeat polymerase chain reaction assay in 3 months to detect parasite clearance but do not need treatment.

## Bibliography

Vannier E, Krause PJ. Human babesiosis. N Engl J Med. 2012 Jun 21;366(25):2397–407. [PMID: 22716978]

## Item 88        Answer:    A

**Educational Objective: Treat a hospitalized patient with pelvic inflammatory disease with antibiotics.**

This patient has clinical evidence of pelvic inflammatory disease (PID) and should be treated with cefoxitin plus

**Answers and Critiques**

**CONT.** doxycycline. Although the ultrasonographic findings excluded a tubo-ovarian abscess, nausea and vomiting and inability to tolerate an oral treatment regimen are indications for hospital admission and initial parenteral therapy. PID occurs primarily in sexually active women, with *Chlamydia trachomatis* and *Neisseria gonorrhoeae* implicated in approximately two thirds of patients. However, PID is considered a polymicrobial infection that may also involve vaginal organisms, including anaerobes, enteric gram-negative rods, and streptococci. Additionally, organisms associated with bacterial vaginosis, such as *Gardnerella vaginalis*, may play a role. Therefore, antibiotic therapy with coverage directed to *C. trachomatis* and *N. gonorrhoeae* is essential, with broader-spectrum coverage to treat other potentially causative organisms. The antibiotic regimen of choice for patients who are hospitalized with PID is cefoxitin or cefotetan (second-generation cephalosporins) plus intravenous doxycycline.

Ceftriaxone plus azithromycin can be used in single-dose regimens for uncomplicated cervicitis, but this regimen is not recommended for treatment of PID. Ceftriaxone as a single-dose intramuscular injection plus a 14-day course of oral doxycycline (with or without metronidazole) can be used to treat PID in patients who do not have an indication for hospitalization. In this patient, symptoms of nausea and vomiting raise concern for the ability to tolerate oral therapy and are an indication for hospitalization. Ciprofloxacin is no longer recommended for an infection requiring coverage for *N. gonorrhoeae* because fluoroquinolone resistance is common with this organism.

Piperacillin-tazobactam does not provide coverage for *C. trachomatis* and would not be appropriate monotherapy in this patient. Additionally, although PID is considered a polymicrobial infection, and piperacillin-tazobactam would provide coverage for Enterobacteriaceae and anaerobes, it is also an antipseudomonal agent and is unnecessarily broad spectrum for this patient.

**KEY POINT**

- Parenteral therapy for pelvic inflammatory disease in a hospitalized patient consists of cefoxitin or cefotetan plus doxycycline.

**Bibliography**

Brunham RC, Gottlieb SL, Paavonen J. Pelvic inflammatory disease. N Engl J Med. 2015 May 21;372(21):2039-48. [PMID: 25992748]

**Item 89        Answer:    D**

**Educational Objective: Treat critically ill patients with oral antimicrobial agents.**

The most appropriate treatment regimen for this patient is oral therapy with ciprofloxacin and metronidazole. Aerobic gram-negative and anaerobic organisms should be considered for empiric coverage in this patient with a community-acquired intra-abdominal abscess pending drainage and fluid Gram stain and culture results. Admission to an ICU or step-down unit does not require that the patient receive intravenous antimicrobial therapy. Oral antimicrobials can be used in critically ill patients who have an intact and functioning gastrointestinal tract (no vomiting, no ileus), if the type of infection being treated does not require intravenous antibiotics (infection involving the central nervous system, *Staphylococcus aureus* bacteremia, endocarditis, osteomyelitis), and if the oral agent(s) with the appropriate spectrum of activity and acceptable bioavailability for the infection being treated is available. This patient has an intact and functioning gastrointestinal tract and is a candidate for oral antimicrobial therapy. Ciprofloxacin and metronidazole have excellent bioavailability and tissue penetration (including abscesses) and provide the necessary spectrum of antimicrobial coverage for aerobic gram-negative and anaerobic bacteria.

Aztreonam provides aerobic gram-negative coverage, and vancomycin adds gram-positive coverage, but the combination does not provide the anaerobic coverage for this patient's empiric therapy.

The combination of vancomycin and clindamycin provides gram-positive and anaerobic coverage but no aerobic gram-negative coverage. Clindamycin has excellent bioavailability and should be considered for oral administration when it is the indicated antibiotic.

Although ampicillin and metronidazole are offered as an oral regimen, they do not provide adequate aerobic gram-negative coverage, including commonly resistant *Escherichia coli*.

**KEY POINT**

- Oral antimicrobial agents can be used in critically ill patients who have an intact and functioning gastrointestinal tract and infection with an organism that does not require intravenous therapy.

**Bibliography**

Cunha BA. Oral antibiotic therapy of serious systemic infections. Med Clin North Am. 2006;90:1197-2222. [PMID: 17116444]

**Item 90        Answer:    C**

**Educational Objective: Diagnose acute HIV-1 infection.**

This patient should be informed that he has acute HIV-1 infection, and further baseline evaluation of new HIV infection with T-cell subset testing and other appropriate laboratory studies should be pursued. The antigen/antibody combination immunoassay is reactive, indicating the presence of HIV-1 or HIV-2 antibody or HIV p24 antigen. The result on a differentiation immunoassay for HIV-1 and HIV-2 antibodies is negative, suggesting that the initial immunoassay was detecting the presence of viral p24 protein. This is confirmed by the nucleic acid amplification test, which had strongly positive results for HIV RNA, indicating the presence of virus even though the patient did not yet have detectable antibodies. These results are most consistent with acute HIV infection presenting in the "window period" before development of a serologic response. His nonspecific febrile illness the previous week may have represented symptoms of acute HIV infection.

The rapid tests for HIV infection, such as a saliva assay, are convenient for patients but are based on detecting HIV antibodies. They would therefore be expected to yield negative or indeterminate results in this patient because he is presenting in the "window period" of acute infection before antibody development.

The Western blot test is no longer recommended for confirmatory HIV testing. Because this patient has early HIV infection, results of Western blot testing for HIV antibody would likely be negative or indeterminate anyway.

Repeating the HIV 1/HIV-2 antibody differentiation immunoassay at a later time is not necessary because acute HIV infection has been diagnosed on the basis of the high level of viral RNA. Antibody testing results will become positive within a few weeks to a few months, but it would not be appropriate to delay further management for HIV until that time.

### KEY POINT

- Positive antigen/antibody immunoassay, negative antibody differentiation assay, and positive nucleic acid amplification test results are consistent results for patients presenting in the "window period" of acute HIV infection before development of a serologic response.

### Bibliography

Branson BM, Owen SM, Wesolowski LG, et al; Centers for Disease Control and Prevention; Association of Public Health Laboratories. Laboratory testing for the diagnosis of HIV infection: updated recommendations. http://stacks.cdc.gov/view/cdc/23447. Published June 27, 2014. Accessed July 21, 2015.

### Item 91     Answer:     A

**Educational Objective: Manage** *Campylobacter* **gastroenteritis.**

This patient, who has spontaneous symptom resolution of *Campylobacter jejuni* infection, requires no further evaluation or treatment. Treatment of bacterial dysentery is controversial; most cases resolve spontaneously, but, in the case of *Salmonella* gastroenteritis, antibiotics may actually prolong bacterial shedding. However, when patients are at risk for extraintestinal complications because of advanced age or immunocompromise, or when symptoms are particularly severe, the benefits of empiric treatment outweigh the risks. For most causes of dysentery, fluoroquinolones, such as levofloxacin, are considered first-line therapy based on limited resistance to most bacterial agents. The exception is *Campylobacter*, which a recent study documented 14% fluoroquinolone resistance in domestically acquired

infections and greater than 50% link to international travel. Consumption of undercooked poultry may raise suspicion for *Campylobacter* infection, but symptoms substantially overlap among the various agents causing dysentery; culture is required to identify the causative agent. Despite treatment with an antibiotic to which the organism was resistant, symptoms completely resolved by the time the culture results were finalized. This underscores the fact that in most cases of bacterial gastroenteritis, infection resolves spontaneously without therapy, and further evaluation or treatment is unnecessary.

Blood cultures are appropriate if symptoms worsen and the patient is at risk for sepsis and extraintestinal infections. However, because this patient's symptoms have resolved, blood cultures would be inappropriate.

Asymptomatic excretion of *Campylobacter* can persist for several weeks following resolution of symptoms; however, person-to-person transmission is uncommon, and surveillance stool cultures are not recommended to document clearance. Considering the patient's occupation, strict attention to hand hygiene would be important to minimize risk for secondary spread.

Macrolides are the preferred treatment for *Campylobacter* infection. This would be an appropriate choice if symptoms had persisted.

Ciprofloxacin would not be a viable option after resistance to levofloxacin is confirmed. *Campylobacter* bacteria resistant to levofloxacin are likely to be resistant to other fluoroquinolones as well.

### KEY POINT

- In most cases of bacterial gastroenteritis, infection resolves spontaneously without therapy, and further evaluation or treatment is unnecessary.

### Bibliography

Ricotta EE, Palmer A, Wymore K, et al. Epidemiology and antimicrobial resistance of international travel-associated Campylobacter infections in the United States, 2005-2011. Am J Public Health. 2014 Jul;104(7):e108-14. [PMID: 24832415]

### Item 92     Answer:     B

**Educational Objective: Manage cryptococcal infection in an otherwise healthy patient.**

This patient has pulmonary cryptococcosis and should undergo lumbar puncture. Whenever *Cryptococcus* is found at a site outside of the central nervous system (CNS), a lumbar puncture should be performed to determine whether CNS infection is also present, even in the absence of CNS symptoms. Patients who are immunocompromised or become immunocompromised following primary infection are at risk for more progressive infection or disseminated infection.

The echinocandins, such as caspofungin, have no activity against *Cryptococcus* and, therefore, play no role in therapy for pulmonary cryptococcosis.

Removal of the pulmonary nodule is not indicated at this time. If radiologic abnormalities and symptoms persist despite antifungal therapy, then surgery should be considered. Because of this patient's smoking history, further histologic investigation might be appropriate if his lung findings do not improve following therapy.

In immunocompetent patients, infection may resolve spontaneously, remain stable for a prolonged duration, or become progressive. Although most immunocompetent patients with primary pulmonary cryptococcosis may be asymptomatic and their infection may resolve without treatment, treatment is indicated to prevent progressive or disseminated disease and usually consists of daily fluconazole for 6 to 12 months. Therefore, providing no additional treatment would not be appropriate.

### KEY POINT

- In patients with pulmonary cryptococcosis, lumbar puncture should be performed to determine if central nervous system (CNS) infection is also present, even in the absence of CNS symptoms.

### Bibliography

Brizendine KD, Baddley JW, Pappas PG. Pulmonary cryptococcosis. Semin Respir Crit Care Med. 2011 Dec;32(6):727-34. [PMID: 22167400]

## Item 93    Answer:    D

**Educational Objective: Diagnose typhoid fever.**

This patient's most likely diagnosis is typhoid fever, also known as enteric fever. It is commonly caused by ingestion of the bacterium *Salmonella enterica* serotype Typhi. Infection is usually acquired via the fecal-oral route either from food or water handled by asymptomatic carriers or by introduction of the organism into sewage-contaminated water systems. Typhoid fever occurs throughout the world but is endemic in the underdeveloped areas of Africa, Asia, and Latin America. In the United States, infection is usually diagnosed in travelers who have come from the Indian subcontinent. The typical clinical presentation of typhoid fever is a progressively rising fever, accompanied by abdominal pain, initial constipation followed by diarrhea, and relative bradycardia. One third of patients develop salmon-colored blanching maculopapular lesions on the trunk or abdominal wall. Tender hepatosplenomegaly is a common finding. Abnormal laboratory results often include anemia, leukopenia with a relative lymphopenia, thrombocytopenia, and elevated liver enzymes and bilirubin levels. The diagnosis may be supported by serologic assays. However, isolation of the organism from blood, stool, urine, and/or bone marrow is required for confirmation.

Brucellosis, another zoonotic infection mostly caused by one of four species named for a specific animal reservoir, occurs through direct contact with infected animals, ingestion of infected animal products, or inhalation. Fever occurs and is often intermittent or undulant. Arthralgia and arthritis, neurologic and psychiatric symptoms, and genitourinary involvement are also common. Gastrointestinal symptoms are infrequent and nonspecific.

Lassa fever is caused by an arenavirus endemic to Western Africa. Infection can be acquired after direct or indirect contact with infected rodent excreta. High fever, abdominal pain, and headache may progress to hemorrhagic manifestations and death.

Leptospirosis is a common zoonotic infection caused by spirochetes found throughout the world. Human infection often follows occupational (farmers, abattoir workers, veterinarians) exposure of damaged skin or mucous membranes to body fluids or environmental sources that have been contaminated with urine from an actively infected animal. However, acquisition of infection related to travel and recreational activities is becoming more common. Disease manifestations include acute fever, muscle pain (typically lumbar and calf regions), redness of the conjunctiva, and, occasionally, aseptic meningitis. Gastrointestinal symptoms are infrequent. Progression to a more severe disease phase of consisting of multisystem damage is rare.

### KEY POINT

- The typical clinical presentation of typhoid fever is a progressively rising fever accompanied by abdominal pain, initial constipation followed by diarrhea, and relative bradycardia; tender hepatosplenomegaly is common.

### Bibliography

Waddington CS, Darton TC, Pollard AJ. The challenge of enteric fever. J Infect. 2014 Jan;68 Suppl 1:S38-50. [PMID: 24119827]

## Item 94    Answer:    A

**Educational Objective: Recognize the clinical presentation of anti-*N*-methyl-D-aspartate receptor (NMDAR) encephalitis.**

Testing this patient's anti-*N*-methyl-D-aspartate receptor (NMDAR) antibodies will confirm her diagnosis. This young woman presents with a subacute alteration in mental status over several weeks, characterized by psychiatric symptoms, seizure activity, and involuntary movements. These features, although individually nonspecific, suggest NMDAR encephalitis when combined. A recently described entity, it is one of the most common autoimmune encephalitides, especially in children and young adults, although it is infrequently diagnosed in older adults. Patients with anti-NMDAR encephalitis classically present with psychiatric symptoms, which can vary from agitation to frank psychosis. Other common signs include autonomic instability, choreoathetoid movements, and seizures or status epilepticus. This syndrome was initially recognized in young women with teratomas but has subsequently been diagnosed in patients without an obvious antigenic trigger, such as tumor or infection. Laboratory confirmation requires detection of anti-NMDAR antibodies in serum or cerebrospinal fluid (CSF).

*Borrelia burgdorferi* is the bacterium that causes Lyme disease. The most common neurologic presentations include cranial neuropathy, meningitis, radiculopathy, and encephalomyelitis, which are inconsistent with this patient's presentation.

Nuchal skin biopsy for immunohistochemistry or polymerase chain reaction may be used to diagnose rabies. Rabies often presents with localized paresthesias at the site of inoculation, with inexorable progression to coma and death over days to weeks. Autonomic instability, muscle spasm, and hydrophobia are commonly present.

VDRL testing of CSF is an indirect test for neurosyphilis. This spirochetal illness causes neurologic symptoms similar to Lyme disease. Early in the disease course, meningitis and cranial neuropathies predominate; however, in late neurosyphilis, dementia or tabes dorsalis may be seen. These symptoms are inconsistent with those distinguishing anti-NMDAR encephalitis.

**KEY POINT**

- Anti-*N*-methyl-D-aspartate receptor encephalitis should be considered in the differential diagnosis of patients with psychiatric symptoms, seizures, autonomic instability, and choreoathetoid movements.

**Bibliography**

Titulaer MJ, McCracken L, Gabilondo I, et al. Treatment and prognostic factors for long-term outcome in patients with anti-NMDA receptor encephalitis: an observational cohort study. Lancet Neurol. 2013 Feb;12(2):157-65. [PMID: 23290630]

## Item 95    Answer:    D

**Educational Objective: Evaluate severe community-acquired pneumonia with sputum cultures.**

Sputum cultures are the most appropriate additional study in this patient. He presents with severe community-acquired pneumonia (CAP) and meets criteria to warrant hospital admission with an age great than 65 years and respiration rate greater than 30/min, which give him a CRB-65 score of 2. Because of his hemodynamic parameters, including hypotension and tachycardia, ICU management is appropriate. In addition to blood cultures, patients with severe CAP should have sputum cultures ordered. The diagnostic yield of sputum cultures varies widely, and culture data for ambulatory patients with uncomplicated CAP do not positively influence outcomes relative to empiric antibiotic therapy. Therefore, sputum cultures are not recommended for these patients. However, in patients being hospitalized and particularly for those with severe disease requiring ICU admission, possible complications of CAP, or multiple underlying comorbidities, sputum cultures may yield diagnostic information useful in guiding treatment. This patient has severe CAP requiring ICU admission; therefore, blood and sputum cultures are indicated.

Although chest CT has higher sensitivity than chest radiography for diagnosing CAP, no evidence shows that CT for initial diagnosis improves clinical outcomes. However, CT is particularly effective for detecting pleural effusion and empyema, cavitary lung lesions, and hilar lymphadenopathy and might be an appropriate diagnostic study if clinical suspicion for one of these complications develops.

C-reactive protein (CRP) is an inflammatory marker that tends to be increased to greater levels in bacterial pneumonia than viral pneumonia and may be helpful in differentiating the cause of pneumonia in patients in whom the diagnosis is unclear. Additional studies regarding use of CRP for this purpose are needed, and it would not be helpful in this patient with a clinical picture consistent with bacterial pneumonia.

Procalcitonin is a circulating molecule produced by cells as a response to bacterial toxins. Therefore, serum procalcitonin levels tend to be elevated in bacterial infections, and this test can be used as an adjunctive test along with other factors to help differentiate viral from bacterial infection. However, this patient has clear evidence of a bacterial cause of his pneumonia, so this study would not yield significant clinical information.

**KEY POINT**

- Patients with severe community-acquired pneumonia should have sputum and blood cultures performed as part of further diagnostic testing.

**Bibliography**

Mandell LA, Wunderink RG, Anzueto A, et al; Infectious Diseases Society of America, American Thoracic Society. Infectious Diseases Society of America/American Thoracic Society consensus guidelines on the management of community-acquired pneumonia in adults. Clin Infect Dis. 2007 Mar 1;44(Suppl 2):S27-72. [PMID: 17278083]

## Item 96    Answer:    A

**Educational Objective: Treat a patient with HIV/AIDS and disseminated *Mycobacterium avium* complex infection.**

The combination of clarithromycin, ethambutol, and rifabutin is the most appropriate treatment for this patient who has AIDS and a disseminated *Mycobacterium avium* complex (MAC) infection. Disseminated MAC infection usually occurs in patients with CD4 cell counts less than 50/µL. Symptoms include fever, night sweats, weight loss, diarrhea, fatigue, and abdominal pain. Laboratory abnormalities often include evidence of bone marrow suppression and an elevated alkaline phosphatase level. The diagnosis is typically made by blood cultures (or cultures from other involved organs). Guidelines for the treatment of MAC in adults with HIV infection recommend clarithromycin as the preferred first agent and ethambutol as the second agent. On the basis of some evidence indicating improved survival and decreased emergence of drug resistance, some experts recommend the addition of rifabutin as a third agent. Primary prophylaxis for MAC prevention with azithromycin or clarithromycin is recommended for patients with HIV whose CD4 cell count is less than 50/µL.

Isoniazid, rifampin, and ethambutol are typically used to treat *Mycobacterium kansasii*, which most commonly causes a lung infection that mimics tuberculosis with cough, fever, weight loss, and cavitary lung disease.

Isoniazid and rifabutin are part of the 4- to 7-month continuation phase of treatment for active tuberculosis, which follows the initial 8-week treatment phase with rifabutin, isoniazid, pyrazinamide, and ethambutol. This patient does not have active tuberculosis.

---

**KEY POINT**

- Treatment with clarithromycin, ethambutol, and rifabutin is recommended for disseminated *Mycobacterium avium* complex infection in patients with HIV/AIDS whose CD4 cell counts are less than 50/µL.

---

**Bibliography**

Panel on Opportunistic Infections in HIV-Infected Adults and Adolescents. Guidelines for the prevention and treatment of opportunistic infections in HIV-infected adults and adolescents: recommendations from the Centers for Disease Control and Prevention, the National Institutes of Health, and the HIV Medicine Association of the Infectious Diseases Society of America. http://aidsinfo.nih.gov/contentfiles/lvguidelines/adult_oi.pdf. Updated April 16, 2015. Accessed July 21, 2015.

---

## Item 97    Answer:    D

**Educational Objective: Manage community-acquired pneumonia with empiric antibiotic therapy.**

This patient should begin outpatient treatment with a respiratory fluoroquinolone, such as levofloxacin; a reasonable alternative would be an oral β-lactam antibiotic in combination with a macrolide or doxycycline. Initial assessment of patients with community-acquired pneumonia (CAP) begins with establishing an appropriate venue of care. Clinical decision tools, such as the modified CRB-65, which omits the blood urea nitrogen (BUN) component of the original CURB-65 (confusion, BUN [>20 mg/dL (7.14 mmol/L)], respiration rate [≥30/min], blood pressure [systolic <90 mm Hg, diastolic <60 mm Hg], and age ≥65 years), can be used in office-based settings to expedite determining the need for hospitalization. This patient has no confusion, is not hypotensive, and does not have significant tachypnea (respiration rate is <30/min), so his CRB-65 score is 0 and he does not require hospitalization. Empiric antibiotic therapy is focused toward the most likely organisms, modified by specific risk factors in a particular patient. Patients with no risk factors for resistant *Streptococcus pneumoniae* are candidates for treatment with either a macrolide or doxycycline. However, in patients with increased risk for resistance (age >65 years, recent [within the past 3-6 months] antimicrobial therapy [with a β-lactam, macrolide, or fluoroquinolone antibiotic], alcoholism, immunosuppression, and certain medical comorbidities [COPD, chronic liver or kidney disease, cancer, diabetes, functional or anatomic asplenia, chronic heart disease]), therapy with a respiratory fluoroquinolone or a β-lactam with a macrolide or doxycycline is appropri-

ate. Because this patient has COPD, his risk for resistant *S. pneumoniae* is increased, and expanded antibiotic coverage is indicated instead of macrolide monotherapy (such as azithromycin).

For patients requiring hospital ward admission for treatment, an empiric regimen of an intravenous β-lactam with a macrolide or doxycycline (such as ampicillin-sulbactam and doxycycline) or a respiratory fluoroquinolone is recommended. However, this patient does not have a clear indication for hospital admission for treatment.

For patients with CAP requiring ICU admission, treatment with an intravenous β-lactam plus either azithromycin or a fluoroquinolone (such as ceftriaxone and azithromycin) is indicated. Because this patient does not require hospitalization or intensive care, this would not be an appropriate empiric treatment regimen.

---

**KEY POINT**

- In patients with increased risk for resistant *Streptococcus pneumoniae*, empiric antibiotic therapy with a respiratory fluoroquinolone, such as levofloxacin, or a β-lactam with a macrolide or doxycycline is most appropriate.

---

**Bibliography**

Mandell LA, Wunderink RG, Anzueto A, et al; Infectious Diseases Society of America, American Thoracic Society. Infectious Diseases Society of America/American Thoracic Society consensus guidelines on the management of community-acquired pneumonia in adults. Clin Infect Dis. 2007 Mar 1;44(Suppl 2):S27-72. [PMID: 17278083]

---

## Item 98    Answer:    B

**Educational Objective: Treat a patient with catheter-associated urinary tract infection.**

This patient likely has a catheter-associated urinary tract infection (CAUTI), and his catheter should be removed and treatment provided for the infection. Fever with no other identifiable cause, suprapubic tenderness, and a urine culture growing $10^3$ or more colony-forming units in a patient with an indwelling urinary catheter are compatible with the diagnosis of CAUTI. Other signs and symptoms that may suggest CAUTI include acute hematuria, costovertebral angle tenderness, pelvic discomfort, malaise, rigors, or confusion. It is not possible to assess for dysuria or urgency while the catheter is in place, but these symptoms may be present if the catheter is removed. Age older than 50 years and diabetes mellitus are two risk factors for CAUTI, as is prolonged catheterization. Catheters inserted in the operating room should be removed within 2 days after surgery to prevent CAUTI, unless the patient has undergone urologic surgery or other surgery on contiguous structures of the genitourinary tract, in which case it may be acceptable to keep the catheter in place longer. Treatment of CAUTI includes removing the urinary catheter if possible because bacteria may be embedded in biofilm and may not be reached by antimicrobial agents. Catheters in place for more than 2 weeks should be removed or changed before a urinalysis and culture are performed;

**CONT.**

otherwise, inaccurate results may be obtained, representing organisms present in biofilm and not necessarily causing UTI.

Although antimicrobial stewardship includes narrowing antibiotic coverage to a specific organism involved, awaiting sensitivity results to guide antimicrobial selection would not be appropriate in this patient with evidence of CAUTI. Empiric antimicrobial coverage based on likely infecting organisms and local resistance patterns with subsequent focused therapy when sensitivities are determined would be indicated in this patient.

The patient's symptoms and urine culture indicate he has a CAUTI; therefore, repeating a urinalysis and culture in 24 hours without treatment would not be appropriate.

No treatment is necessary for patients with asymptomatic bacteriuria, defined as bacteriuria of $10^3$ colony-forming units or greater without signs or symptoms of UTI. However, this patient has evidence of active infection, so treatment is indicated.

**KEY POINT**

- Patients with probable catheter-associated urinary tract infection should have the catheter removed and appropriate antimicrobial treatment provided for the infection, based on results of a urine culture.

**Bibliography**

Hooton TM, Bradley SF, Cardenas DD, et al; Infectious Diseases Society of America. Diagnosis, prevention, and treatment of catheter-associated urinary tract infection in adults: 2009 International Clinical Practice Guidelines from the Infectious Diseases Society of America. Clin Infect Dis. 2010;50:625-63. [PMID: 20175247]

## Item 99  Answer:  D

**Educational Objective: Diagnose *Vibrio vulnificus*-associated necrotizing fasciitis.**

This patient has necrotizing fasciitis caused by *Vibrio vulnificus*. Patients who are immunocompromised, particularly those with liver disease, are at increased risk for infection with this gram-negative bacillus. Infection usually occurs after consumption of raw shellfish (such as oysters) or skin trauma incurred in contaminated warm (>20 °C [68.0 °F]) sea water or brackish water where the organism thrives. Hemorrhagic bullae are the classic cutaneous manifestation. Guideline recommendations for the management of these infections include antibiotic therapy with doxycycline plus ceftazidime in addition to surgery.

*Erysipelothrix rhusiopathiae* is a gram-positive bacillus that can infect animals, including swine and poultry, and is a saprophyte associated with fish, crustaceans, and molluscs. Exposures to these types of animals or their secretions can be occupationally acquired (fisherman, fish and shellfish handlers, veterinarians, and butchers). Classically, a painful localized violaceous cutaneous infection of the hand or fingers (known as erysipeloid) develops at the site of trauma or a preexisting wound. Fever is not often present. More diffuse skin infections and systemic infections including bacteremia and endocarditis are well-described but are much less common.

Methicillin-resistant *S. aureus* can cause a monomicrobial necrotizing fasciitis and should be empirically covered by the initial antibiotic regimen while awaiting microbiologic confirmation. However, the intraoperative tissue specimen from this patient reveals gram-negative bacilli and not gram-positive cocci in clusters that would herald a MRSA infection.

*Mycobacterium marinum* skin infections typically develop at sites of skin injury that have been exposed to salt or fresh water, such as in fish tanks (fish tank granuloma). The upper extremity is often involved and lesions are usually papular before becoming ulcerative. Systemic toxicity is not usually seen in skin infections caused by this nontuberculous acid-fast bacillus. The Gram stain of infected tissue would be negative.

**KEY POINT**

- Patients who are immunocompromised, particularly those with liver disease, are at increased risk for infection with *Vibrio vulnificus*.

**Bibliography**

Horseman MA, Surani S. A comprehensive review of Vibrio vulnificus: an important cause of severe sepsis and skin and soft-tissue infection. Int J Infect Dis. 2011 Mar;15(3):e157-66. [PMID: 21177133]

## Item 100  Answer:  C

**Educational Objective: Diagnose Middle East respiratory syndrome.**

This patient has Middle East respiratory syndrome (MERS), which was first reported in Saudi Arabia in 2012 and is caused by a novel β-coronavirus (MERS-CoV). This virus is similar to but distinct from the severe acute respiratory syndrome–coronavirus (SARS-CoV) outbreak originally identified in China in 2002. Close contact with a patient infected with MERS appears to be necessary for transmission. All cases of MERS have been directly or indirectly linked to travel or residence in countries of the Arabian Peninsula but have also been imported to areas of Europe and the United States by travelers; therefore, clinical suspicion for this diagnosis must be maintained in patients with respiratory illness who have traveled in these areas. Severe disease with MERS occurs primarily in older persons with comorbidities such as diabetes mellitus, end-stage kidney disease, and obesity and has an overall mortality rate of more than 40%.

After an average incubation period of 5 days, patients report a typical viral-like syndrome. In severe illness, the patient often progresses to pneumonia and significant respiratory distress, often necessitating mechanical ventilation. Gastrointestinal manifestations and acute kidney injury may also occur. Treatment consists of supportive care. Standard care precautions using personal protective equipment and contact and airborne isolation are crucial infection control measures when MERS is suspected or diagnosed.

Although this patient traveled to Liberia, where Ebola is endemic, Ebola is not a primary respiratory infection. Additionally, no coagulopathy, which is usually seen with Ebola infection, is evident in this patient.

Influenza infection as a cause of this patient's clinical presentation would not be likely during the summer months, and primary pneumonia is a less common presentation of influenza infection.

Respiratory syncytial virus is associated with seasonal outbreaks and may affect children and adults. It may also cause upper and lower respiratory tract illness. However, except in patients who are immunocompromised, the clinical manifestations of this infection are usually milder than those seen in this patient.

> **KEY POINT**
>
> • Middle East respiratory syndrome should be suspected in any person presenting with respiratory illness following travel in or around the Arabian Peninsula.

**Bibliography**

Sampathkumar P. Middle East respiratory syndrome: what clinicians need to know. Mayo Clin Proc. 2014;89(8):1153-8. [PMID: 25034307]

## Item 101    Answer:    B

**Educational Objective: Manage central line-associated *Staphylococcus aureus* bloodstream infection.**

Vancomycin should be changed to a penicillinase-resistant semisynthetic penicillin antibiotic (oxacillin or nafcillin). The patient's blood cultures indicate infection with a methicillin-sensitive *Staphylococcus aureus* (MSSA) isolate. The β-lactam antibiotics are more rapidly bactericidal than vancomycin and are therefore the preferred class of antibiotics for treating serious *S. aureus* infections. Because this patient is not allergic to penicillin, oxacillin or nafcillin are the best choices. Vancomycin is associated with worse outcomes when used to treat MSSA infections. Empiric therapy with vancomycin is appropriate for patients in whom infection with methicillin-resistant *S. aureus* is a consideration. However, therapy should be modified as appropriate as soon as culture and antimicrobial susceptibility results are available.

Combination antimicrobial therapy (such as vancomycin and rifampin) for the treatment of *S. aureus* bacteremia does not improve clinical outcomes. Therefore, it would not be the most appropriate management choice for this patient.

Vancomycin therapy is monitored by serum trough levels, not serum peak levels. When vancomycin is used in the appropriate setting, the usual goal for the serum trough level is 15 to 20 µg/mL.

Definite or probable thrombosis occurs in approximately 70% of patients who have central venous catheter–associated *S. aureus* bacteremia. Imaging of the previous intravenous site is not necessary unless suspicion

exists for suppurative thrombophlebitis (pain, swelling, palpable cord) or a fluid collection that would require drainage.

> **KEY POINT**
>
> • Methicillin-susceptible *Staphylococcus aureus* should be treated with a penicillinase-resistant semisynthetic penicillin.

**Bibliography**

Thwaites GE, Edgeworth JD, Gkrania-Klotsas E, et al; UK Clinical Infections Research Group. Clinical management of *Staphylococcus aureus* bacteraemia. Lancet Infect Dis. 2011 Mar;11(3):208-22. [PMID: 21371655]

## Item 102    Answer:    A

**Educational Objective: Manage infection control practices for a patient suspected of having tuberculosis.**

This patient comes from a country with a high prevalence of tuberculosis and is at increased risk for infection with *Mycobacterium tuberculosis*. Her symptoms of fever, cough, decreased appetite, night sweats, and weight loss, as well as the location of chest infiltrates in the apical area of the upper lobes, are characteristic of pulmonary tuberculosis. *M. tuberculosis* spreads by airborne particles known as droplet nuclei, which are 5 µm or smaller in size. These airborne particles are expelled when an infected patient sneezes or coughs. Transmission of infection can occur when these airborne particles are inhaled into the lung alveoli. Consequently, this patient should be placed in empiric negative-pressure airborne isolation while further evaluation is pursued. Negative-pressure isolation prevents airborne droplets from escaping the room, and at least 6 to 12 air changes of the room air are provided per hour. Doors to isolation rooms must remain closed, and all persons entering must wear a respirator that has a filtering capacity of 95% and a tight seal over the nose and mouth. Patients in airborne isolation who require transport outside of their isolation room for medical procedures should wear surgical masks that cover their nose and mouth during transport.

Contact isolation is instituted for patients who have a suspected or known illness transmitted by direct contact (such as *Clostridium difficile*, vancomycin-resistant enterococci, *Shigella* species, hepatitis A virus).

Droplet isolation is instituted for patients who have a suspected or known illness transmitted by large-particle droplets (>5 µm in size) (for example, *Neisseria meningitidis*, influenza virus, adenovirus, *Bordetella pertussis*, *Mycoplasma pneumoniae*). Droplet precautions involve a face mask without high-level respirator masks or special air handling.

Standard precautions, which include hand hygiene, respiratory hygiene, injection safety measures, use of personal protective equipment (gloves, gowns, face masks/shields, respirators), and appropriate environmental and

CONT.

disinfection measures, are instituted for all patients in a health care setting regardless of illness.

- Patients with pulmonary tuberculosis, or infections with other organisms transmitted by small droplet nuclei, should be placed in airborne isolation to prevent the spread of infection.

**Bibliography**

Siegel JD, Rhinehart E, Jackson M, Chiarello L; Health Care Infection Control Practices Advisory Committee. 2007 Guideline for Isolation Precautions: Preventing Transmission of Infectious Agents in Health Care Settings. Am J Infect Control. 2007 Dec;35(10 Suppl 2):S65-164. [PMID: 18068815]

## Item 103     Answer:   D

**Educational Objective: Treat a patient with a furuncle without antibiotic therapy.**

Clinical follow-up with no additional treatment is indicated at this time for this patient who has undergone incision and drainage of a furuncle (boil). Usually, incision and drainage alone is the primary treatment recommended for a patient with a simple furuncle. Antibiotics generally are recommended only when the response to incision and drainage is inadequate, when involved areas are challenging to drain (such as the genitalia, hands, or face); when disease is extensive or rapidly progressive with associated cellulitis; in immunodeficiency and other comorbidities; for very young or very old patients; those with clinical signs of systemic illness; and in the presence of associated septic phlebitis. Furuncles are typically due to community-acquired methicillin-resistant *Staphylococcus aureus* (CA-MRSA). Empiric use of adjunctive antibiotics with CA-MRSA activity after incision and drainage of a furuncle is generally reserved for patients who are immunosuppressed, who do not respond adequately to incision and drainage or antibiotics without MRSA activity, or who have systemic signs of infection.

Oral dicloxacillin has activity against methicillin-sensitive *S. aureus* (MSSA), but not MRSA. It would be recommended for adjunctive use when culture of purulent material from a furuncle demonstrates MSSA.

Because of the high likelihood that MRSA may be the causative agent, when antibiotics are used, empiric treatment with agents with activity against MRSA is recommended. Doxycycline has activity against MRSA and would be a reasonable choice, but it is not indicated for this patient who has undergone incision and drainage of his furuncle. Trimethoprim-sulfamethoxazole is another reasonable option for empiric MRSA therapy if antibiotic therapy is needed, although this agent would be contraindicated in this patient with a known allergy to this medication.

Although it is bactericidal against some strains of MRSA, rifampin monotherapy is not recommended because of the development of resistance.

- No antibiotic treatment is needed after incision and drainage of a simple furuncle, except in patients who are immunosuppressed, who do not respond adequately to incision and drainage or antibiotics without MRSA activity, or who have systemic signs of infection.

**Bibliography**

Liu C, Bayer A, Cosgrove SE, et al; Infectious Diseases Society of America. Clinical practice guidelines by the Infectious Diseases Society of America for the treatment of methicillin-resistant Staphylococcus aureus infections in adults and children [erratum in Clin Infect Dis. 2011 Aug 1;53(3):319]. Clin Infect Dis. 2011 Feb 1;52(3):e18-55. [PMID: 21208910]

## Item 104     Answer:   A

**Educational Objective: Treat a patient with appropriate antibiotic therapy who is admitted to the hospital with community-acquired pneumonia with suspected *Pseudomonas aeruginosa* infection.**

Empiric antibiotic therapy with cefepime, levofloxacin, and gentamicin is the most appropriate regimen for this patient. She presents with severe community-acquired pneumonia (CAP) requiring ICU treatment and, therefore, requires appropriate antibiotics for this setting (typically, a β-lactam plus either azithromycin or a fluoroquinolone, such as cefepime, levofloxacin, or ciprofloxacin). Patients at increased risk for *Pseudomonas aeruginosa* infection include those with structural lung disease (such as bronchiectasis) and recent or frequent glucocorticoid and antibiotic use. Because this patient has bronchiectasis and recent glucocorticoid use, she is at increased risk for *Pseudomonas* infection and should be treated with a β-lactam with antipseudomonal activity (such as cefepime) as part of her regimen with the addition of another antipseudomonal agent, such as gentamicin.

A β-lactam in combination with a macrolide or doxycycline, such as ceftriaxone and azithromycin, is an appropriate empiric regimen for patients requiring inpatient treatment in a medical ward setting. However, it does not provide adequate coverage for *P. aeruginosa* infection and thus would not be an appropriate regimen for this patient. A respiratory fluoroquinolone plus aztreonam is an alternative regimen to empiric treatment with a β-lactam plus either azithromycin or a fluoroquinolone in patients requiring treatment in the ICU for CAP, particularly for patients who are allergic to penicillin. However, this regimen does not provide adequately robust coverage against *P. aeruginosa*.

The combination of ceftriaxone and levofloxacin provides some coverage against *P. aeruginosa* but would not be the best choice for an antibiotic regimen targeting suspected *P. aeruginosa* CAP because of ceftriaxone's inadequate coverage against *P. aeruginosa*.

Meropenem, a broad-spectrum carbapenem β-lactam antibiotic, would be an appropriate component of an empiric regimen for treatment of possible *Pseudomonas*

**H**
**CONT.**

infection only if given in combination with a respiratory fluoroquinolone or another agent providing pseudomonal coverage. Meropenem monotherapy would not provide adequate coverage against *Pseudomonas* infection and thus would not be an appropriate empiric treatment regimen for this patient.

> **KEY POINT**
>
> - Patients admitted to the hospital with community-acquired pneumonia thought be caused by *Pseudomonas aeruginosa* require broad coverage empiric antibiotic therapy that includes an antipseudomonal β-lactam, an aminoglycoside, and a respiratory fluoroquinolone, which offer coverage of gram-negative organisms.

**Bibliography**

Mandell LA, Wunderink RG, Anzueto A, et al; Infectious Diseases Society of America, American Thoracic Society. Infectious Diseases Society of America/American Thoracic Society consensus guidelines on the management of community-acquired pneumonia in adults. Clin Infect Dis. 2007 Mar 1;44(Suppl 2):S27-72. [PMID: 17278083]

## Item 105     Answer:   B

**Educational Objective: Provide preexposure prophylaxis for HIV to a person at ongoing risk.**

This patient is at risk for HIV infection because of regular sexual activity with an infected person and should be considered for preexposure prophylaxis (PrEP). Daily combination tenofovir-emtricitabine therapy is FDA approved for prevention of HIV infection in persons considered at ongoing risk for infection. Studies have shown efficacy in men who have sex with men, heterosexual couples, and injection drug users. Rates of effectiveness in prevention depend on adherence to the medication, and prophylaxis should always be accompanied by safer-sex counseling. Testing for HIV and other sexually transmitted diseases, pregnancy, and kidney function should be performed before initiation of prophylaxis and every 2 to 3 months during preventive therapy.

Reduction in viral load with antiretroviral therapy does reduce transmission of HIV, although transmission may still occur even with undetectable blood levels. Although consistent condom use can reduce the risk for HIV transmission, the addition of PrEP can further reduce rates of acquisition of HIV and should be considered in those at high risk. Such preventive therapy should be taken daily, however, and not episodically only with exposure.

Studies on which FDA approval was based used a two-drug combination of tenofovir-emtricitabine alone without additional medication. Therefore, no clear indication exists for exposing the patient to the additional cost and risk of a third drug. The three-drug regimen of combination tenofovir-emtricitabine and raltegravir is the preferred regimen for postexposure prophylaxis. Whereas tenofovir alone has shown some benefit in reducing acquisition of HIV because of concerns about resistance, combination tenofovir-emtricitabine is preferred for PrEP.

> **KEY POINT**
>
> - Combination tenofovir-emtricitabine should be considered as preexposure prophylaxis to prevent HIV infection in all persons considered at ongoing risk of infection.

**Bibliography**

Centers for Disease Control and Prevention (CDC). Interim guidance: preexposure prophylaxis for the prevention of HIV infection in men who have sex with men. MMWR Morb Mortal Wkly Rep. 2011 Jan 28;60(3):65-8. [PMID: 21270743]

## Item 106     Answer:   E

**Educational Objective: Manage a patient with prolonged fever of unknown origin.**

This patient has classic fever of unknown origin (FUO), defined as a temperature greater than 38.3 °C (100.9 °F) for at least 3 weeks that remains undiagnosed after two visits in the ambulatory setting or 3 days of in-hospital assessment. She has undergone a reasonable evaluation for the most common causes of FUO, which include infection (endocarditis, tuberculosis, abscesses, complicated urinary tract infection), neoplasm, and connective tissue disease; therefore, she should be observed carefully, and further diagnostic or therapeutic interventions should be based on changes in history or physical examination. Histopathologic examination of tissue obtained by aspiration or biopsy can provide a definitive diagnosis in some cases of FUO if the clinical evaluation suggests disease in a particular organ. An exception to performing blind biopsies is biopsy of the temporal artery, which may be indicated in older adult patients with FUO and an elevated erythrocyte sedimentation rate even if localizing signs are absent.

A bone marrow aspirate and biopsy would be indicated if hematologic abnormalities were seen and are helpful in diagnosing disseminated granulomatoses, such as tuberculosis and histoplasmosis, or malignancies, such as leukemia and lymphoma. Because the patient's blood counts are normal and she has no other clinical findings suggesting a process with bone marrow involvement, performing a bone marrow aspirate and biopsy is not indicated.

Therapeutic trials of antibiotics, glucocorticoids, or NSAIDs are rarely indicated in patients with FUO. They may be successful in eliminating fever, or fever may remit spontaneously, and the correct diagnosis may be delayed. Empiric therapy should be reserved for patients who are seriously ill or when a specific diagnosis is reasonably likely. In general, this occurs most often when disseminated tuberculosis is suspected and an empiric therapeutic trial of antibiotics is indicated.

In the absence of any new localizing signs or symptoms, repeat or more extensive imaging is likely to be low-yield and not cost-effective. The longer the duration of FUO, the less likely it is to have an infectious cause.

**Answers and Critiques**

**KEY POINT**

- When a patient has been reasonably evaluated (laboratory studies, repeat blood cultures, imaging studies) for ongoing fever, a diagnosis of fever of unknown origin should be reached and the patient should be observed in case further interventions would be appropriate later.

**Bibliography**

Hayakawa K, Ramasamy B, Chandrasekhar PH. Fever of unknown origin: an evidence-based review. Am J Med Sci. 2012 Oct;344(4):307-16. [PMID: 22475734]

## Item 107    Answer:    C

**Educational Objective: Diagnose postinfluenza community-acquired pneumonia caused by *Staphylococcus aureus*.**

This patient mostly likely has postinfluenza pneumonia caused by *Staphylococcus aureus*. She presents with recurrent cough and dyspnea after recently being diagnosed with influenza pneumonia, and her chest radiograph shows cavitary lesions, which are most consistent with S. *aureus*. Secondary bacterial pneumonia following influenza is a significant cause of morbidity and mortality, particularly in patients aged 65 years or older. Influenza virus affects the tracheobronchial epithelium, impairing normal mucociliary clearance mechanisms and predisposing to bacterial infection. The most common clinical presentation in patients with secondary bacterial pneumonia is the exacerbation of respiratory symptoms and fever after a period of initial improvement of acute influenza symptoms. Patients with secondary bacterial pneumonia typically develop higher fevers than were present with influenza and a cough productive of purulent sputum. Chest radiography will show pulmonary infiltrates.

*Legionella* species are an uncommon cause of secondary pneumonia associated with influenza infection compared with *Streptococcus pneumoniae* and *S. aureus*. Additionally, this patient has no additional risk factors predisposing her to developing CAP from *Legionella*, such as exposure to a community outbreak or contaminated water source.

Pneumonia due to *Pseudomonas aeruginosa* is an uncommon cause of CAP, and generally occurs in patients with chronic lung disease. It would, therefore, be an unlikely cause of secondary pneumonia in this patient.

Although *S. pneumoniae* is more common than S. *aureus* in postinfluenza pneumonia, it does not typically produce the radiographic picture of cavitary lesions, so it is unlikely to be the causative pathogen in this patient.

**KEY POINT**

- A patient with recently diagnosed influenza pneumonia and cavitary lesions on chest radiograph most likely has *Staphylococcus aureus* postinfluenza community-acquired pneumonia.

**Bibliography**

Mandell LA, Wunderink RG, Anzueto A, et al; Infectious Diseases Society of America, American Thoracic Society. Infectious Diseases Society of America/American Thoracic Society consensus guidelines on the management of community-acquired pneumonia in adults. Clin Infect Dis. 2007 Mar 1;44(Suppl 2):S27-72. [PMID: 17278083]

## Item 108    Answer:    A

**Educational Objective: Manage recurrent urinary tract infection with low-dose antimicrobial prophylaxis.**

This patient should begin low-dose antimicrobial prophylaxis. She has recurrent urinary tract infection (UTI), which is defined as three UTIs in the previous 12 months or two UTIs in the previous 6 months. Recurrent UTI affects 20% to 30% of women. She has already tried a modifiable behavioral practice by voiding after sexual intercourse. Scientific evidence is lacking for most behavioral strategies, but they are low risk and worth attempting. Low-dose antimicrobial prophylaxis is an effective intervention to manage frequent, recurrent, acute, uncomplicated UTI. It may be administered daily or every other day, generally at bedtime, or as postcoital prophylaxis. The initial duration of prophylaxis is generally 6 months; however, 50% of women experience recurrence by 3 months after discontinuation of prophylaxis. If this occurs, prophylaxis should be reinstated for 1 or 2 years with reassessment after that time. Because continuous prophylaxis may result in unnecessary antimicrobial use, an alternative strategy is patient self-diagnosis and self-treatment at the start of symptoms.

Methenamine salts produce formaldehyde, which acts as a bacteriostatic agent without affecting microbial susceptibility to antibiotic agents. They are well tolerated and effective. However, carcinogenic potential is a concern if they are used at high doses for a prolonged duration. They can be used for up to 1 week to prevent UTI in patients without urinary tract abnormalities, but not long term.

Vitamin C (ascorbic acid) has not been shown to be effective and is therefore not recommended for the prevention of UTI based on current evidence.

Anatomic or functional abnormalities of the urinary tract should be excluded as a cause of recurrent UTI in men and postmenopausal women. In premenopausal women, however, the yield for this indication is low. Therefore, urethroscopic assessment of this patient would not be indicated.

**KEY POINT**

- Low-dose antimicrobial prophylaxis is an effective intervention to manage frequent, recurrent, acute, uncomplicated urinary tract infection.

**Bibliography**

Prevention of recurrent urinary tract infections in women. Drug Ther Bull. 2013 Jun;51(6):69-72. [PMID: 23766394]

## A  NAME AND ADDRESS (Please complete.)

Last Name _____ First Name _____ Middle Initial

Address _____

Address cont. _____

City _____ State _____ ZIP Code

Country _____

Email address _____

## B  Order Number

(Use the Order Number on your MKSAP materials packing slip.)

| | | | | | | | | | | | | | | | |
|---|---|---|---|---|---|---|---|---|---|---|---|---|---|---|---|

## C  ACP ID Number

(Refer to packing slip in your MKSAP materials for your ACP ID Number.)

| | | | | | | | | | | | | | | | |
|---|---|---|---|---|---|---|---|---|---|---|---|---|---|---|---|

---

**ACP®** American College of Physicians
Leading Internal Medicine, Improving Lives

**Medical Knowledge Self-Assessment Program® 17**

### TO EARN *AMA PRA CATEGORY 1 CREDITS™* YOU MUST:

1. Answer all questions.
2. Score a minimum of 50% correct.

==================================================

### TO EARN *FREE* INSTANTANEOUS *AMA PRA CATEGORY 1 CREDITS™* ONLINE:

1. Answer all of your questions.
2. Go to **mksap.acponline.org** and enter your ACP Online username and password to access an online answer sheet.
3. Enter your answers.
4. You can also enter your answers directly at **mksap.acponline.org** without first using this answer sheet.

### To Submit Your Answer Sheet by Mail or FAX for a $15 Administrative Fee per Answer Sheet:

1. Answer all of your questions and calculate your score.
2. Complete boxes A-F.
3. Complete payment information.
4. Send the answer sheet and payment information to ACP, using the FAX number/address listed below.

---

## COMPLETE FORM BELOW ONLY IF YOU SUBMIT BY MAIL OR FAX

Last Name _____ First Name _____ MI

| | | | | | | | | | | | | | | | | | | | | | | | | | | | | | | | |
|---|---|---|---|---|---|---|---|---|---|---|---|---|---|---|---|---|---|---|---|---|---|---|---|---|---|---|---|---|---|---|---|---|

**Payment Information. Must remit in US funds, drawn on a US bank.**

**The processing fee for each paper answer sheet is $15.**

☐ Check, made payable to ACP, enclosed

Charge to  ☐ **VISA**  ☐ **MasterCard**  ☐ **AMERICAN EXPRESS**  ☐ **DISCOVER**

Card Number _____

Expiration Date _____ / _____
                       MM          YY

Security code (3 or 4 digit #s) _____

Signature _____

**Fax to:** 215-351-2799

**Mail to:**
Member and Customer Service
American College of Physicians
190 N. Independence Mall West
Philadelphia, PA 19106-1572

**D**

## TEST TYPE

| | Maximum Number of CME Credits |
|---|---|
| ○ Cardiovascular Medicine | 21 |
| ○ Dermatology | 12 |
| ○ Gastroenterology and Hepatology | 16 |
| ○ Hematology and Oncology | 22 |
| ○ Neurology | 16 |
| ○ Rheumatology | 16 |
| ○ Endocrinology and Metabolism | 14 |
| ○ General Internal Medicine | 26 |
| ○ Infectious Disease | 19 |
| ○ Nephrology | 19 |
| ○ Pulmonary and Critical Care Medicine | 19 |

**E**

## CREDITS CLAIMED ON SECTION
### (1 hour = 1 credit)

Enter the number of credits earned on the test to the nearest quarter hour. Physicians should claim only the credit commensurate with the extent of their participation in the activity.

**F**

### Enter your score here.

Instructions for calculating your own score are found in front of the self-assessment test in each book.

You must receive a minimum score of 50% correct.

_____ %

Credit Submission Date: _____

1 (A) (B) (C) (D) (E)
2 (A) (B) (C) (D) (E)
3 (A) (B) (C) (D) (E)
4 (A) (B) (C) (D) (E)
5 (A) (B) (C) (D) (E)

6 (A) (B) (C) (D) (E)
7 (A) (B) (C) (D) (E)
8 (A) (B) (C) (D) (E)
9 (A) (B) (C) (D) (E)
10 (A) (B) (C) (D) (E)

11 (A) (B) (C) (D) (E)
12 (A) (B) (C) (D) (E)
13 (A) (B) (C) (D) (E)
14 (A) (B) (C) (D) (E)
15 (A) (B) (C) (D) (E)

16 (A) (B) (C) (D) (E)
17 (A) (B) (C) (D) (E)
18 (A) (B) (C) (D) (E)
19 (A) (B) (C) (D) (E)
20 (A) (B) (C) (D) (E)

21 (A) (B) (C) (D) (E)
22 (A) (B) (C) (D) (E)
23 (A) (B) (C) (D) (E)
24 (A) (B) (C) (D) (E)
25 (A) (B) (C) (D) (E)

26 (A) (B) (C) (D) (E)
27 (A) (B) (C) (D) (E)
28 (A) (B) (C) (D) (E)
29 (A) (B) (C) (D) (E)
30 (A) (B) (C) (D) (E)

31 (A) (B) (C) (D) (E)
32 (A) (B) (C) (D) (E)
33 (A) (B) (C) (D) (E)
34 (A) (B) (C) (D) (E)
35 (A) (B) (C) (D) (E)

36 (A) (B) (C) (D) (E)
37 (A) (B) (C) (D) (E)
38 (A) (B) (C) (D) (E)
39 (A) (B) (C) (D) (E)
40 (A) (B) (C) (D) (E)

41 (A) (B) (C) (D) (E)
42 (A) (B) (C) (D) (E)
43 (A) (B) (C) (D) (E)
44 (A) (B) (C) (D) (E)
45 (A) (B) (C) (D) (E)

46 (A) (B) (C) (D) (E)
47 (A) (B) (C) (D) (E)
48 (A) (B) (C) (D) (E)
49 (A) (B) (C) (D) (E)
50 (A) (B) (C) (D) (E)

51 (A) (B) (C) (D) (E)
52 (A) (B) (C) (D) (E)
53 (A) (B) (C) (D) (E)
54 (A) (B) (C) (D) (E)
55 (A) (B) (C) (D) (E)

56 (A) (B) (C) (D) (E)
57 (A) (B) (C) (D) (E)
58 (A) (B) (C) (D) (E)
59 (A) (B) (C) (D) (E)
60 (A) (B) (C) (D) (E)

61 (A) (B) (C) (D) (E)
62 (A) (B) (C) (D) (E)
63 (A) (B) (C) (D) (E)
64 (A) (B) (C) (D) (E)
65 (A) (B) (C) (D) (E)

66 (A) (B) (C) (D) (E)
67 (A) (B) (C) (D) (E)
68 (A) (B) (C) (D) (E)
69 (A) (B) (C) (D) (E)
70 (A) (B) (C) (D) (E)

71 (A) (B) (C) (D) (E)
72 (A) (B) (C) (D) (E)
73 (A) (B) (C) (D) (E)
74 (A) (B) (C) (D) (E)
75 (A) (B) (C) (D) (E)

76 (A) (B) (C) (D) (E)
77 (A) (B) (C) (D) (E)
78 (A) (B) (C) (D) (E)
79 (A) (B) (C) (D) (E)
80 (A) (B) (C) (D) (E)

81 (A) (B) (C) (D) (E)
82 (A) (B) (C) (D) (E)
83 (A) (B) (C) (D) (E)
84 (A) (B) (C) (D) (E)
85 (A) (B) (C) (D) (E)

86 (A) (B) (C) (D) (E)
87 (A) (B) (C) (D) (E)
88 (A) (B) (C) (D) (E)
89 (A) (B) (C) (D) (E)
90 (A) (B) (C) (D) (E)

91 (A) (B) (C) (D) (E)
92 (A) (B) (C) (D) (E)
93 (A) (B) (C) (D) (E)
94 (A) (B) (C) (D) (E)
95 (A) (B) (C) (D) (E)

96 (A) (B) (C) (D) (E)
97 (A) (B) (C) (D) (E)
98 (A) (B) (C) (D) (E)
99 (A) (B) (C) (D) (E)
100 (A) (B) (C) (D) (E)

101 (A) (B) (C) (D) (E)
102 (A) (B) (C) (D) (E)
103 (A) (B) (C) (D) (E)
104 (A) (B) (C) (D) (E)
105 (A) (B) (C) (D) (E)

106 (A) (B) (C) (D) (E)
107 (A) (B) (C) (D) (E)
108 (A) (B) (C) (D) (E)
109 (A) (B) (C) (D) (E)
110 (A) (B) (C) (D) (E)

111 (A) (B) (C) (D) (E)
112 (A) (B) (C) (D) (E)
113 (A) (B) (C) (D) (E)
114 (A) (B) (C) (D) (E)
115 (A) (B) (C) (D) (E)

116 (A) (B) (C) (D) (E)
117 (A) (B) (C) (D) (E)
118 (A) (B) (C) (D) (E)
119 (A) (B) (C) (D) (E)
120 (A) (B) (C) (D) (E)

121 (A) (B) (C) (D) (E)
122 (A) (B) (C) (D) (E)
123 (A) (B) (C) (D) (E)
124 (A) (B) (C) (D) (E)
125 (A) (B) (C) (D) (E)

126 (A) (B) (C) (D) (E)
127 (A) (B) (C) (D) (E)
128 (A) (B) (C) (D) (E)
129 (A) (B) (C) (D) (E)
130 (A) (B) (C) (D) (E)

131 (A) (B) (C) (D) (E)
132 (A) (B) (C) (D) (E)
133 (A) (B) (C) (D) (E)
134 (A) (B) (C) (D) (E)
135 (A) (B) (C) (D) (E)

136 (A) (B) (C) (D) (E)
137 (A) (B) (C) (D) (E)
138 (A) (B) (C) (D) (E)
139 (A) (B) (C) (D) (E)
140 (A) (B) (C) (D) (E)

141 (A) (B) (C) (D) (E)
142 (A) (B) (C) (D) (E)
143 (A) (B) (C) (D) (E)
144 (A) (B) (C) (D) (E)
145 (A) (B) (C) (D) (E)

146 (A) (B) (C) (D) (E)
147 (A) (B) (C) (D) (E)
148 (A) (B) (C) (D) (E)
149 (A) (B) (C) (D) (E)
150 (A) (B) (C) (D) (E)

151 (A) (B) (C) (D) (E)
152 (A) (B) (C) (D) (E)
153 (A) (B) (C) (D) (E)
154 (A) (B) (C) (D) (E)
155 (A) (B) (C) (D) (E)

156 (A) (B) (C) (D) (E)
157 (A) (B) (C) (D) (E)
158 (A) (B) (C) (D) (E)
159 (A) (B) (C) (D) (E)
160 (A) (B) (C) (D) (E)

161 (A) (B) (C) (D) (E)
162 (A) (B) (C) (D) (E)
163 (A) (B) (C) (D) (E)
164 (A) (B) (C) (D) (E)
165 (A) (B) (C) (D) (E)

166 (A) (B) (C) (D) (E)
167 (A) (B) (C) (D) (E)
168 (A) (B) (C) (D) (E)
169 (A) (B) (C) (D) (E)
170 (A) (B) (C) (D) (E)

171 (A) (B) (C) (D) (E)
172 (A) (B) (C) (D) (E)
173 (A) (B) (C) (D) (E)
174 (A) (B) (C) (D) (E)
175 (A) (B) (C) (D) (E)

176 (A) (B) (C) (D) (E)
177 (A) (B) (C) (D) (E)
178 (A) (B) (C) (D) (E)
179 (A) (B) (C) (D) (E)
180 (A) (B) (C) (D) (E)